AF333025

Microsurgical Reconstruction
of the
Cancer Patient

Microsurgical Reconstruction of the Cancer Patient

EDITOR

Mark A. Schusterman, M.D.

Professor and Chairman
Department of Plastic Surgery
The University of Texas
M.D. Anderson Cancer Center
Houston, Texas

With illustrations by Peg Gerrity

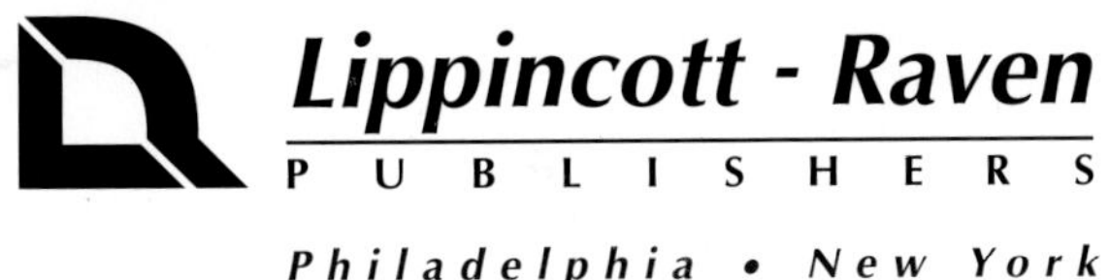

Philadelphia • New York

Acquisitions Editors: Danette Knopp and James Ryan
Developmental Editor: Rhoda Dunn
Manufacturing Manager: Dennis Teston
Production Manager: Jodi Borgenicht
Production Editor: Raeann Touhey
Cover Designer: Ede Dreikers
Indexer: Linda Van Pelt
Compositor: Lippincott–Raven Electronic Production
Color Separator/Prepress: Chroma Graphics (overseas), Pte Ltd.
Printer: Toppan Printers, Pte Ltd., Singapore

© 1997, by Lippincott–Raven Publishers. All rights reserved. This book is protected by copyright. No part of it may be reproduced, stored in a retrieval system, or transmitted, in any form or by any means—electronic, mechanical, photocopy, recording, or otherwise—without the prior written consent of the publisher, except for brief quotations embodied in critical articles and reviews. For information write Lippincott–Raven Publishers, 227 East Washington Square, Philadelphia, PA 19106-3780.

Materials appearing in this book prepared by individuals as part of their official duties as U.S. Government employees are not covered by the above-mentioned copyright.

Printed and bound in Singapore

9 8 7 6 5 4 3 2 1

Library of Congress Cataloging-in-Publication Data

Microsurgical reconstruction of the cancer patient / editor, Mark A.
    Schusterman; with illustrations by Peg Gerrity.
        p. cm.
    Includes bibliographical references and index.
    ISBN 0-397-51391-7
    1. Cancer—Surgery. 2. Microsurgery. 3. Surgery, Plastic.
    4. Flaps (Surgery) I. Schusterman, Mark A.
    [DNLM: 1. Neoplasms—surgery. 2. Surgical Flaps—methods.
    3. Microsurgery—methods.   QZ 268 M626 1997]
    RD651.M53   1997
    616.99'4059—dc21
    DNLM/DLC
    for Library of Congress

Care has been taken to confirm the accuracy of the information presented and to describe generally accepted practices. However, the authors, editor, and publisher are not responsible for errors or omissions or for any consequences from application of the information in this book and make no warranty, express or implied, with respect to the contents of the publication.

The authors, editor, and publisher have exerted every effort to ensure that drug selection and dosage set forth in this text are in accordance with current recommendations and practice at the time of publication. However, in view of ongoing research, changes in government regulations, and the constant flow of information relating to drug therapy and drug reactions, the reader is urged to check the package insert for each drug for any change in indications and dosage and for added warnings and precautions. This is particularly important when the recommended agent is a new or infrequently employed drug.

Some drugs and medical devices presented in this publication have Food and Drug Administration (FDA) clearance for limited use in restricted research settings. It is the responsibility of the health care provider to ascertain the FDA status of each drug or device planned for use in their clinical practice.

To my children, Asher and Elizabeth, who are my continual source of inspiration

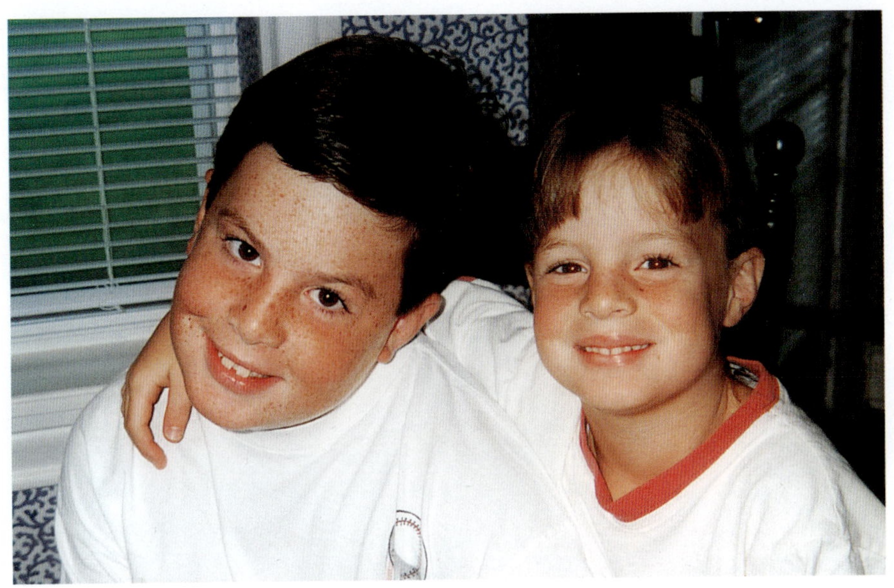

Contents

III. Extremities

Contributing Authors

L. Franklyn Elliott II, M.D., *Clinical Instructor, Department of Plastic Surgery, Emory University School of Medicine, 1365 Clifton Road, Northeast, Atlanta, Georgia 30322; and Atlanta Plastic Surgery, P.A., Suite 500, 975 Johnson Ferry Road, Northeast, Atlanta, Georgia 30342*

Gregory R. D. Evans, M.D., *Associate Professor, Department of Plastic Surgery, The University of Texas, M.D. Anderson Cancer Center, 1515 Holcombe Boulevard, Box 062, Houston, Texas 77030*

Giulio Gherardini, M.D., *Fellow in Reconstructive Microvascular Surgery, Department of Plastic Surgery, The University of Texas, M.D. Anderson Cancer Center, 1515 Holcombe Boulevard, Box 062, Houston, Texas 77030*

Daniel P. Goldberg, M.D., *Assistant Professor, Department of Surgery, Division of Plastic and Reconstructive Surgery, Case Western Reserve University, 11100 Euclid Avenue, Cleveland, Ohio 44106-5044*

Stephen S. Kroll, M.D., *Professor, Department of Plastic Surgery, The University of Texas, M.D. Anderson Cancer Center, 1515 Holcombe Boulevard, Box 062, Houston, Texas 77030*

Michael J. Miller, M.D., *Assistant Professor, Department of Plastic Surgery, The University of Texas, M.D. Anderson Cancer Center, 1515 Holcombe Boulevard, Box 062, Houston, Texas 77030*

Foad Nahai, B.Sc., M.B., Ch.B., F.A.C.S., *Professor, Department of Surgery, Emory University School of Medicine, 1365 Clifton Road, Northeast, Atlanta, Georgia 30322*

Christian E. Paletta, M.D., *Associate Professor, Department of Plastic Surgery, St. Louis University Medical Center, 3635 Vista, P.O. Box 15250, St. Louis, Missouri 63110*

Gregory P. Reece, M.D., *Associate Surgeon and Assistant Professor, Department of Plastic Surgery, The University of Texas, M.D. Anderson Cancer Center, 1515 Holcombe Boulevard, Box 062, Houston, Texas 77030*

Geoffrey L. Robb, M.D., *Deputy Division Head, Division of Surgery and Anesthesiology; Director, Graduate Education Program; and Deputy Chairman and Associate Professor, Department of Plastic Surgery, The University of Texas, M.D. Anderson Cancer Center, 1515 Holcombe Boulevard, Box 062, Houston, Texas 77030*

Mark A. Schusterman, M.D., *Professor and Chairman, Department of Plastic Surgery, The University of Texas, M.D. Anderson Cancer Center, 1515 Holcombe Boulevard, Box 062, Houston, Texas 77030*

John M. Shamoun, M.D., *Newport Institute of Plastic Surgery, 360 San Miguel, Suite 406, Newport Beach, California 92660*

Preface

The purpose of this book is to provide a simple step-by-step description of how the reconstructive microsurgical procedures now performed in the Department of Plastic Surgery at The University of Texas/M.D. Anderson Cancer Center are performed. When the reconstructive microsurgery program began in 1988, I used standard techniques that were taught to me during my residency and fellowship to reconstruct cancer defects. As the techniques evolved and the educational program at our institution progressed, I realized that our approach was fairly unique. This book, therefore, describes the "M.D. Anderson" approach to free flap reconstruction of the cancer patient.

The "M.D. Anderson" approach in terms of plastic surgery is done with one primary goal in mind—reliability. This is due to the high volume of immediate reconstructions performed by our service. The plastic surgeon's role is to provide a reliable reconstruction with minimal complications so that adjuvant therapy is not delayed. The plastic surgeon in essence must be transparent. Function and aesthetics are important goals as well, but they cannot take precedence over reliability. Thus, there is a paradox of using the most complex procedure because it is the most reliable. This book will explain how we perform free flaps simply, quickly, and with a success rate over 96%.

This book is designed to be easily used by plastic surgeons faced with a patient who has a difficult cancer defect. The plastic surgeon's standard thought process is as follows: assess the defect, establish the clinical goal, list the possible flaps that might address the defect and accomplish the goal, evaluate the advantages and disadvantages of each flap, and then select and implement the appropriate flap.

This book is divided into three sections based on recipient or defect site—Head and Neck, Breast, and Extremities. In our practice free flaps are most commonly used from these regions. There is no section on trunk reconstruction, since most of these defects are closed with pedicle flaps.

The first chapter of each section discusses principles pertinent to all defect sites in the region. These common principles include patient evaluation, room setup, instrumentation, and microsurgical technique. The following chapters in each section address specific defect type, and discuss all of the flaps utilized for that defect. The rationale for flap selection, details on anatomy, flap evaluation, and inset are also provided. The reader can choose a chapter on a specific defect, and learn how we address the defect, why we use specific flaps, when each flap is appropriate, and the technical details of flap elevation and inset.

One problem with designing the book in this format is that many flaps, such as the rectus abdominis and latissimus dorsi muscle flaps, are used in several different areas. To make the book easier to use, the flap anatomy and harvest technique are shown in each chapter where the flap is described. Why describe flap elevation in more than one chapter? This book was not designed to be read cover-to-cover, but rather as a technical guide for the practicing plastic surgeon or trainee.

The Breast section is the only section that does not follow this format. Most people believe that the free transverse rectus abdominis myocutaneous (TRAM) flap is most frequently chosen for breast reconstruction. The other flaps are used a distant second or third. As a result, most of our faculty has limited experience with the other flaps. Still, there are situations when they may be necessary, so I recruited contributors from outside the institution to describe these other flaps.

In most of the chapters, the number of flaps discussed is limited. This was done intentionally. This book is not designed to give the reader an encyclopedic review of all the flaps used for a specific defect. Furthermore, commonly used flaps are described in greater detail than those less commonly used. For example, the osteocutaneous radial forearm flap for mandibular reconstruction is discussed only modestly, whereas the discussion of the fibula flap is extensive.

This book is meant to be used as a tool and handbook, so that the busy practitioner or resident can keep it in his or her operating room locker to be available when tough cases present themselves. My hope is that this book will be a handy reference guide that is easy to use.

Mark A. Schusterman, M.D.

Acknowledgments

My appreciation for help with this book goes first to my collaborators, especially my fellow plastic surgeons at The University of Texas/M.D. Anderson Cancer Center: Stephen S. Kroll, Geoffrey L. Robb, Gregory R. Reece, Michael J. Miller, Bonnie J. Baldwin, and Gregory R. Evans. I would also like to thank Christian E. Paletta, Foad Nahai, Frank Elliot, and John Shamoun for their help in the breast reconstruction section. In addition, I would like to thank the microsurgery fellows who helped with the preparation of many of the chapters in this book, and the illustrator, Peg Gerrity, for her outstanding artwork throughout this volume.

Finally a well-deserved thank you goes to Lippincott–Raven Publishers for their help and patience, especially Jim Ryan for initiating this project and Danette Knopp for helping to complete it.

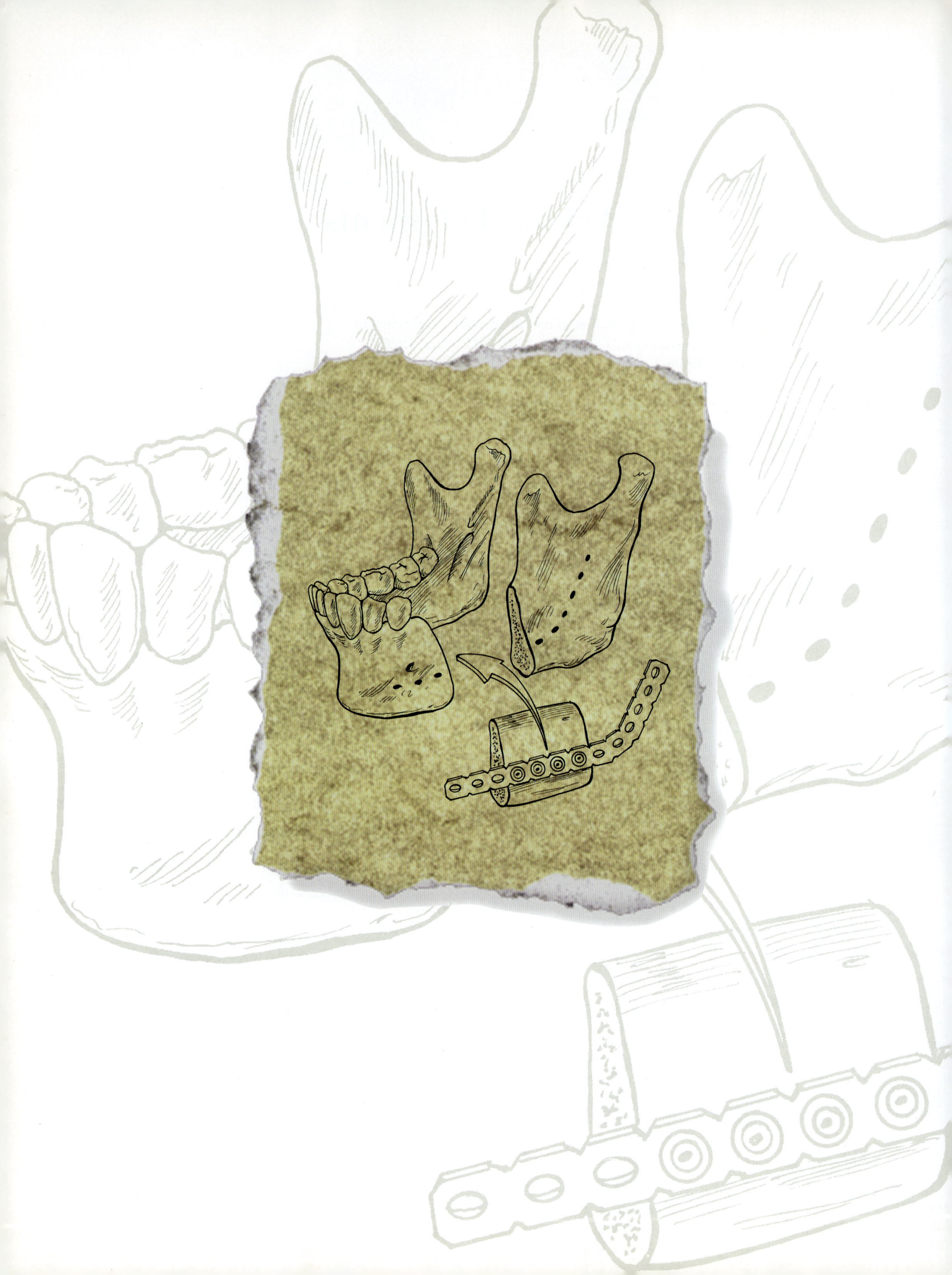

Microsurgical Reconstruction of the Cancer Patient, edited by M.A. Schusterman.
Lippincott-Raven Publishers, Philadelphia © 1997.

1

General Principles of Free Flap Reconstruction of the Head and Neck

Mark A. Schusterman

The development of free tissue transfer has revolutionized reconstruction for head and neck cancer defects by making available to the plastic surgeon a wide spectrum of tissues of varying composition and size that allow for better reconstruction of the challenging defects encountered after head and neck cancer ablation. Because the tissue is vascularized, wound healing is enhanced, even in the hostile environment often present in head and neck cancer defects as a result of oral cavity contamination and irradiation. The goal of reconstructive surgery in the oncology patient is to repair the defect at the time of ablative surgery so that the wound heals primarily, function is maintained, and normal cosmesis is achieved. The reconstructive procedure must not prolong the hospitalization, increase the complication rate, or cause any delay in adjuvant therapy. Specifically, what is required is a one-stage, immediate reconstruction with well-vascularized tissue and a low complication rate. These requirements are met, paradoxically, by free tissue transfer, often considered a complex, time-consuming, and risky procedure. Later chapters describe in detail how various flaps are used for specific defects of the head and neck after cancer ablation. This chapter describes general principles common to all head and neck free flaps, and gives some insight into how these procedures can be performed with a high degree of reliability and consistency.

M. A. Schusterman: Department of Plastic Surgery, The University of Texas, M.D. Anderson Cancer Center, Houston, Texas 77030.

PATIENT EVALUATION

The most common cancer of the upper aerodigestive tract is squamous cell carcinoma. The cause of this disease is usually a genetic predisposition influenced by factors such as tobacco and alcohol abuse, which often contributes to the patients' poor health. Patients frequently have cardiovascular and/or pulmonary disease, and they may have impaired hepatic and renal function or diabetes.

Because such a background is the norm, a meticulous patient history should be taken, and a comprehensive physical examination should include special attention to the vascular system. The neck vessels must be palpated and auscultated to assess their adequacy as recipient vessels. The adequacy of the vessels at the donor site should also be thoroughly assessed, if possible. A complete review of systems is essential since many diseases can influence flap selection. Respiratory status should be reviewed, not only for routine presurgical concerns but also because a patient with a respiratory disability may have serious ventilatory compromise after harvest of an abdominal wall flap. Gastrointestinal disease with or without previous surgery also may preclude use of abdominal donor sites. The presence of advanced hepatic disease, with ascites, may disallow the use of a free jejunal segment for transfer. Diseases of the nervous system with resultant paralysis or dysesthesia preclude use of muscle flaps from the affected areas.

FLAP CHOICE

Once the extent of the defect is accurately defined and characterized, donor sites are evaluated, and the most appropriate and reliable flap is selected. Craniofacial resections that leave exposed dura and require soft tissue coverage can best be managed with a large muscle or myocutaneous flap, such as the latissimus dorsi or rectus abdominis flaps.

The extent of a potential oral cavity defect is assessed by estimating the amount of soft tissue and measuring the quantity of bone to be excised in the planned operation. In most cases of squamous cell carcinoma, replacement of the soft tissue should take precedence over the bony restitution since oral function is generally more dependent on tongue mobility and function.

After a partial glossectomy, the goal of surgical reconstruction is to promote tongue mobility, and this is often best and most reliably accomplished with a free radial forearm flap. For total or subtotal glossectomies, the surgical objective is replacement of tongue bulk to deter aspiration and preserve the larynx. A bulky flap is used in these circumstances, and several choices are available: the rectus abdominis (either a vertical or transverse configuration), the latissimus dorsi, or the scapular flap.

Segmental resections of the mandible can cause significant disfigurement and loss of function. Mandibular dysfunction increases as more of the mandibular body is excised, and resections of the anterior arch result in the most severe morbidity and the greatest need for reconstruction. Since most intraoral tumors arise in the mucosa, a tumor large enough to involve the mandible will by definition also involve a significant amount of soft tissue. It is important to address the soft tissue defect as well as the bony defect, and use of a composite flap is required. The fibula osteocutaneous flap has become the workhorse for repair of these defects at this center. A resection of the posterior body and ramus of the mandible may require soft tissue replacement only.

The hypopharynx and cervical esophagus are reconstructed with either a free jejunal transfer or a tubed free radial forearm flap, depending on the patient's health and history. We prefer to use the free jejunal transfer unless the patient's condition discourages intraabdominal surgery.

EQUIPMENT

The operating microscope should be of high quality, with good optics and a strong light source. The Wild Leitz 680 is an excellent operating microscope since there are separate focus and zoom controls for the surgeon and the assistant (Fig. 1). An

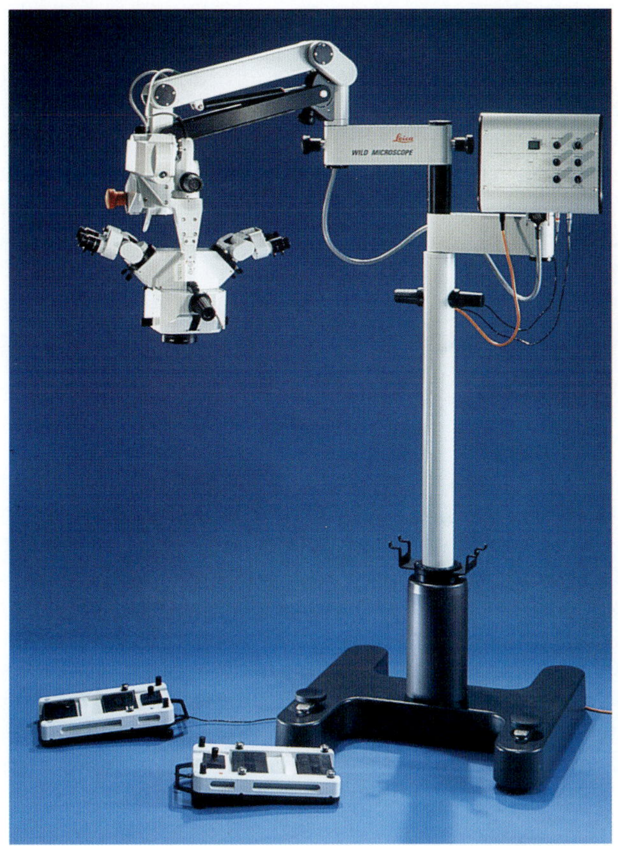

FIG. 1. The Wild Leitz 680 operating microscope with dual focus and zoom controls allows the surgeon and the assistant to operate their views separately.

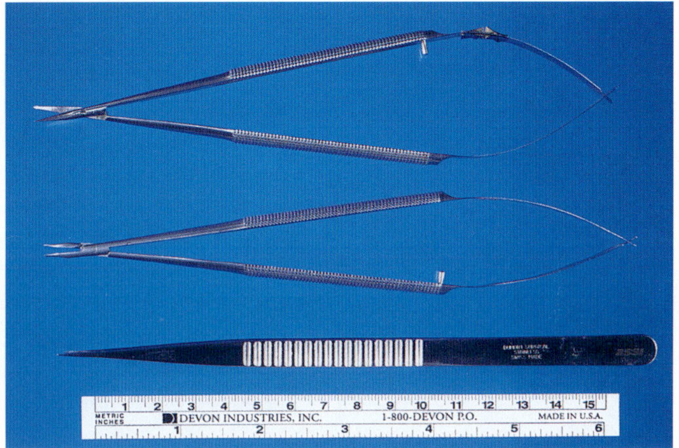

FIG. 2. The microsurgical instruments used for head and neck free flaps need to be long-handled to allow easier reach of the deep structures of the neck.

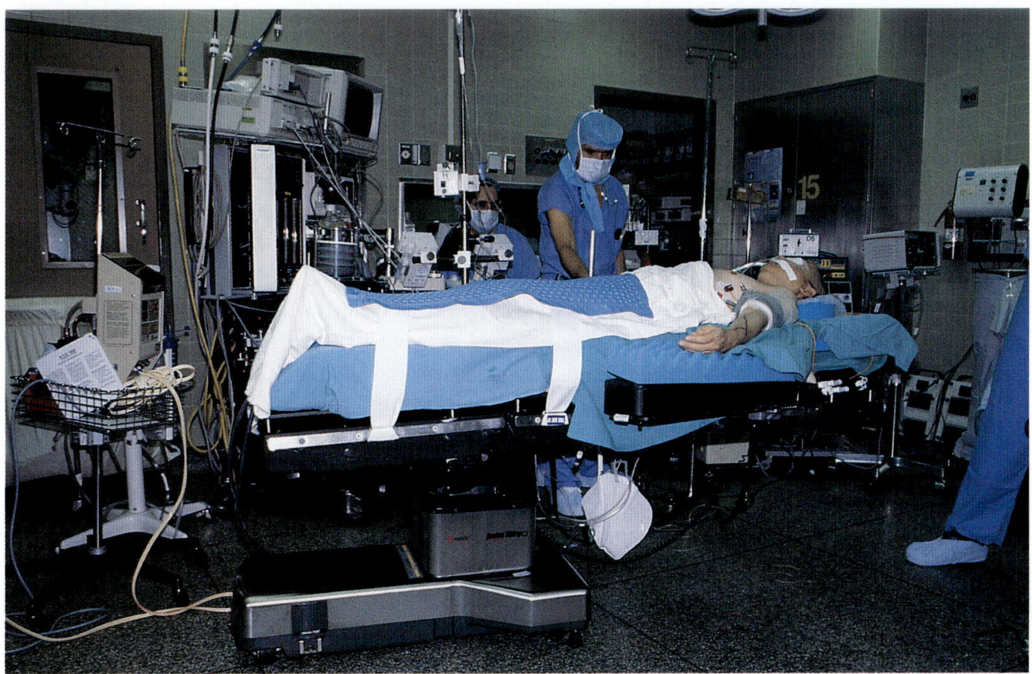

FIG. 3. The operating table should be turned so that the head of the patient is placed at the foot of the bed, thus allowing room for the operating microsurgeon's knees if the surgeon wishes to sit when performing the anastomosis.

attached video camera allows the scrub nurses to view the anastomosis as well; this allows them to anticipate the need to pass instruments. A 200-mm lens is optimal for keeping the microscope at the proper working distance. Microinstruments 18 cm long should be used since the structures in the neck are difficult to reach, particularly from the assistant's side of the table (Fig. 2). Some of the larger vessels can be anastomosed under loupe magnification, but this prevents an assistant from helping and should be done only when a microscope is not available. Loupes are, however, essential for flap elevation particularly during dissection of the pedicle and during preparation of the recipient vessels. Loupe magnification of 2.5× is the minimum; a 3.2× wide field is the optimal power for flap dissection, and a 4.5× wide field is the minimum power if one desires to do use loupes for the anastomosis.

ROOM SETUP

In preparing the operating room for head and neck reconstruction with a free flap, several measures are beneficial. The operating table should be turned so that the patient's head is positioned at the foot, thus giving space under the table for the surgeon's legs during microsurgery (Fig. 3). There should also be adequate foam padding on the table and extra padding at all pressure points to prevent injuries to the patient. In addition, if the patient can be positioned so that both the ablative and the reconstructive teams can work simultaneously, the operating time and the duration of anesthesia will be reduced. Central venous access is recommended for intraoperative monitoring and fluid replacement, and a urethral catheter with a temperature probe should be placed to monitor urine output and core temperature. Sequential pneumatic compression boots should be used for prophylaxis against deep venous thrombosis.

RECIPIENT VESSELS AND REVASCULARIZATION

The key factor in promoting reliability of free tissue transfer is achieving a high rate of blood flow into and out of the flap. To accomplish this goal, we use large recipient vessels, principally the external carotid artery and the internal jugular vein. If functional neck dissections are routinely done, these major vessels will generally be available. The vessels are isolated with vessel loops, which allow the surgeon to elevate the recipient vessels from the vascular bed for better access.

An end-to-side anastomosis is used routinely on both the artery and vein and, again, we believe that this technique promotes reliability. The vein is usually anastomosed first in order to prevent engorgement of the flap. The venotomy is made by grasping the vessel wall, pulling upward, and then using curved microscissors to cut the vessel wall from either side (Fig. 4). The recipient and donor vessels are irrigated with a solution of 100 units of heparin per milliliter of saline. The donor vessels are spatulated, and a running suture is used from each end of the anastomosis: one suture closing the posterior wall and the other closing the anterior wall (Fig. 5). Once the venous anastomosis is completed, the arteriotomy in the external carotid artery is made using microknife and a coronary artery punch 2.5 mm in diameter (Fig. 6). If the situation mandates an end-to-end anastomosis, a running, spatulated technique should be used to promote patency and speed (Fig. 7).

Number 8-0 or 9-0 sutures are used routinely, depending on the vessel size, with the larger suture used most often for the artery, particularly when the vessel walls are thickened. A cutting needle such as the Ethicon™ micropoint or the Sharpoint™ microedged taper is helpful in preventing dulling of the point and difficulty in passing the needle multiple times through the vessel wall as is needed in a running anastomosis.

When the preferred recipient vessels are not present, a vein graft to the opposite side can be done. Adequate preoperative evaluation of the patient including a detailed history with thorough analysis of operative notes describing any previous neck surgery

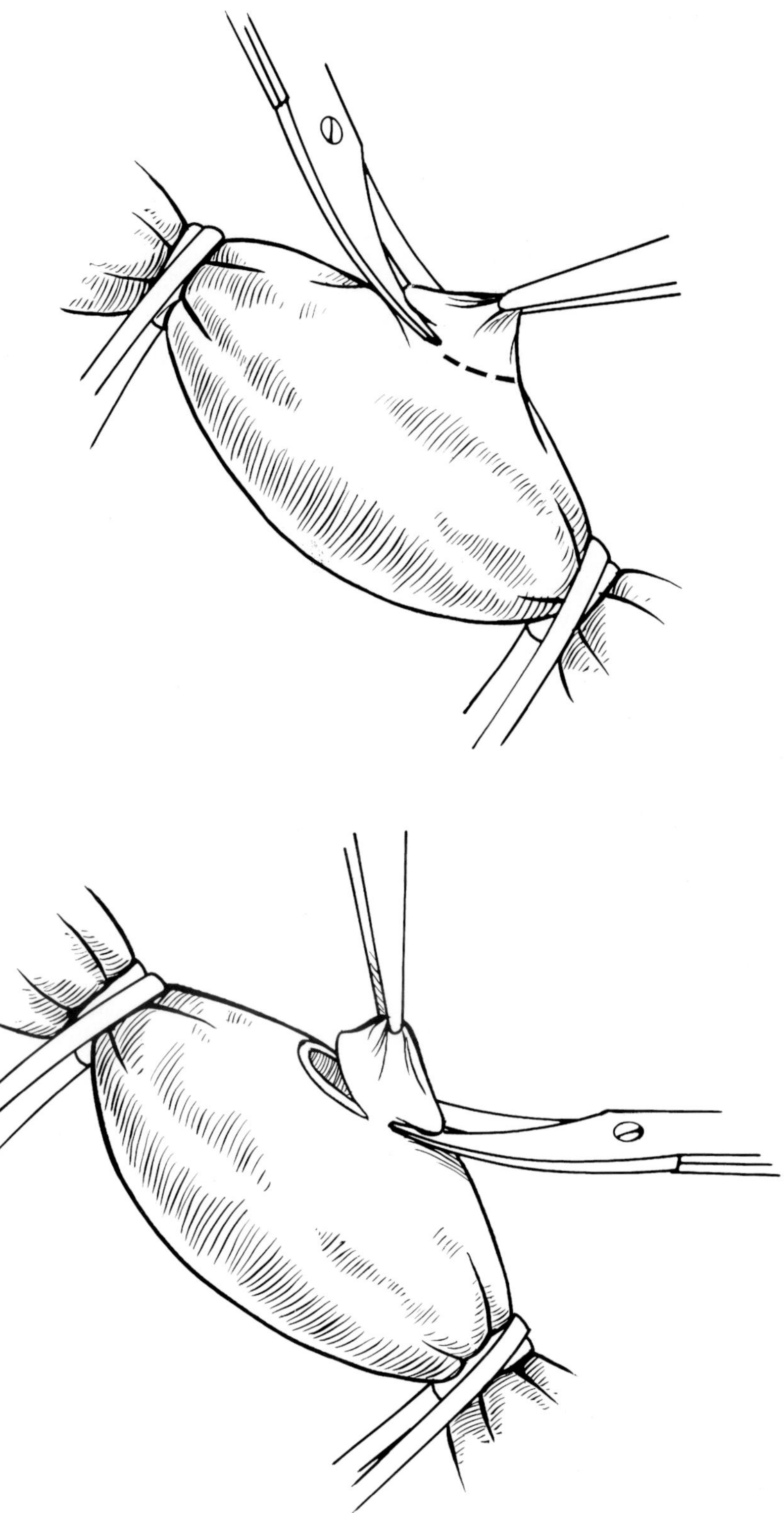

FIG. 4. The venotomy is made in the internal jugular vein by grasping the vein wall, pulling upward, and cutting out a segment of vessel wall with the curved microscissors making one cut from either end.

should reveal whether there is a need for a vein graft. The saphenous vein is the most common donor vein used as a vein graft. Large-caliber vessels such as the great vessels in the contralateral neck or the axillary vessels are used as recipient vessels. An arteriovenous fistula is temporarily created with the vein graft. This high-flow situation serves to dilate and untwist the vein graft prior to its division and anastomosis to the appropriate arterial and venous segments. If a venous recipient vessel is missing (as is often the case in patients who have undergone a conventional radical neck dissection), the cephalic vein can be harvested from the arm and rotated into the neck as the recipient vein.

When the flap is transferred, it should be inset at least partially prior to revascularization, since once the flap is revascularized, bleeding due to postischemic hyperemia makes insetting more difficult. In addition, insetting the flap before revascularization minimizes the risk of inadvertent avulsion of the anastomosis caused by pedicle traction. Transferring an insetting of the flap usually results in an ischemia period of less than 2 hours, which is well tolerated by free flaps. However, if the flap insetting requires a longer time, revascularization should proceed at the 3-hour point no matter what the stage of flap inset.

TEAMWORK

Free flaps are the key to successful, reliable, and consistent results when used for immediate reconstruction for head and neck defects. To facilitate use of these complex procedures in the immediate setting, it is imperative for the ablative and reconstructive surgeons to work as a team. It is essential to discuss the nature of the ablative surgery and whether tissue from the proposed donor site is adequate or appropriate to repair the anticipated defect. Issues such as how much soft tissue is to be removed, whether the mandible will be involved, whether the larynx or surrounding structures will be affected, whether there is a possibility of facial nerve sacrifice, and whether brain or any other vital structure will be exposed and to what extent may be ascertained only during a detailed discussion with the ablative team. Many of the details outlined above, particularly in the section on room setup, may be foreign to the ablative surgeon, and it is important to communicate these issues and issues concerning skin preparation and draping of the donor site well before the surgical procedure is to take place, so that both parties are in agreement at the time of surgery. It is always distressing for the reconstructive surgeon to come into the operating room the morning of surgery to find an intravenous line in the extremity he or she was planning to use as a donor site. Although the ablative and reconstructive teams perform separate functions, the final outcome is dependent on a collegial and supportive interaction between the teams.

SUMMARY

General concepts and principles have been presented that should help the reader perform free flaps for head and neck reconstruction reliably and safely. The basic tenets are the following: perform a detailed analysis of the patient preoperatively, use large caliber recipient vessels, use a running end-to-side anastomosis, inset the flap prior to revascularization, and communicate effectively with the ablative team. The flaps that are used most often are the radial forearm free flap, the rectus abdominis free flap, the latissimus dorsi free flap, the fibula osteocutaneous flap, the iliac crest free flap, the scapula flap (with and without bone), and the free jejunal flap. The details of flap harvest and inset are presented in the following chapters.

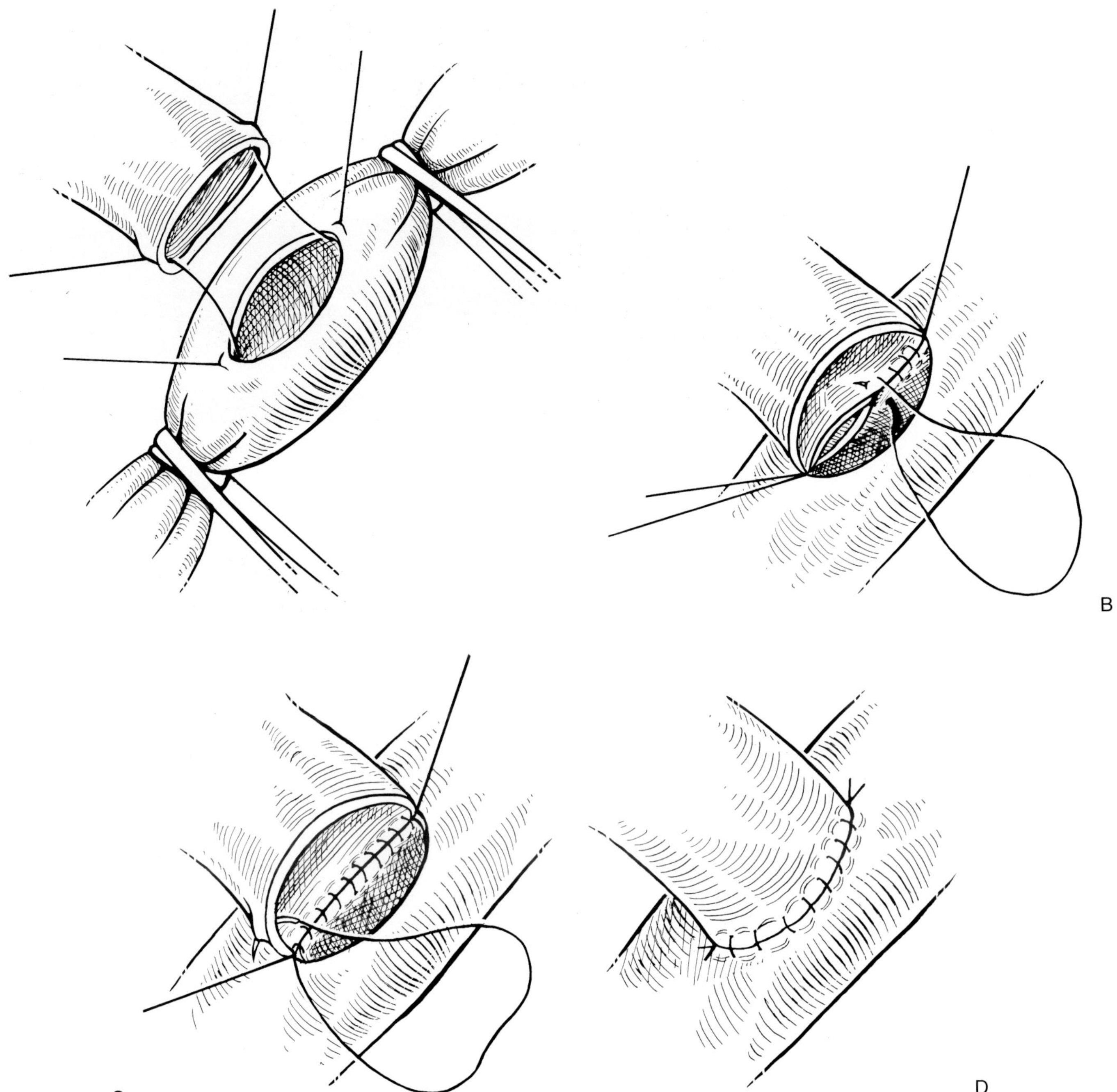

FIG. 5A–D. The end-to-side anastomosis is done by placing one suture at either end of the anastomosis and suturing first the front then the back wall. The back wall can usually be sutured from an external approach simply by retracting the donor vessel away from the surgeon.

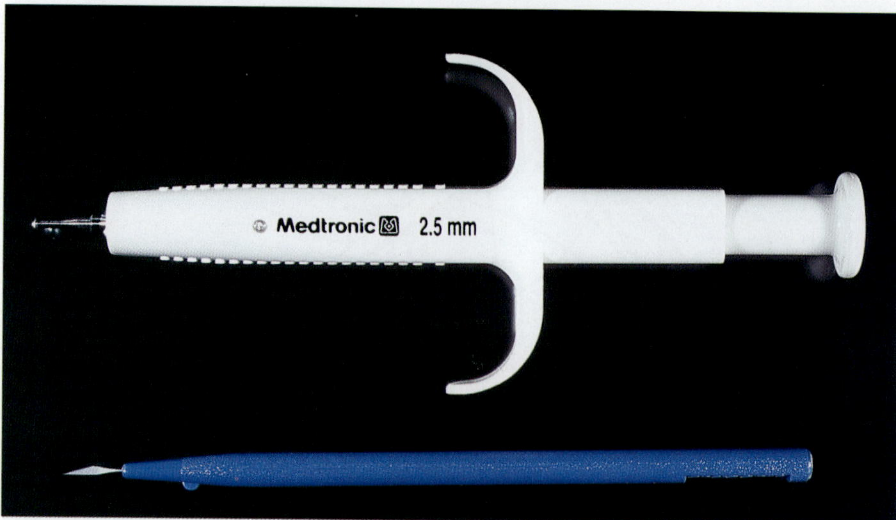

FIG. 6. The microknife used to make the incision in the external carotid artery. The 2.5-mm arterial punch used to make the arteriotomy in the external carotid artery.

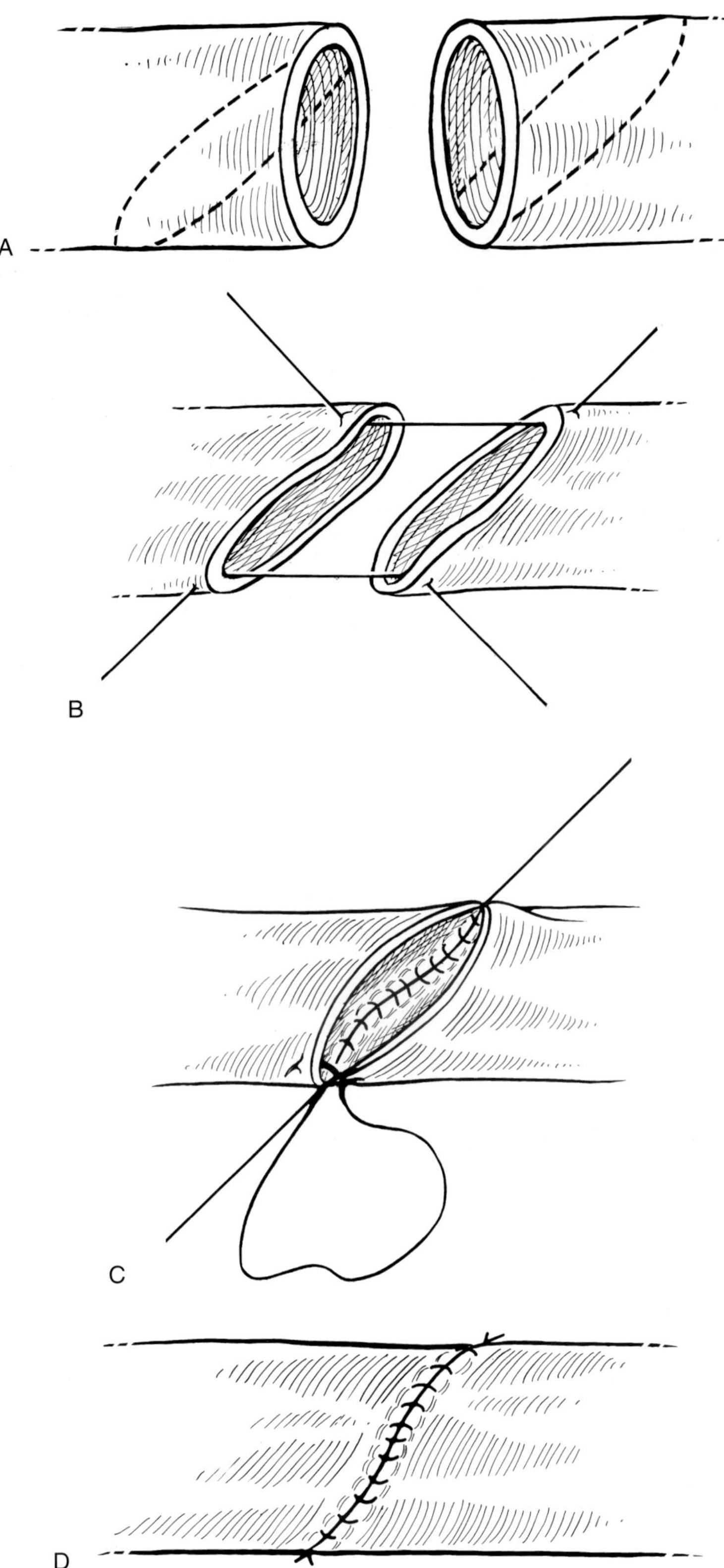

FIG. 7A–D. If an end-to-end anastomosis is required, the vessels should be cut obliquely, and a running spatulated anastomosis is performed. This technique is fast and promotes patency.

SELECTED READINGS

Achauer BM, Salibian AH, Furnas DW. Free flaps to the head and neck. *Head Neck Surg* 1982;4:315–323.

Bengtson BP, Schusterman MA, Baldwin BJ, Miller MJ, Reece GP, Kroll SS, et al. Influence of prior radiotherapy on the development of postoperative complications and success of free tissue transfers in head and neck cancer reconstruction. *Am J Surg* 1993;166:326–330.

Blair EA, Callender DL. Head and neck cancer: the problem. In: Schusterman MA, editor. *Clinics in plastic surgery*. Philadelphia: W. B. Saunders, 1994;1–7.

Duncan MJ, Manktelow RT, Zuker RM, Rosen IB. Mandibular reconstruction in the radiated patient: the role of osteocutaneous free tissue transfers. *Plast Reconstr Surg* 1985;76:829–840.

Fisher J. Microvascular reconstruction of the head and neck. *Mayo Clin Proc* 1986;61:451–458.

Harashina T, Fujino T, Aoyagi F. Reconstruction of the oral cavity with a free flap. *Plast Reconstr Surg* 1976;58: 412–414.

Hardesty RA, Jones NF, Swartz WM, Ramasastry SS, Heckler FD, Newton ED, et al. Microsurgery for macrodefects: microvascular free-tissue transfer for massive defects of the head and neck. *Am J Surg* 1987;154: 399–405.

Hidalgo DA, Jones CS. The role of emergent exploration in free-tissue transfer: a review of 150 consecutive cases. *Plast Reconstr Surg* 1990;86:492–498.

Knoll SS, Reece GP, Miller MJ, Schusterman MA. Comparison of the rectus abdominis free flap with the pectoralis major myocutaneous flap for reconstructions in the head and neck. *Am J Surg* 1992;164:615–618.

Miller MJ, Schusterman MA, Reece GP, Knoll SS. Interposition vein grafting in head and neck reconstructive microsurgery. *J Reconstr Microsurg* 1993;9:245–251.

Mulholland S, Boyd JB, McCabe S, Gullane P, Rotstein L, Brown D, et al. Recipient vessels in head and neck microsurgery: radiation effect and vessel access [see comments]. *Plast Reconstruct Surg* 1993;92:628–632.

al Qattan MM, Boyd JB. Complications in head and neck microsurgery. [Review]. *Microsurgery* 1993;14: 187–195.

Rosen IB, Bell MSG, Barron PT, Zuker RM, Manktelow RT. Use of microvascular flaps including free osteocutaneous flaps in reconstruction after composite resection for radiation-recurrent oral cancer. *Am J Surg* 1979; 138:544–549.

Schusterman MA, Kroll SS, Weber RS, Byers RM, Guillamondegui OM, Goepfert H. Intraoral soft tissue reconstruction after cancer ablation: a comparison of the pectoralis major flap and the free radial forearm flap. *Am J Surg* 1991;162:397–399.

Schusterman MA, Miller MJ, Reece GP, Kroll SS, Marchi M, Goepfert H. A single center's experience with 308 free flaps for repair of head and neck cancer defects. *Plast Reconstr Surg* 1994;93(3):472–478.

Shestak KC, Myers EN, Ramasastry SS, Jones NF, Johnson JT. Vascularized free-tissue transfer in head and neck surgery. [Review]. *Am J Otolaryngol* 1993;14:148–154.

Soutar DS, McGregor IA. The radial forearm flap in intraoral reconstruction: the experience of 60 consecutive cases. *Plast Reconstr Surg* 1986;78:1–8.

Tabah R, Flynn M, Acland R, Banis JC. Microvascular free tissue transfer in head and neck and esophageal surgery. *Am J Surg* 1984;148:498–504.

Urken ML, Weinberg H, Buchbinder D, Moscoso JF, Lawson W, Catalano PJ, et al. Microvascular free flaps in head and neck reconstruction. Report of 200 cases and review of complications. *Arch Otolaryngol Head Neck Surg* 1994;120:633–640.

Wells MD, Edwards AL, Luce EA. Intraoral reconstructive techniques. [Review]. *Clin Plast Surg* 1995;22: 91–108.

Wells MD, Luce EA, Edwards AL, Vasconez HC, Sadove RC, Bouzaglou S. Sequentially linked free flaps in head and neck reconstruction. *Clin Plast Surg* 1994;21:59–67.

Zuker RM, Manktelow RT, Palmer JA, Rosen IB. Head and neck reconstruction following resection of carcinoma, using microvascular free flaps. *Surgery* 1980;88:461–466.

Zuker RM, Rosen IB, Palmer JA, Sutton FR, McKee NH, Manktelow RT. Microvascular free flaps in head and neck reconstruction. *Can J Surg* 1980;23:157–162.

Microsurgical Reconstruction of the Cancer Patient, edited by M.A. Schusterman.
Lippincott-Raven Publishers, Philadelphia © 1997.

2

Intraoral Soft Tissue Reconstruction

Gregory R. D. Evans and Stephen S. Kroll

NATURE OF THE DEFECT

Squamous cell carcinoma frequently arises in the oral cavity. Contact of the oral mucosa with alcohol and tobacco is a contributing factor in the development of head and neck cancer. Reconstructive surgeons commonly encounter defects of the oral cavity and base of tongue, the floor of the mouth, and the retromolar trigone. In some cases, the defects are composite and extensive, including the mandible, skin of the cheek and/or neck, and even the orbit. In most cases, however, the defects are confined to the intraoral mucous membranes and require replacement lining and a variable quantity of underlying soft tissue for repair.

FLAP SELECTION

Although a variety of free flaps are available for repair of any given intraoral defect, each surgeon usually has a few favorite flaps used frequently because of their reliability. For us, these flaps would include the radial forearm and the rectus abdominis free flap. One of these two flaps will be suitable for almost any intraoral defect not requiring bone. The goals of intraoral reconstruction are first to ensure good speech and swallowing, and second to obtain good cosmesis. Oral function is determined by tongue function. If there is 20% or more of the native tongue remaining, one should use a thin pliable flap to ensure mobility of the remaining tongue segment. If, however there is less tongue remaining, one needs to replace tongue bulk by using a thicker, less pliable flap.

G. E. Evans and S. S. Kroll: Department of Plastic Surgery, The University of Texas, M.D. Anderson Cancer Center, Houston, Texas 77030.

The thin, pliable flap of choice for us is the free radial forearm flap. This flap not only has the optimal characteristics to ensure tongue mobility, but is highly reliable due to the large diameters of its recipient vessels. A patient with a floor of mouth cancer requiring marginal mandibulectomy and coverage with soft tissue would be a typical example of a defect best served by the radial forearm flap (Fig. 1A–F). In this particular case, the remaining native mandible has been reinforced with a reconstruction plate.

For total or subtotal defects of the tongue, the bulky flap of choice is the rectus abdominis flap. This flap can be harvested either in the vertical or transverse orientation, depending on the amount of tissue that is needed. Thus, thorough mastery of these two flaps will enable a surgeon to repair almost any intraoral defect that might be encountered. We will first describe the use of the radial forearm flap.

RADIAL FOREARM FREE FLAP

Anatomy

The anatomic basis of the radial forearm free flap lies with the vascularity supplied by the radial artery (Fig. 2A, B). This artery runs longitudinally along the volar aspect of the forearm and gives off perforating branches to the skin, subcutaneous tissue, muscle, and bone. The flap's cutaneous septal perforators lie between the flexor carpi radialis and the brachioradialis muscles. The entire flap may be raised on this septal stalk with maintenance of vascularity. Reconstruction of the radial artery with vein grafts is usually not required. However, if necessary due to insufficient flow to the radial side of the hand through the palmar arch, radial artery replacement can be achieved by using one of the many forearm veins.

Three separate venous systems provide drainage for the flap. These systems are the cephalic vein, the basilic vein, and the venae comitantes that run adjacent to the artery. The venae comitantes are the veins most frequently utilized for flap transfer, but are occasionally too small. Consequently, it is advisable to elevate a cephalic or basilic vein with the flap in case an alternative venous drainage pathway is required (Fig. 2C).

Sensory innervation of the flap is provided by the medial and lateral cutaneous nerves of the forearm. If a sensate flap is desired, one of these branches can be harvested with the flap and sutured to the lingual or superficial sensory nerves in the neck.

Technique of Dissection: Fasciocutaneous Flaps

Variations in anatomy may divide the vascular distribution of the ulnar and radial side of the hand, requiring a preoperative Allen's test. It is essential that any obstruction within the radial, ulnar, or digital arteries be known prior to flap elevation. Absence of collateral circulation precludes the use of the radial forearm flap, or at least requires vascular reconstruction.

Defect type and tissue requirements dictate the design of the flap. The territory of the flap may be extended from the lower third of the anterior aspect of the arm proximally to the wrist flexion crease distally. Distal width is from the extensor carpi radialis longus muscle to the extensor carpi ulnaris muscle. Proximal width may vary from the lateral to the medial humeral epicondyle. If pedicle length is desired, flap design is placed distally on the extremity. If pedicle length is not an issue, dissection places the distal edge of the flap 2.0 to 5.0 cm proximal to the wrist crease. This offers thicker flap skin for reconstruction and less exposure of the flexor tendons after flap elevation. A tourniquet is placed on the upper arm and once the limb is exsanguinated with an Esmarch, the tourniquet pressure is maintained at 250 mm Hg (tourniquet time averages 1 hour). Several techniques have been reported for flap elevation. We prefer to identify structures at the distal border first. The flexor tendons, radial artery and vena comitantes, cephalic vein, brachioradialis, and median nerve are all identified. Elevation can begin on either the radial or ulnar side of the forearm; however, we pre-

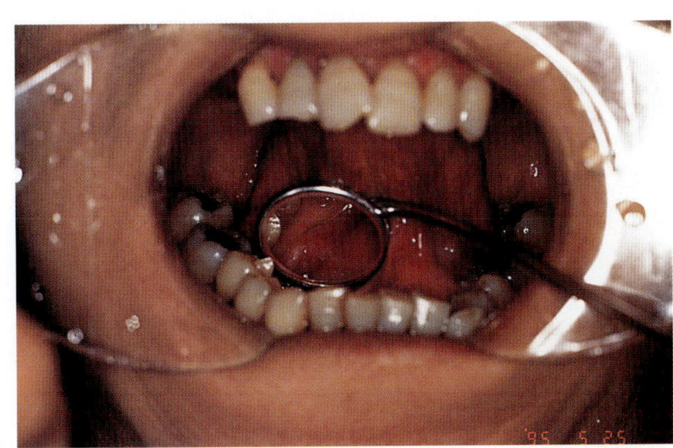

FIG. 1A. A patient with a squamous cell carcinoma of the floor of mouth impinging on the gingiva.

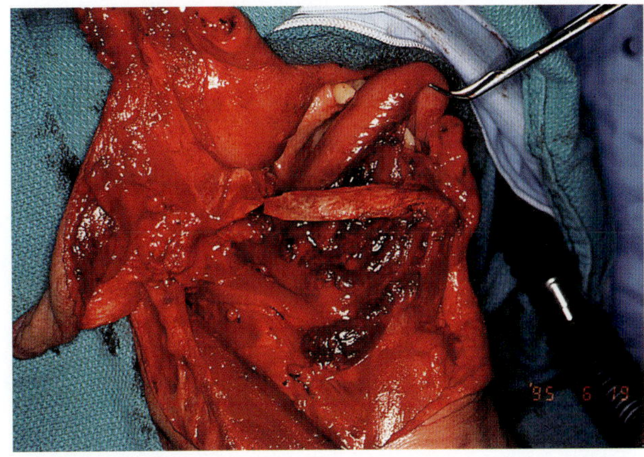

FIG. 1B. The defect after soft tissue resection and marginal mandibulectomy.

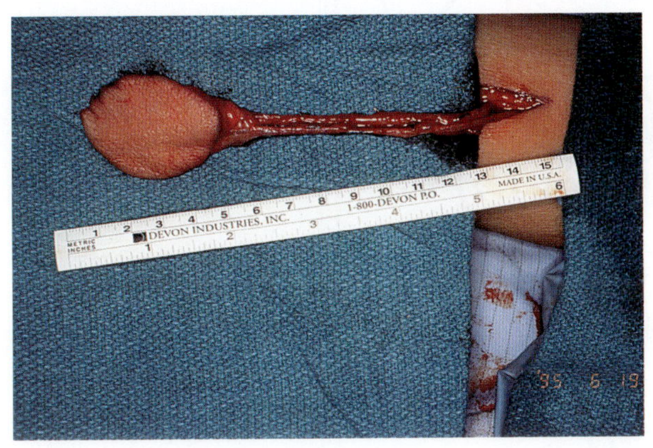

FIG. 1C. The radial forearm flap after elevation. Note the length of the pedicle.

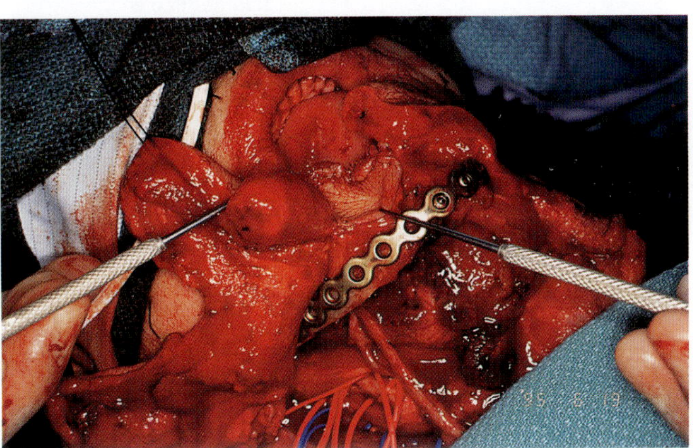

FIG. 1D. Flap after partial inset. Note that the flap is inset prior to revascularization. A reconstruction plate has been placed to reinforce the mandible.

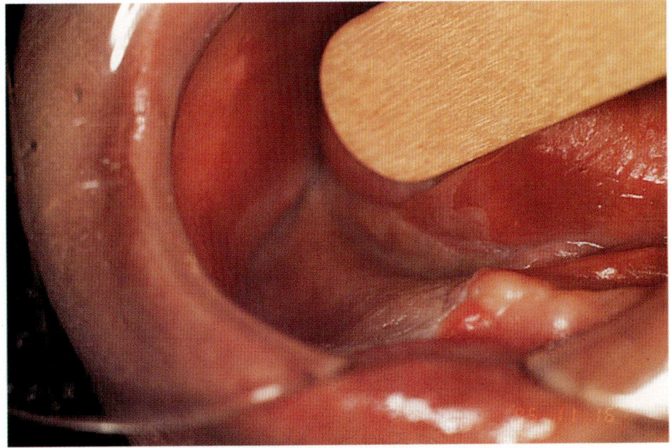

FIG. 1E. Final result. Note how the flap reapproximates the normal soft tissue contours.

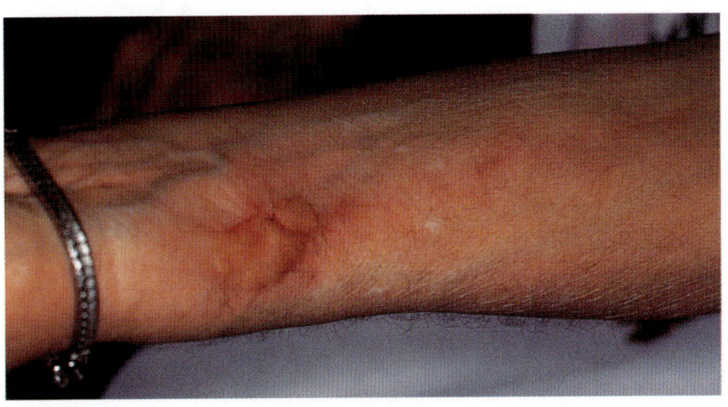

FIG. 1F. A full-thickness graft from the groin has been used to close the donor defect. Use of full-thickness grafts improves the donor site aesthetics.

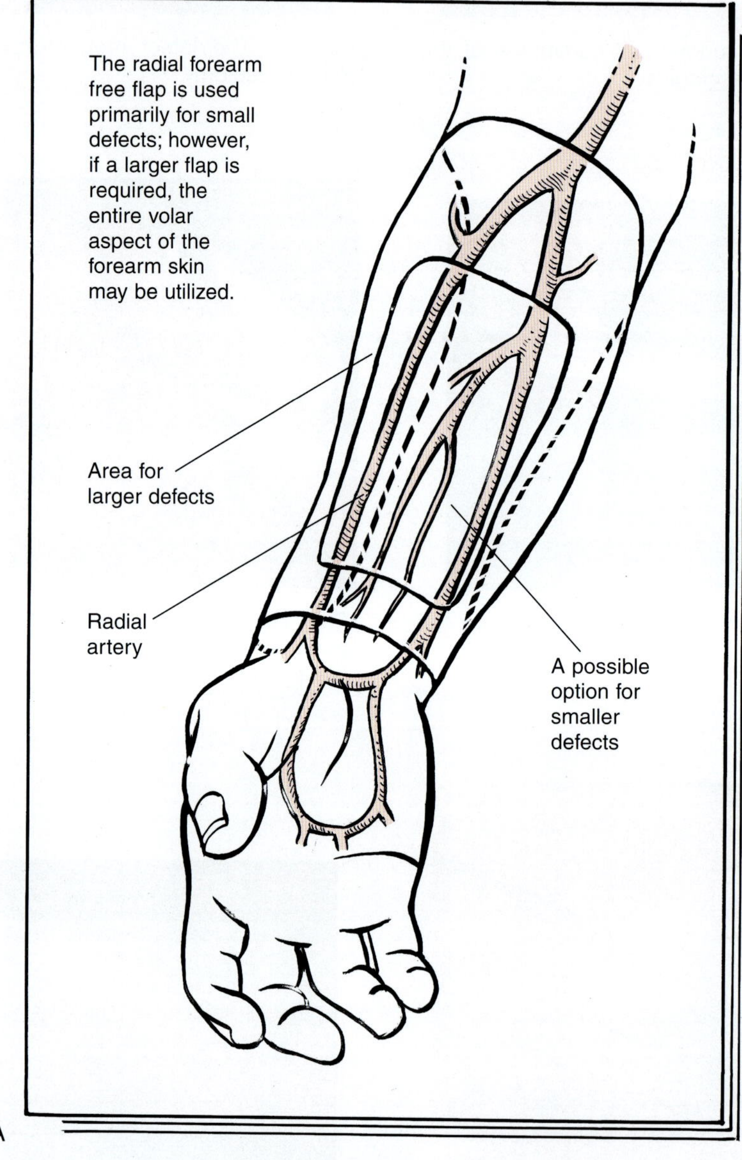

FIG. 2A. The anatomy of the radial forearm flap. Note the flap should be located over the the route of the radial vessels.

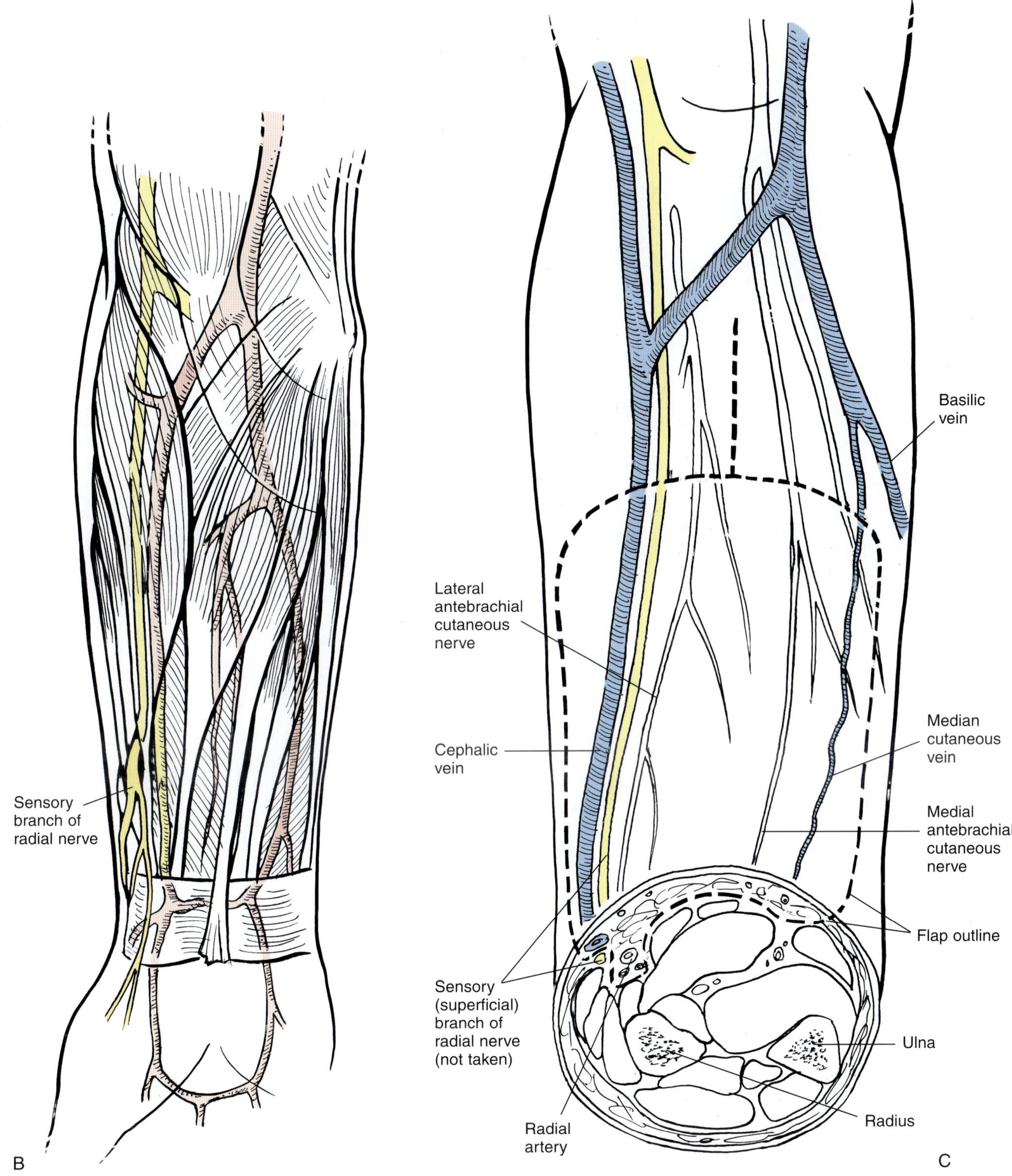

FIG. 2B. The radial sensory nerve exits at the lower portion of the brachioradialis muscle. This must be preserved when elevating the flap.

FIG. 2C. A diagram of the venous anatomy showing the flap design so that the cephalic vein is included in the flap.

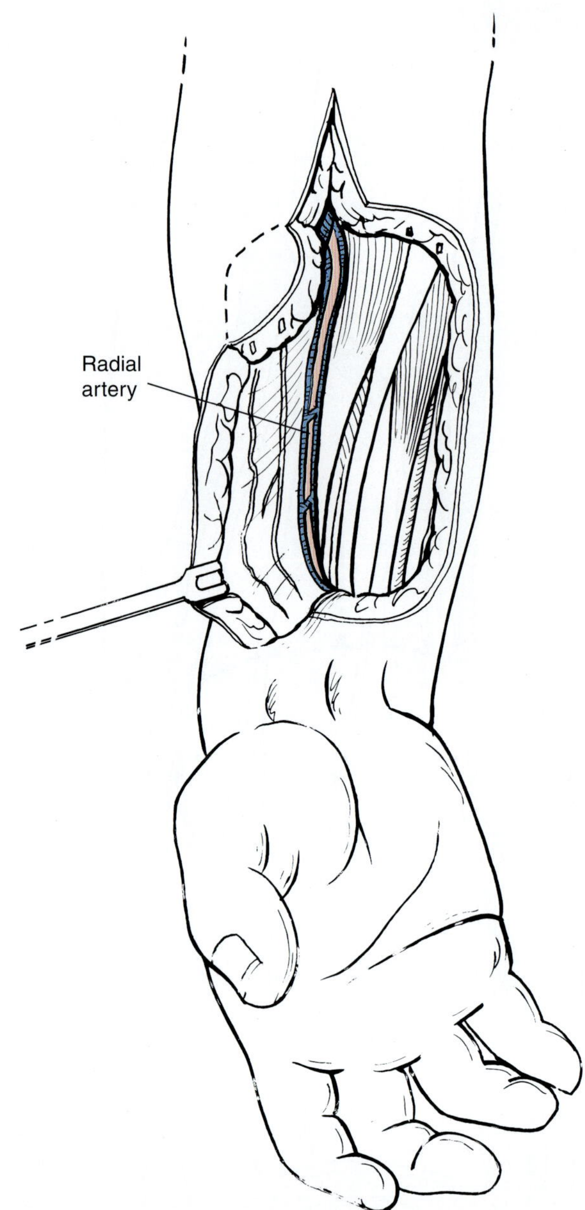

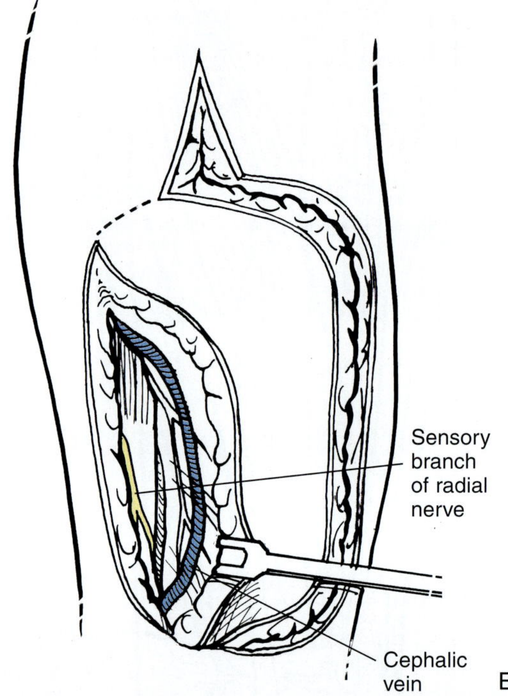

FIG. 3A. Flap harvest is started by first elevating the ulnar side of the flap.

FIG. 3B. The radial incision is then made, and the cephalic vein is identified, ligated distally, and the superficial radial nerve is then dissected free from the fascia.

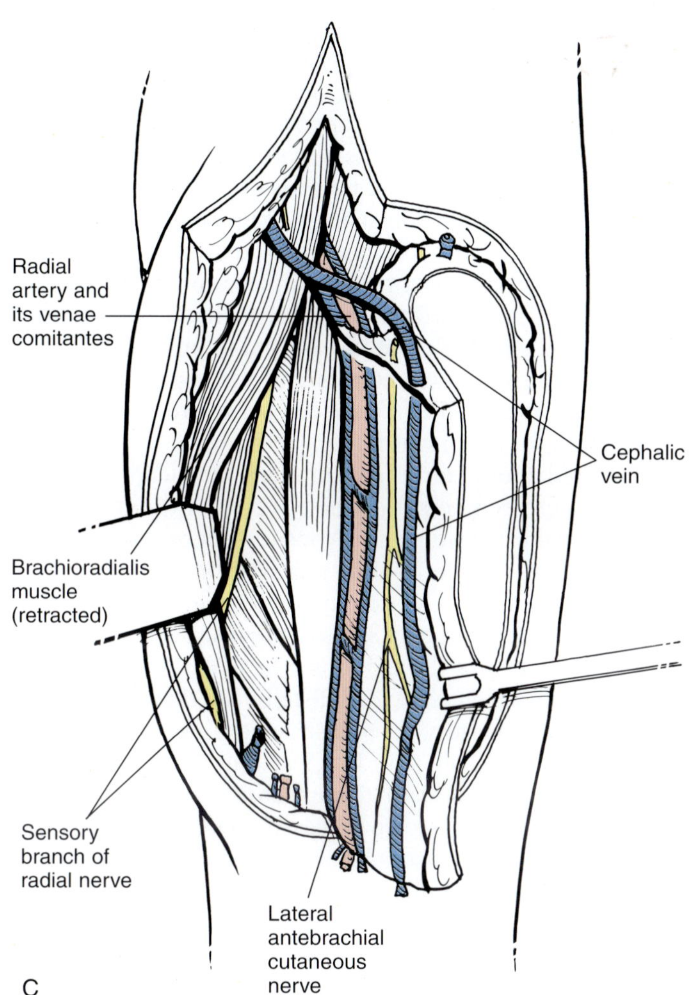

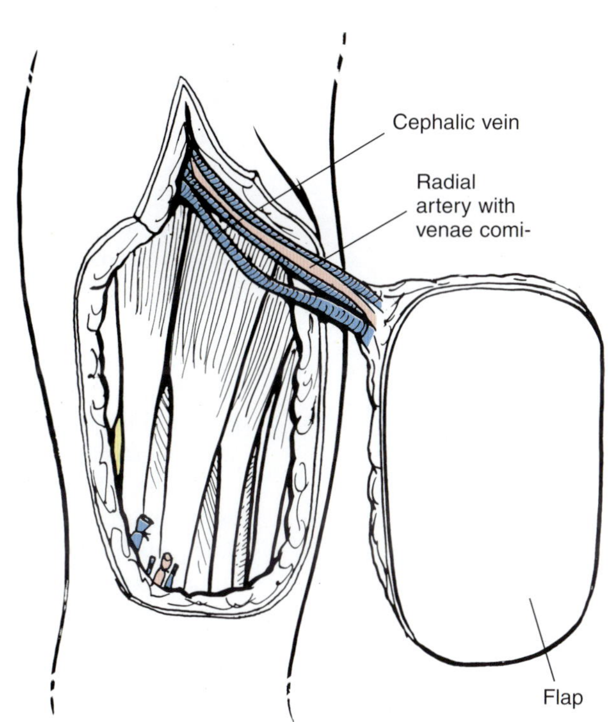

FIG. 3C. The radial artery and venae comitantes are then identified and ligated distally.

FIG. 3D. The flap is then elevated from distal to proximal. Once the proximal aspect of the flap has been reached, an incision is made up to the antecubital fossa, and the cephalic vein and radial vessels are dissected toward their origin. Care should be taken to avoid injury to the ulnar vessels.

fer initial ulnar elevation (Fig. 3A). The antebrachial fascia is incised, and dissection proceeds just below this fascia along the flexor tendons. Care must be taken to preserve the paratenon for adequate skin graft take. Suturing the antebrachial fascia to the skin can prevent shearing; however, we have not had this difficulty. Dissection is continued radially under the antebrachial fascia until the radial vessels are identified (Fig. 3B). Special attention should be paid to prevent damage to the fasciocutaneous branches as they emerge from the intermuscular septum. The radial vessels are divided distally and the dissection continues toward the extensor carpi radialis longus muscle. The antebrachial fascia is incised over the brachioradialis muscle, if the flap design extends this far. Care must be taken to preserve the superficial branches of the radial sensory nerve (Fig. 3B, C). The sensory radial nerve lies superficial to the radial artery and arborizes after reaching its superficial location. This nerve runs from below the fascia to the subcutaneous plane, emerging between the tendons of the extensor carpi radialis longus and those of the brachioradialis tendon at about the juncture of the distal third and middle third of the forearm (Fig. 2B). The nerve may exit anywhere from the midportion of the forearm to as far distally as a few centimeters proximal to the radial styloid. If dissected with the flap, the superficial veins (cephalic or basilic) are also divided distally (Fig. 3C). The flap is then elevated in a distal to proximal direction on its radial artery pedicle with the venae comitantes and the superficial vein intact (Fig. 3D). The lateral and medial antebrachial cutaneous nerve provides sensation to the forearm and can be elevated for attempted flap innervation.

If a long vascular pedicle is required, the forearm incision may be extended to the bifurcation of the ulnar artery. The increased vessel diameter (2–4 mm) around the antecubital fossa facilitates microvascular anastomoses. After dissection, tourniquet compression is released and the vascularity of the hand is assessed. If arterial reconstruction is required, any of the numerous upper extremity superficial veins can be used. Alternatively, the flap may be elevated from both sides to the fascial septum over the radial artery, allowing continued blood flow through this artery until the defect is prepared for flap transfer. The radial artery is then divided distally, the flap is elevated with the radial artery pedicle, and the radial artery is reconstructed if necessary.

Closure of the forearm proceeds simultaneously with flap insetting. Reactive hyperemia requires 5 to 10 minutes of pressure on the forearm to compensate for this reaction. Adequate hemostasis is essential if the skin graft is to be successful. Dermal absorbable sutures are used to close as much of the forearm as possible. Skin sutures (4-0 nylon) or staples may also be used for skin approximation. Full- or split-thickness unmeshed skin grafts are placed over the remaining open wound (Fig. 1F). The paratenon must be intact, and every effort to advance muscle over the tendons should be made before skin grafting. Dressings and a volar split are applied with the hand in neutral or position of function. This provides stabilization to prevent shearing until neovascularization of the skin graft can occur (by postoperative day 5). Dressings are usually maintained for 5 days. Active and passive motion are begun after these 5 days if the graft appears to be viable and adherent. Skin grafts are kept moist with cream or bacitracin ointment.

Three-dimensional defects are easily filled, as the flap can be folded on itself for insetting (Fig. 4A). Insetting requires adequate exposure, frequently necessitating lip-splitting incisions along with mandibulotomies. Mattress sutures (Vicryl, Ethicon Inc., Somerville, New Jersey) are required to secure a "water-tight" closure. Insetting is usually completed before performing the anastomosis to allow for accurate placement of sutures without bleeding or flap edema (Fig. 4B). In irradiated tissue, blood flow of the recipient vessels must be assessed before the anastomosis. Arterial and venous dissection should proceed with care in these irradiated patients and excessive manipulation should be limited.

Donor Defects

The fear of significant donor defects has prevented some reconstructive surgeons from using the radial forearm free flap. We have not found donor defects to be a sig-

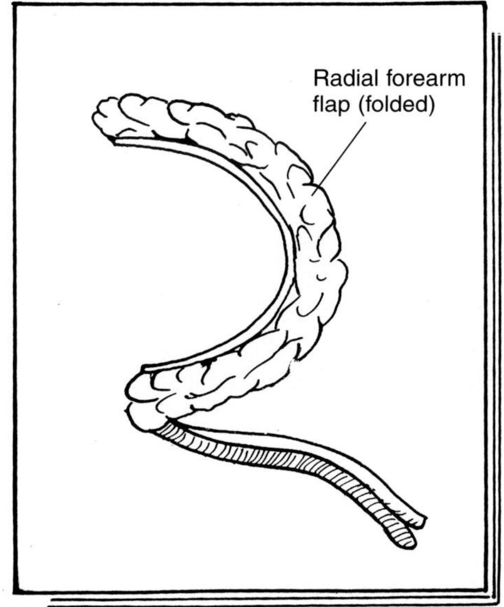

A

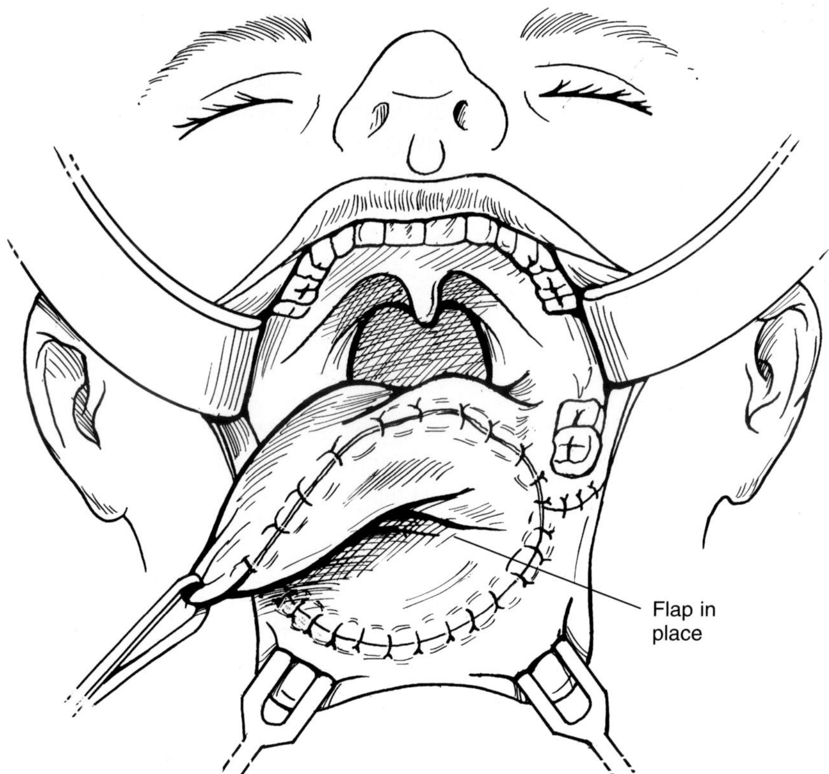

B

FIG. 4A,B. The flap is inset into the floor of the mouth. Note that the thinness of the flap allows it to follow the contours of the oral cavity and better approximate the native soft tissue configuration.

nificant deterrent to the use of this flap, provided certain guidelines are followed. The paratenon must be preserved over the tendon for the skin graft to be successful. Exposed tendons after skin graft coverage, although bothersome, have not led to long-term problems in mobility of the wrist or arm. If an osseous component is harvested, beveling the osteotomy sites and limiting bony resection to one-third of the radius diameter reduces the risk of fracture. Immobilization for 6 to 8 weeks has been our routine. If reconstruction of the radial artery is necessary, or if the radial sensory nerve is exposed, rotational flaps may be required to cover these exposed structures. We have avoided meshing split-thickness skin grafts utilized for coverage.

The radial forearm free flap offers, in our opinion, the single best form of oral lining replacement, provided that bulk or bone is not required. With the flap's versatility and ease of execution, it has become a workhorse for intraoral reconstruction of cancer-related defects.

RECTUS ABDOMINIS FREE FLAP

The rectus abdominis free flap is both versatile and useful when used for intraoral soft tissue reconstruction. It has a long pedicle with large-caliber vessels, and the donor site is easily hidden by clothing. The flap can carry a skin paddle for large defects and enough tissue volume for breast reconstruction. Although often thick and bulky, in some patients the flap is thin enough to be used to reconstruct the floor of the mouth. The rectus abdominis flap is technically easy to execute, so failure of the flap is distinctly uncommon. For these reasons, it has become a commonly used flap in our reconstructive practice.

In most cases, the rectus abdominis free flap is raised with a vertical skin paddle (Fig. 5), based on the part of the rectus abdominis muscle closest to the umbilicus. The flap is elevated off the external oblique fascia from lateral to medial until perforating vessels are seen entering the flap from the underlying rectus abdominis muscle. These vessels, located in a lateral row, are usually equidistant from the midline (Fig. 6A). Consequently, once one vessel is found, the others are usually easily located.

The fascia is incised just lateral to the perforators, then reflected laterally to expose the rectus muscle. The fascial incision extends to below the lowest perforator, then turns and heads superiorly, circumscribing the fascia that includes the perforating vessels that will be removed with the flap (Fig. 6B). The fascial incision is then extended inferiorly to facilitate retraction of the abdominal wall and exposure of the deep inferior epigastric vessels, allowing direct visual dissection and the ability to obtain a long vascular pedicle (Fig. 6B,C).

Once the pedicle has been isolated, the muscle is divided above and below the flap. These fibers of the rectus muscle lateral to the perforating vessels, like the fascia, can be preserved in situ. If most of the perforators are lateral, muscle can be preserved medially as well. The surgeon should only include as much muscle as is necessary to maintain the blood supply in the flap, because excess muscle bulk tends to interfere with flap insertion. The muscle should not be relied on for restoration of missing bulk, except perhaps in reconstruction of the tongue, because of the risk of future muscle atrophy.

The rectus abdominis flap can be folded (Fig. 7A–C) to maximize the amount of volume and fill the oral cavity as completely as possible while still allowing mouth closure. The excess volume is needed to compensate for muscle atrophy during the first 6 months after surgery. In most cases, the final result will be adequate to permit reasonable function, but only if the surgeon has tried diligently to make the tongue as large as possible during the reconstruction itself.

If the oral defect is limited to one-half to two-thirds of the tongue, an excellent reconstruction can often be accomplished by using a rectus abdominis muscle without a skin paddle. Split-thickness skin grafts may be used directly on the muscle, or the anterior fascial coverage of the muscle can be used. Although this reconstruction

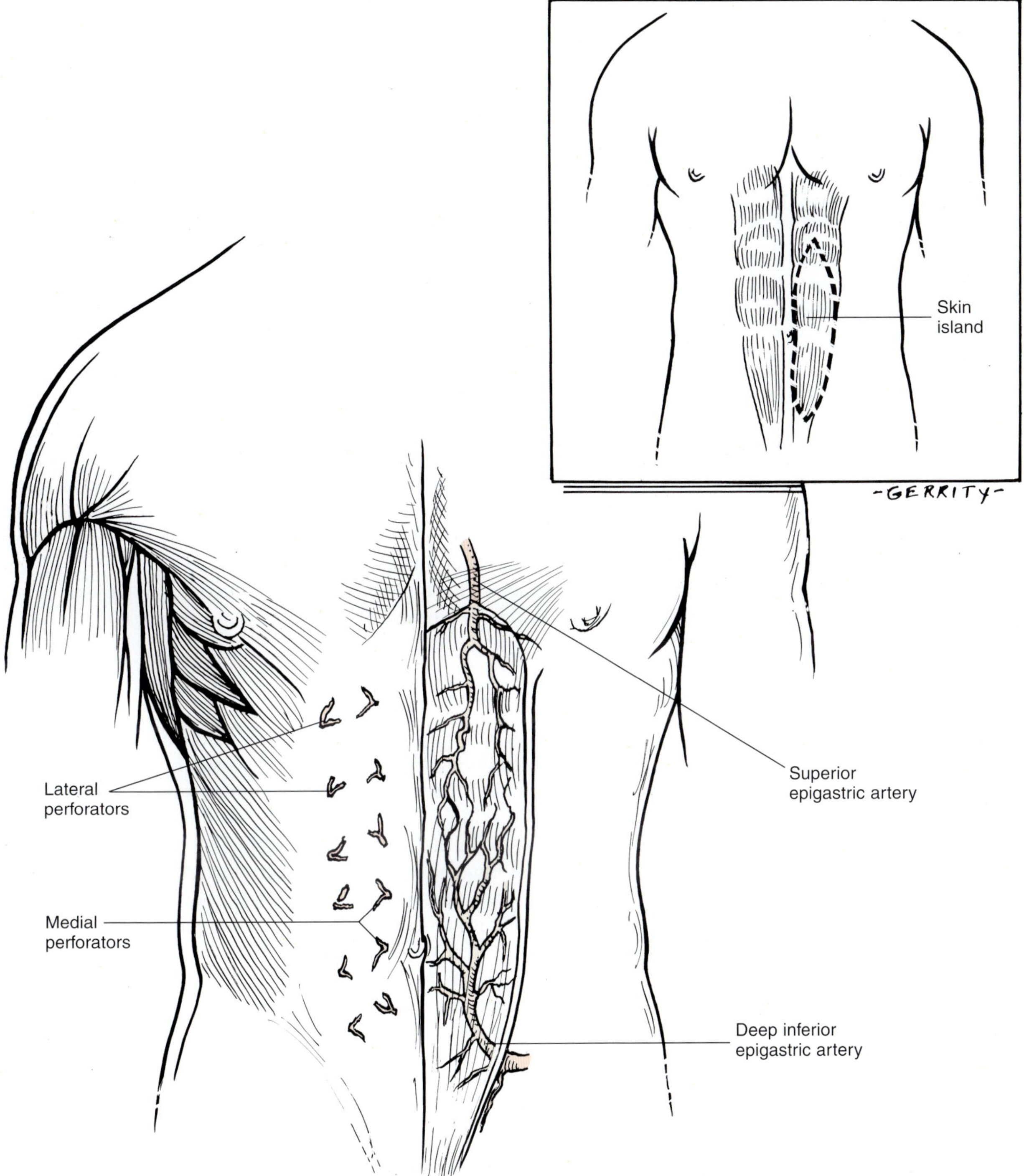

FIG. 5. The anatomy of the rectus abdominis muscle. The vertical orientation of the perforators allow for vertical orientation of the skin paddle.

will use denervated muscle that is susceptible to atrophy, it often maintains more of its bulk than might be expected, perhaps because of the influence of adjacent innervated muscle.

Another common indication for the rectus abdominis flap is a posterior mandibular defect. In such cases, restoration of the large oral lining defect contributes more to the restoration of function than does replacement of the bone. Unilateral absence of the posterior mandible alone, unaccompanied by a lining defect, creates relatively little morbidity. Provided that the remaining mandible is in the normal position, both function and appearance can be almost normal. For this reason, posterior mandibular defects in patients who are not good surgical candidates for reconstruction with vascularized bone can be alternatively managed with a rectus abdominis free flap (Fig. 8).

The flap is raised in the usual way, and the anastomoses performed to the great vessels in the neck. The lining defect is then measured, and the flap is trimmed to fit the intraoral defect. The flap is then inset with absorbable sutures (usually 3-0 Vicryl) using the subcutaneous fatty tissue bulk of the flap to substitute for the absent mandible. This soft-tissue substitution can prevent lateral drift of the residual jaw. The appearance of the neck will be improved if the muscle volume in the flap is minimized. However, if muscle must be included, it should be sutured superiorly to prevent drift into the lower part of the neck (Fig. 9). Although occlusion will be imperfect, the appearance and function of the patient can be very acceptable (Fig. 10A–C). Although considered a compromise compared to replacement of the absent mandible with vascularized bone, the technique does have the advantages of reduced donor site morbidity, shorter operative time, and a high success rate. This alternative can be a useful solution to an otherwise difficult problem.

CONCLUSION

Although a wide variety of options are available for reconstruction of the oral cavity, a radial forearm or rectus abdominis free flap is usually the best choice when defects larger than 3 cm are encountered. These techniques have high success rates, acceptable donor site morbidity, and lower complication rates than comparable regional flaps, and can usually achieve the reconstructive goals in one stage. The development of free tissue transfer has revolutionized the repair of oral cavity defects, and dramatically improved the outcomes of surgical treatment by making more extensive resections feasible. With the radial forearm and the rectus abdominis free flaps, the reconstructive surgeon can repair almost any soft-tissue oral defect that might be encountered. Once a surgeon has truly mastered these flaps, he or she will inevitably come to believe that there are few indications for the more traditional alternatives.

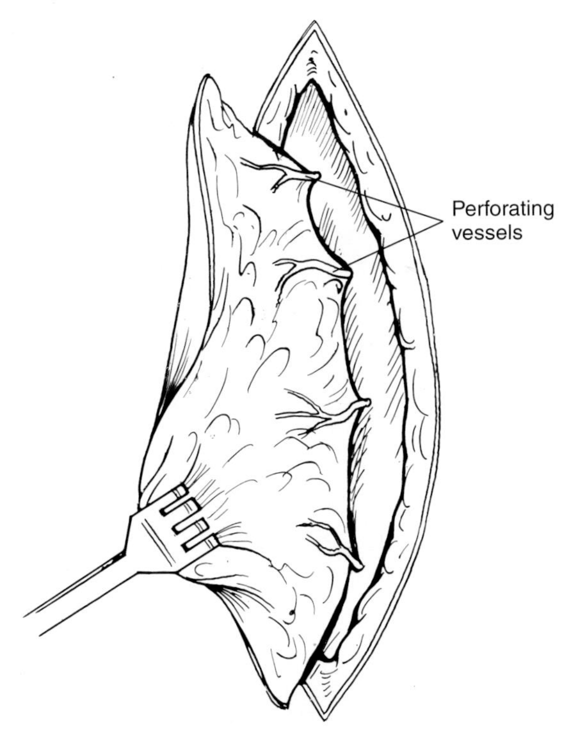

A

FIG. 6A. The lateral row of perforators entering the rectus abdominis flap equidistant from the midline.

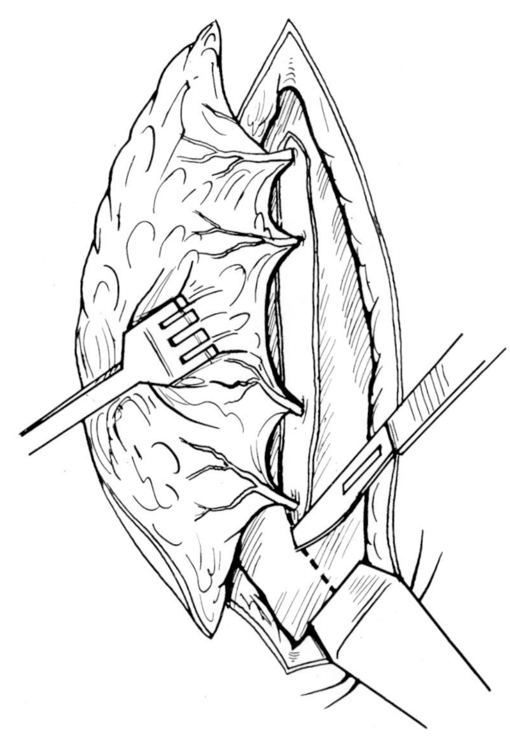

B

FIG. 6B. The incision through the anterior rectus sheath, designed to include all perforators with the rectus abdominis flap.

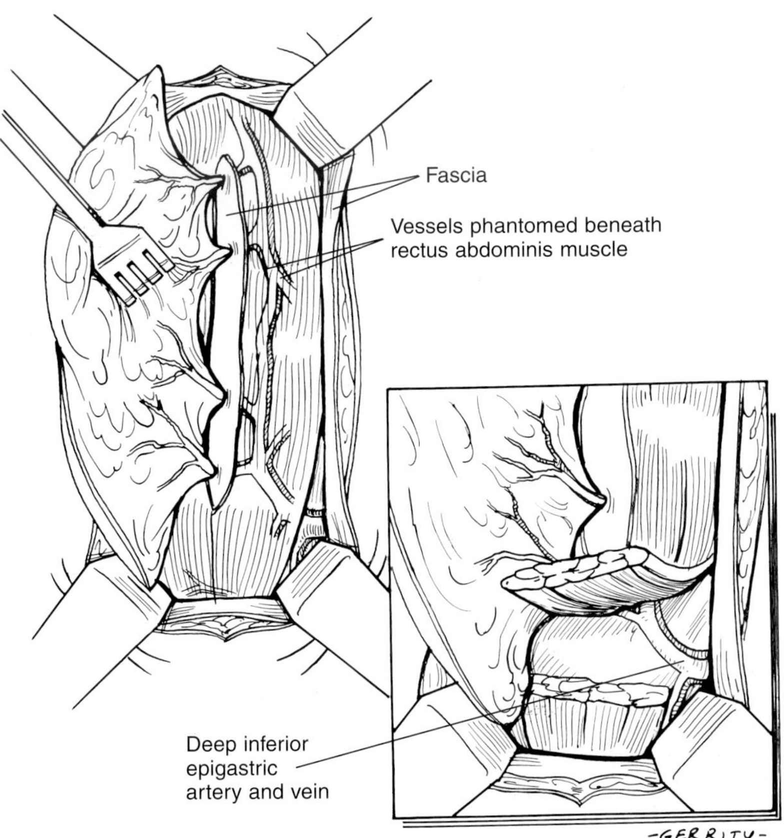

C

FIG. 6C. The inferior fascial extension, which improves exposure of the deep inferior epigastric vessels. The exposure of the deep inferior epigastric vessels allows easy dissection of a long flap pedicle.

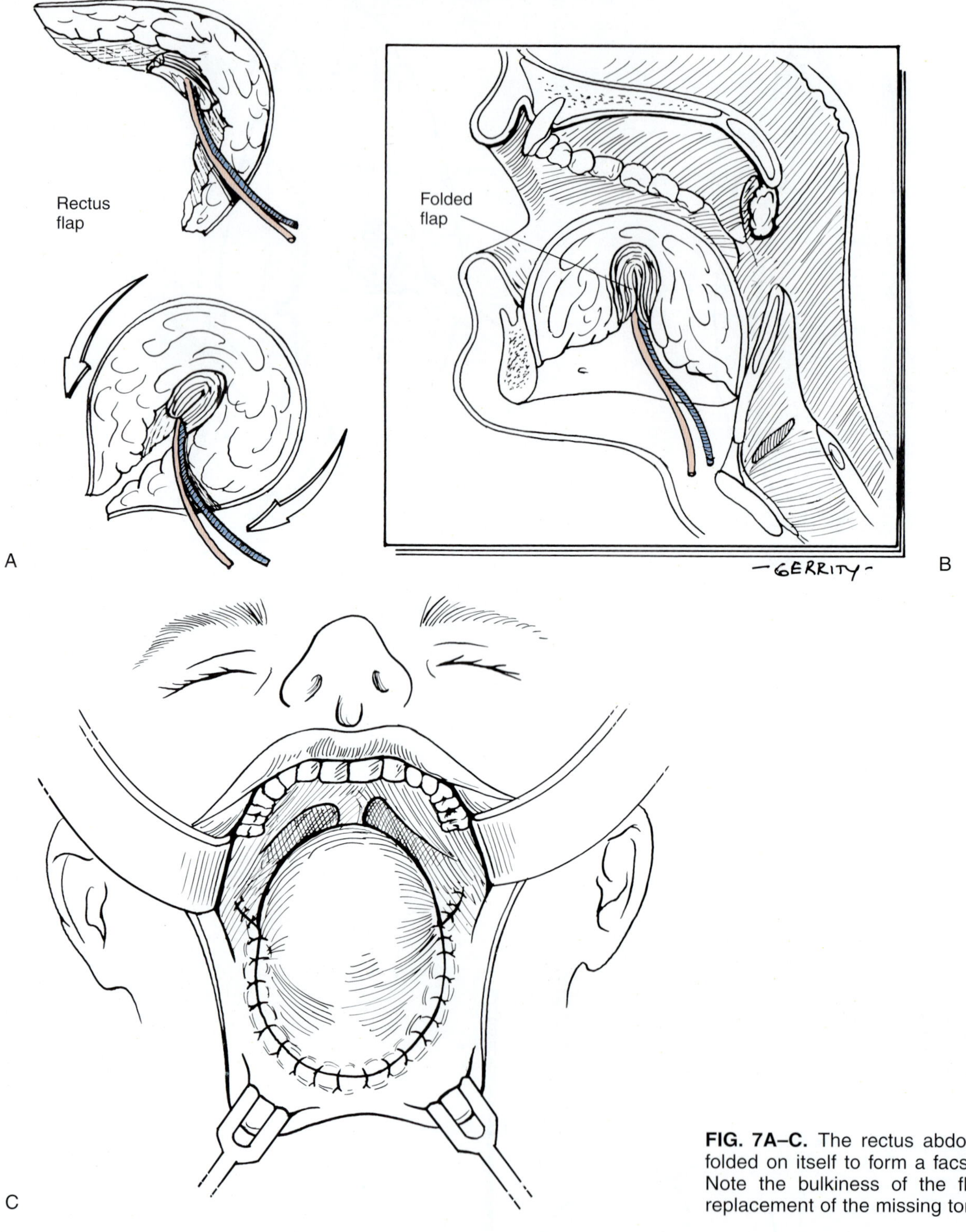

FIG. 7A–C. The rectus abdominis flap can be folded on itself to form a facsimile of a tongue. Note the bulkiness of the flap is optimal for replacement of the missing tongue bulk.

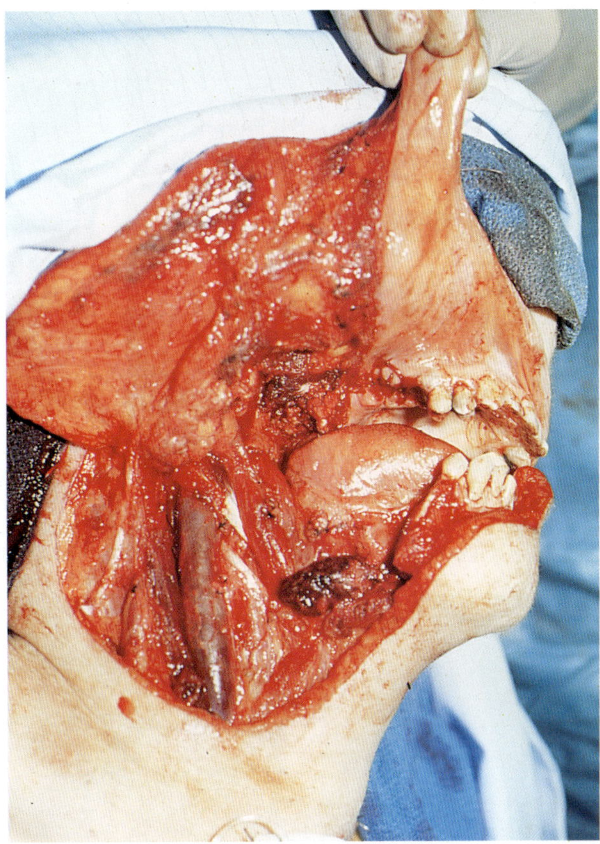

FIG. 8. A posterior mandibular defect following composite resection for an intraoral squamous cell carcinoma.

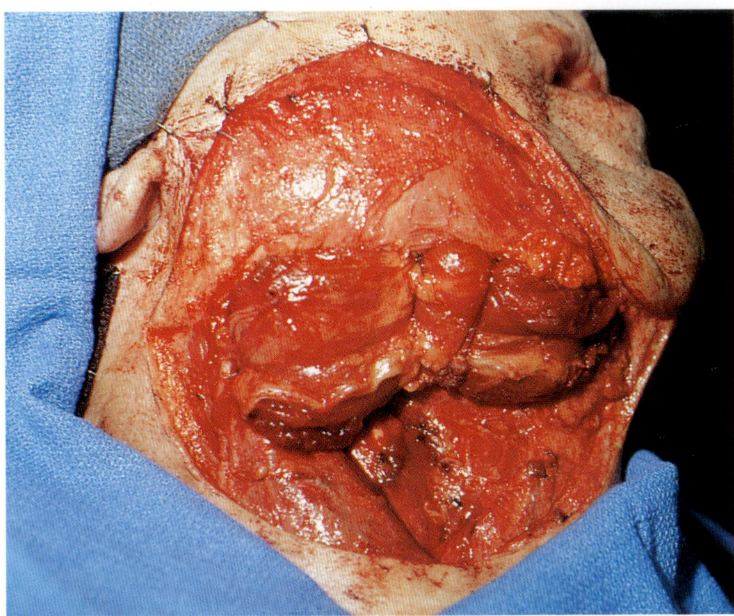

FIG. 9. The muscular portion of a rectus abdominis free flap being retained in the upper neck with sutures.

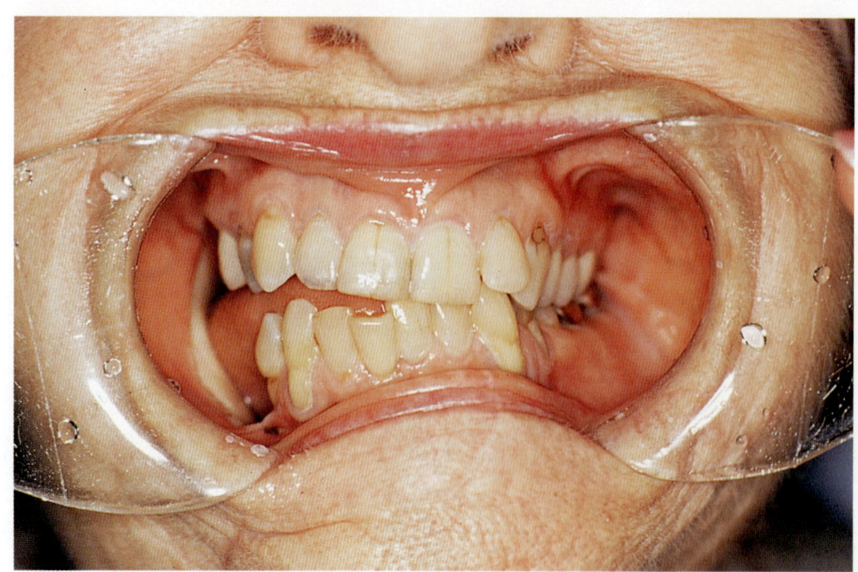

A

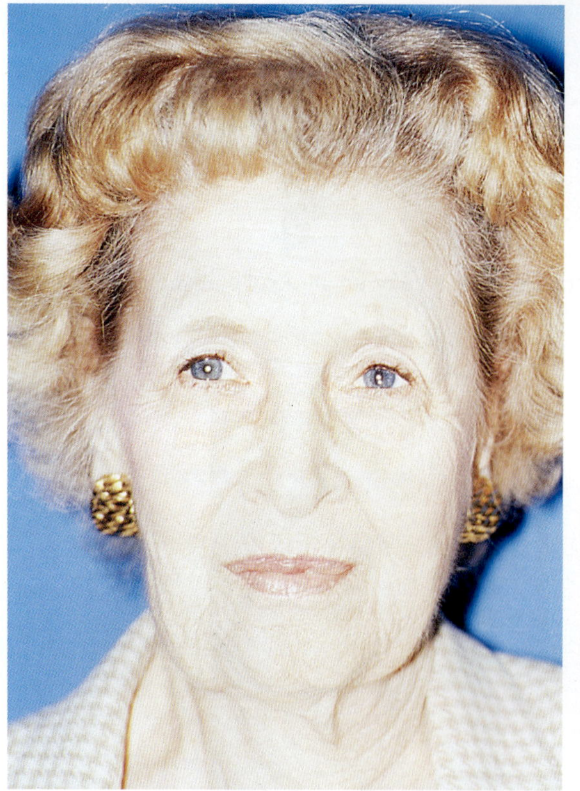

B

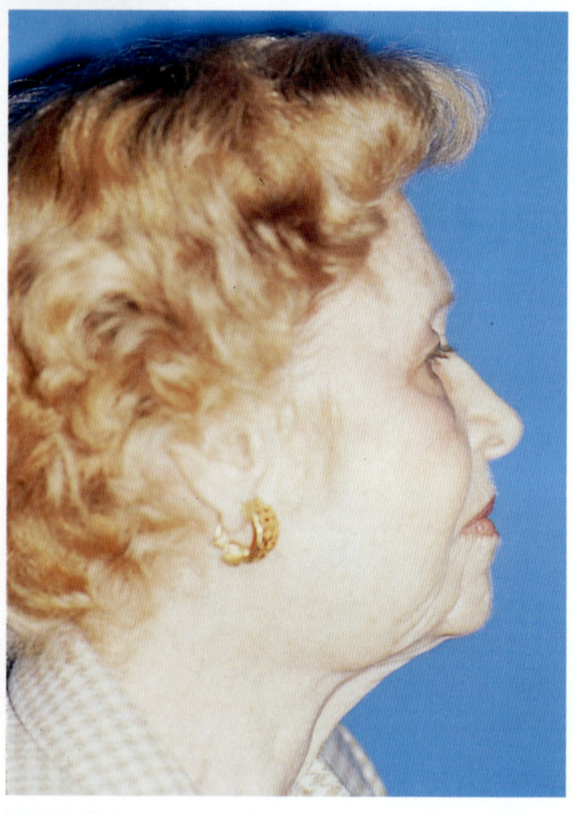

C

FIG. 10A–C. The appearance of the patient in Fig. 8 1 year later is almost normal, despite the absence of bone posteriorly.

SELECTED READINGS

Anthony JP, Singer MI, Mathes SJ. Pharyngoesophageal reconstruction using the tubed free radial forearm flap. *Clin Plast Surg* 1994;21:137–147.

Bardsley AF, Soutar DS, Elliot D, Batchelor AG. Reducing morbidity in the radial forearm flap donor site. *Plast Reconstr Surg* 1990;86:287–294.

Buncke HJ: *Microsurgery: transplantation-replantation. An atlas text*. Philadelphia: Lea and Febiger, 1991.

Cormack GC, Lamberty BGH. A classification of fascio-cutaneous flaps according to their patterns of vascularization. *Br J Plast Surg* 1984;37:80–87.

Evans GRD, Schusterman MA, Kroll SS, Miller MJ, Reece GP, Robb GL, Ainslie N. The radial forearm free flap for head and neck reconstruction: a review. *Am J Surg* 1994;168:446–450.

Evans HB, Lampe HB. The radial forearm flap in head and neck reconstruction. *J Otolaryngol* 1987;16:382.

Hentz VR, Pearl RM, Grossman JAI, Wood MB, Cooney WP. The radial forearm flap: a versatile source of composite tissue. *Ann Plast Surg* 1987;19:485–498.

Juretic M, Car M, Zambelli M. The radial forearm free flap: our experience in solving donor site problems. *J Craniomaxillofac Surg* 1992;20:184–186.

Mackinnon SE, Dellon AL. *Surgery of the peripheral nerve*. New York: Thieme, 1988.

Michiwaki Y, Ohno K, Imai S, Yamashita Y, Suzuki N, Yoshida H, Michi K. Functional effects of intraoral reconstruction with a free radial forearm flap. *J Craniomaxillofac Surg* 1990;18:164–168.

Song R, Gao T, Song Y, Yu Y, Song Y. The radial forearm flap. *Clin Plast Surg* 1982;9:21.

Strauch B, Yu HL. *Atlas of microvascular surgery: anatomy and operative approaches*. New York: Thieme, 1993.

Urken ML, Weinberg H, Vickery C, Biller HF. The neurofasciocutaneous radial forearm flap in head and neck reconstruction: a preliminary report. *Laryngoscope* 1990;100:161–173.

Vaughan ED. The radial forearm free flap in orofacial reconstruction. Personal experience in 120 consecutive cases. *J Craniomaxillofac Surg* 1990;18:2–7.

Yang G, Chen B, Gad Y. Forearm free skin flap transplantation. *Chung-Hua I Hsueh Tsa Chih* 1981;61:139.

Microsurgical Reconstruction of the Cancer Patient, edited by M.A. Schusterman.
Lippincott-Raven Publishers, Philadelphia © 1997.

3

Free Flap Reconstruction of the Mandible

Mark A. Schusterman

Reconstruction of the mandible presents a unique challenge to the oncologic reconstructive surgeon. Essential functions of deglutition, mastication, speech, and retention of saliva are all inherently incumbent on a functioning and intact mandibular arch. Use of vascularized bone by means of free tissue transfer has facilitated our ability to reconstruct large segmental losses of the mandible. Bony union is complete in 6 weeks and very little resorption occurs; thus, the amount of bone placed at the time of the reconstruction is the amount that will remain.

Several different types of flaps from a variety of donor sites have been described. The determination of flap choice is based on the defect location and size. The mandible is resected most commonly due to invasion by large soft tissue tumors originating in the oral cavity mucosa; thus, the bony defect is usually accompanied by a significant soft tissue deficit. It is therefore important to address the soft tissue deficit as well as the bony deficit. For this reason, it is important to choose a flap that can be used reliably as a composite flap. Four composite flaps presently are in common use: the fibular osteocutaneous flap, the iliac crest flap based on the deep circumflex iliac artery (DCIA), the scapular osteocutaneous flap, and the radial forearm osteocutaneous flap.

FLAP CHOICE

The free fibular flap has become the workhorse for mandibular reconstruction. This flap has the longest segment of bone available, up to 25 cm, so condyle-to-condyle reconstructions are possible. The skin paddle derives its blood supply from the septo-

M. A. Schusterman: Department of Plastic Surgery, The University of Texas, M.D. Anderson Cancer Center, Houston, Texas 77030.

cutaneous and musculocutaneous perforators originating on the peroneal vessels and it is highly reliable. The location of the donor site on the lower extremity allows for flap harvest simultaneously with the ablative surgery and for dissection under tourniquet control. There is minimal donor site morbidity, particularly when compared to the iliac crest and scapular flaps. The free fibular flap has become our flap of choice in most instances of mandibular replacement, particularly for repair of anterior mandibular defects (Fig. 1A–K).

The iliac crest flap is based on the DCIA and can be configured to include bone, the internal oblique muscle, and the overlying flank skin, or any combination thereof. The main advantage of this flap is that the donor site scar is well hidden. Additionally, the bone portion of this flap is quite thick and readily accepts osseointegrated dental implants. The pedicle is large and consistent. The disadvantages of the flap are several. First, it is a bulky flap, particularly when the skin paddle is used intraorally. This may impede tongue mobility and therefore negatively influence oral function. There is also quite a bit of donor site morbidity; because the entire thickness of abdominal wall and bone are harvested, hernia formation is significant, particularly in older, debilitated patients. To remedy this situation, the split iliac crest flap, using only the inner cortex, has been advocated. Another donor site issue is the pain that patients experience with this procedure, including the chronic thigh paresthesia that may result if the lateral femoral cutaneous nerve is injured during the dissection (see below). Because of these problems, the iliac crest flap is used most commonly for cases in which the fibula is not available, because of trauma or vascular insufficiency, or in situations in which the amount of bone required is limited and the split iliac crest flap will suffice.

Use of the scapular osteocutaneous flap for mandibular reconstruction was popularized by Swartz. The flap has the unique advantage of having three separate vascular stalks with two skin paddles and one paddle of bone; these allow for easier shaping and insetting of the flap. The disadvantages of the scapular flap are several. First, there is a limited quantity of bone available for harvest. The maximum length of bone that can be harvested is 12 cm, and the width is adequate for placement of osseointegrated implants in only 70% to 80% of the specimens. Second, there is some limitation of shoulder mobility resulting from flap harvest. This can be especially problematic in patients who have had standard radical neck dissections with sacrifice of the spinal accessory nerve. Finally, the patient needs to be turned in order to harvest the flap, so the harvest cannot be performed at the same time as the ablation; this adds operative time to an already lengthy procedure. The scapular flap is best indicated for cases in which two skin paddles are required, specifically large through-and-through defects.

The radial forearm osteocutaneous flap is mentioned only for the sake of completeness. We have found very few instances in which the radial forearm osteocutaneous flap would be our flap of choice for mandibular replacement. The free radial forearm flap has already been described for soft tissue replacement; however, a segment of the lateral aspect of the radius can be included in the flap to create an osteocutaneous flap. This flap has two serious problems: first, the amount of bone is the smallest of any of the flaps described, and second, there is a significant reduction in structural strength of the radius after harvest, making the remaining radius susceptible to fracture. The wrist must be immobilized for a minimum of 6 weeks for donor site rehabilitation, and in some patients, plating and bone grafting are required. With such a small amount of bone harvested at such a high cost, and with other excellent flaps available, we believe that the radial forearm flap is rarely if ever indicated for reconstruction of the mandible. However, for certain other defects of the craniofacial skeleton, particularly those involving the orbit and midface, the radial forearm osteocutaneous flap is ideal.

BONE FIXATION

Several methods of bone fixation have been described: miniplates, interosseous wires, and reconstruction plates. The disadvantage of the first two methods is that they

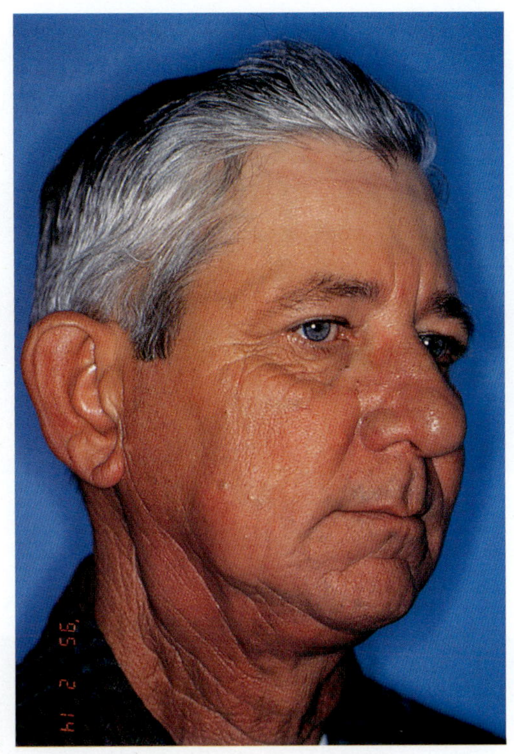

FIG. 1A. Preoperative view of patient with anterior floor of mouth cancer.

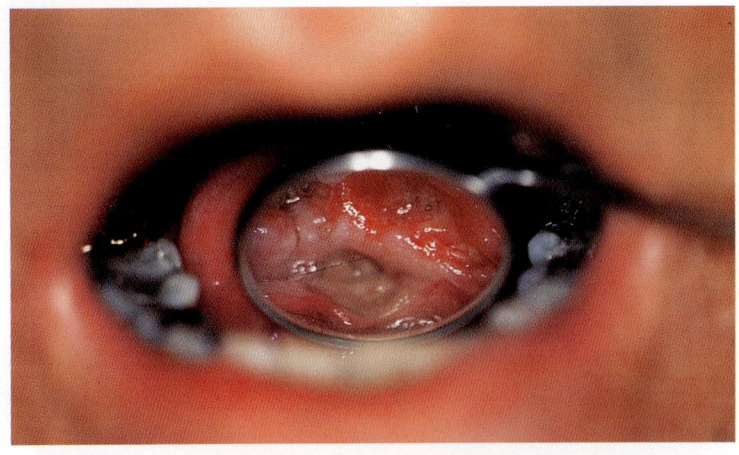

FIG. 1B. Preoperative intraoral view of squamous cell carcinoma of the floor of mouth cancer invading the mandible.

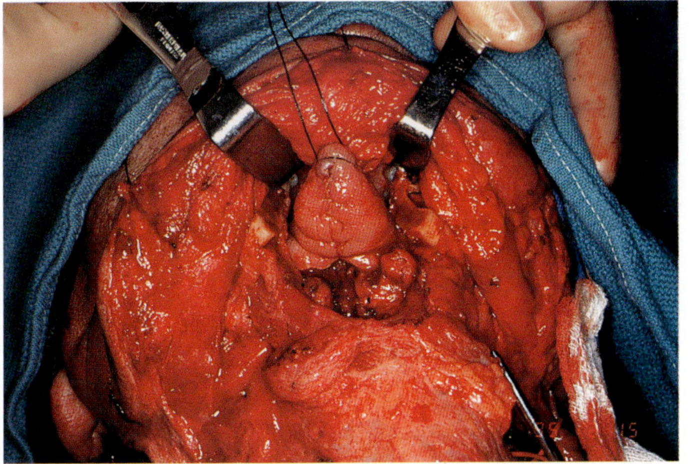

FIG. 1C. Defect after tumor resection as viewed from below.

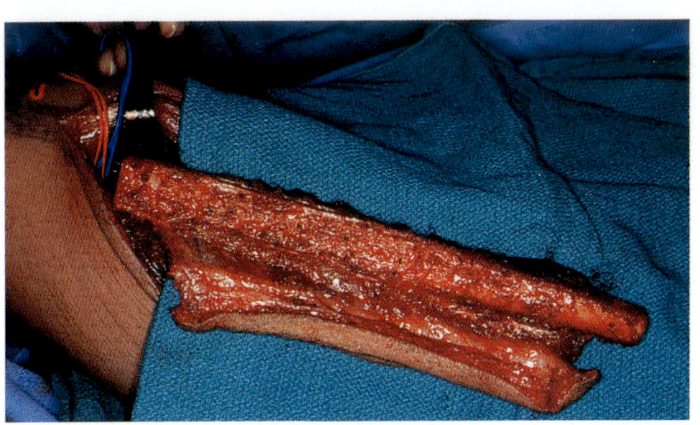

FIG. 1D. The osteocutaneous fibula flap after elevation.

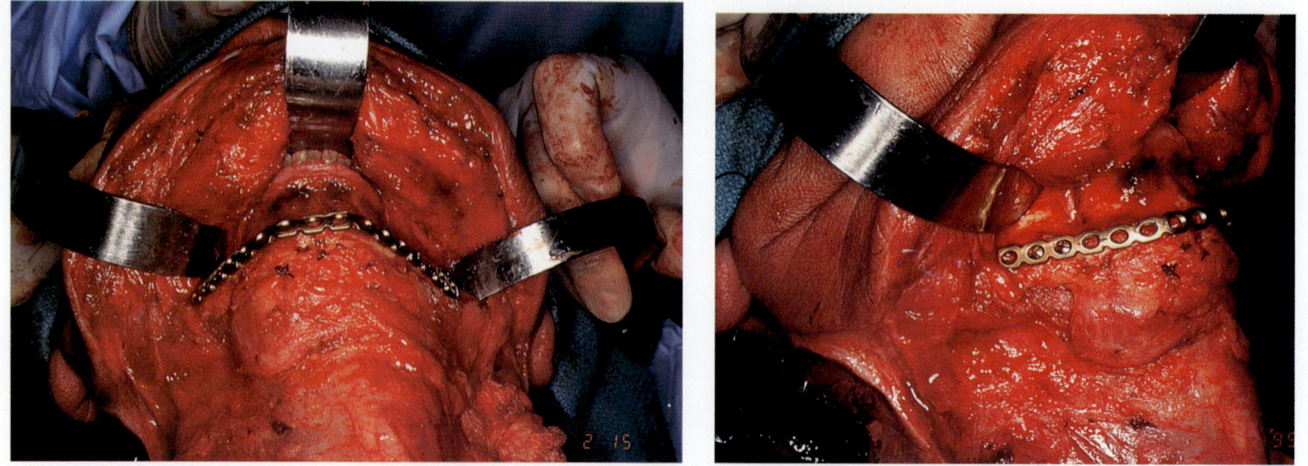

FIG. 1E,F. Prebending the reconstruction plate prior to performing the osteotomies and removing the specimen.

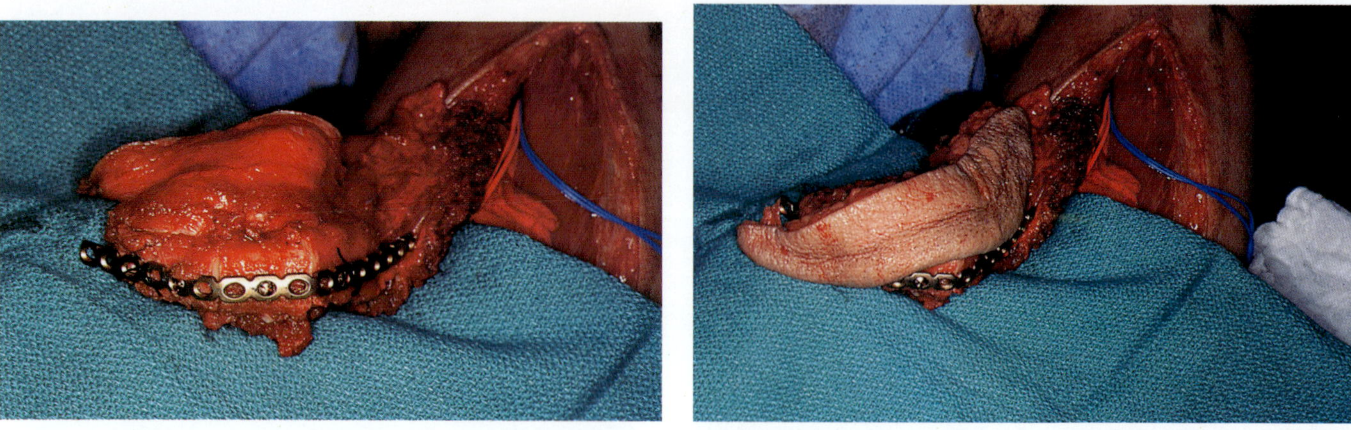

FIG. 1G,H. The plate is then taken to the donor site where closing wedge osteotomies are performed in order to shape the fibula, and the entire unit is fixed to the prebent plate in situ. The bone shaping is done while the fibula is being perfused in order to limit the ischemia time.

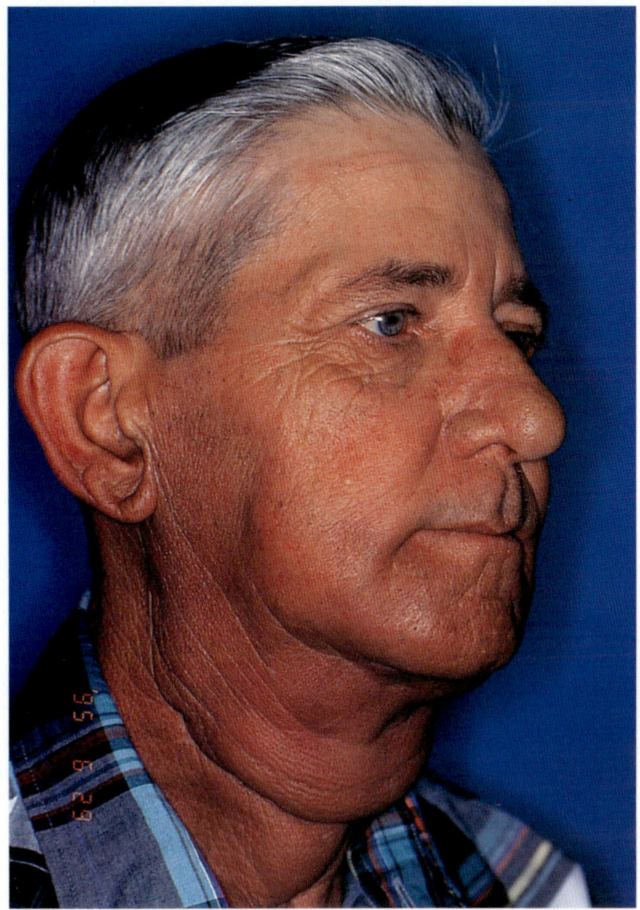

FIG. 1I. Postoperative appearance of patient.

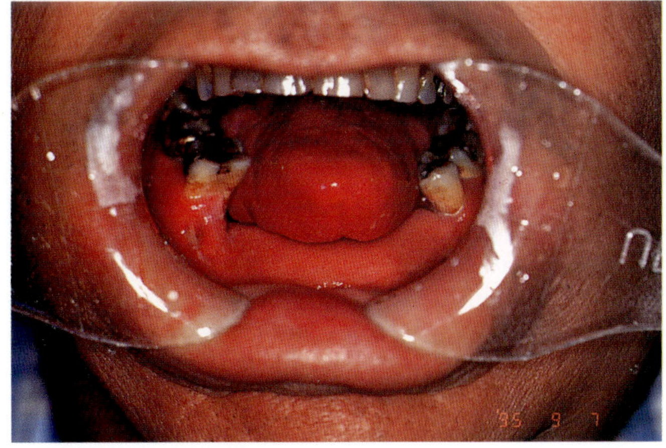

FIG. 1J. Postoperative intraoral view demonstrating the excellent reapproximation of the resected mucosa by the skin paddle of the fibula.

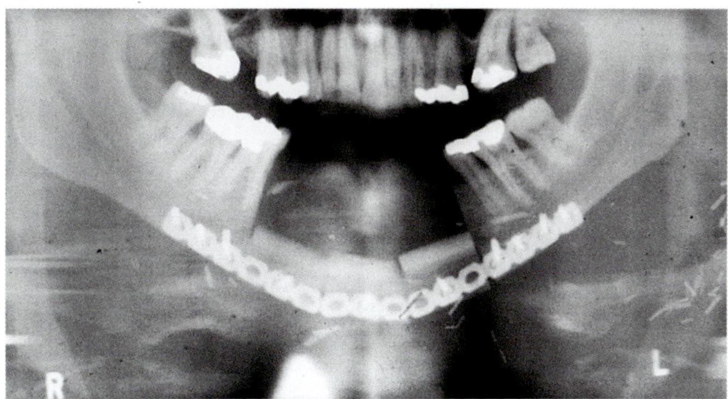

FIG. 1K. Radiograph of the reconstructed mandible.

provide no model or template of the resected mandible nor the ability to control the position of the condyles, something that is particularly critical in an anterior resection/reconstruction. It is imperative when reconstructing the mandible to maintain precise occlusal relationships between the mandible and maxillary dentition. In a posterior resection, this can be readily accomplished by use of intermaxillary fixation. In an anterior resection, however, the dentition is often sacrificed, making proper orientation of the remaining condylar segments difficult.

Use of a reconstruction plate remedies all these issues. The plate is bent over the mandible prior to the segmental resection and fixed into place with screws (Figs. 1F and 2A). The location of the screws is noted, and the screws and plate are then removed and saved for later fixation of the bone flap. By placing the plate on the mandible prior to resection, the reconstructive surgeon obtains an accurate template of the shape, and the proper occlusal relationships can be maintained. The reconstruction plate is taken to the recipient site for bone shaping and fixation to the plate. This is done while the flap is being perfused, thus limiting ischemia time (Fig. 1F,G). The bone-plate unit is then returned to the recipient site, where the bone is trimmed to its final shape and the unit is fixed into place with the original screws (Figs. 1H and 2B,C). The reconstruction plate thus provides a good mechanism for fixation of the bone and an accurate template of the original mandibular shape and occlusal/condylar relationships. This technique simplifies and facilitates free flap reconstruction of the mandible.

FIBULAR OSTEOCUTANEOUS FLAP

Anatomic Considerations

The fibular flap is based on the peroneal vein and artery, which is one of three terminal branches of the popliteal artery. As the popliteal artery enters the leg, it gives rise to the anterior tibial artery and then bifurcates into the posterior tibial and peroneal arteries approximately 7 cm below the knee joint (Fig. 3A,B). The peroneal artery then courses along the medial aspect of the fibula. The fibula itself lies in the deep posterior compartment along the lateral aspect of the leg. It is bordered laterally by the peroneal muscles, anteriorly by the extensor digitorum longus muscle, laterally by the posterior tibialis muscle, and inferiorly by the flexor hallucis longus muscle. The blood supply to the skin arises from the inferolateral intermuscular septum and consists of septocutaneous branches as well as musculocutaneous branches arising from the flexor hallucis longus and the soleus muscles (Fig. 4).

At the superior aspect of the fibula, the peroneal nerve crosses just below the head, and care must be taken to avoid injury to this nerve during the dissection. Inferiorly, the fibula is an important contributor to the ankle joint; thus, to preserve ankle joint integrity, the inferior 8 cm of the fibula must not be damaged or sacrificed.

Preoperative assessment of the vascular supply to the lower extremities is essential prior to utilizing the free fibular flap. Although preoperative angiography is not mandatory, it should be considered if there is clinical evidence of vascular compromise such as diminished pulses or atrophy of the skin. Using these clinical criteria for assessment of the lower extremity, we have not had any complications due to vascular compromise of the foot or lower leg.

Operative Technique

If no skin paddle is required, the fibula is harvested from the ipsilateral leg. If skin is needed in the reconstruction, the contralateral leg is selected (Fig. 5). The mandibular area being resected determines whether the proximal or distal part of the fibula is used. A posterior mandibular reconstruction requires the creation of a ramus; the proximal fibula provides a pedicle that is near the midpoint of the flap, with the peroneal vessels positioned optimally for the anastomoses (Fig. 6A). In an anterior arch recon-

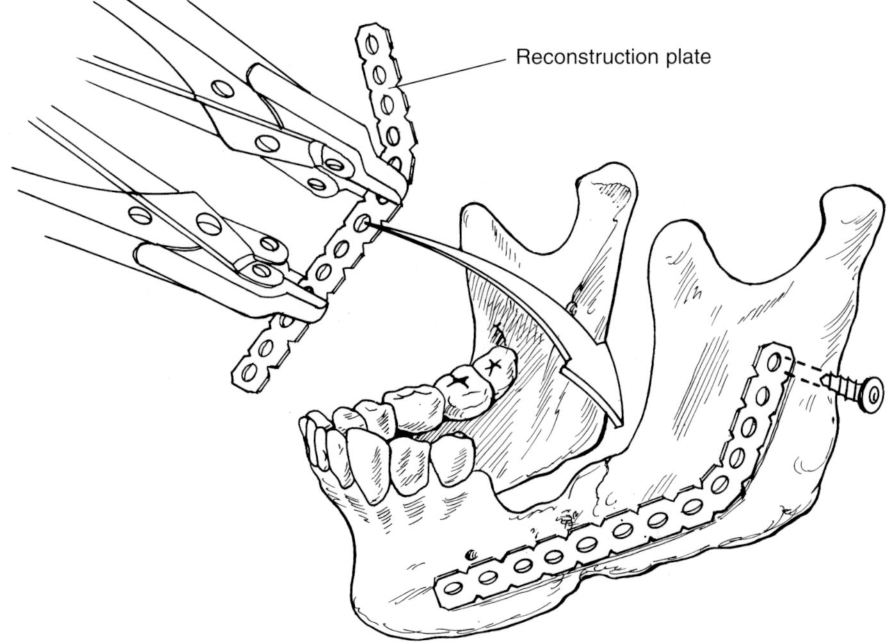

FIG. 2A. The reconstruction plate is prebent over the native mandible prior to tumor resection.

A

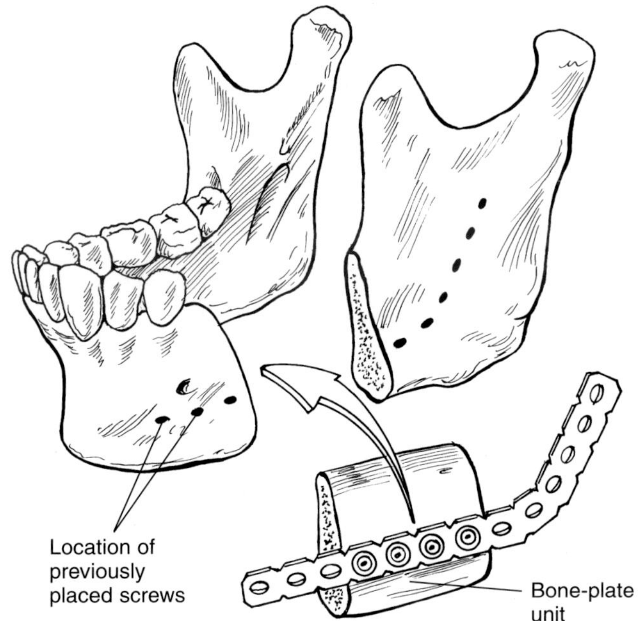

B

FIG. 2B. The vascularized bone graft is then fixed to the plate, and the bone-plate unit is then returned to the recipient site for fixation.

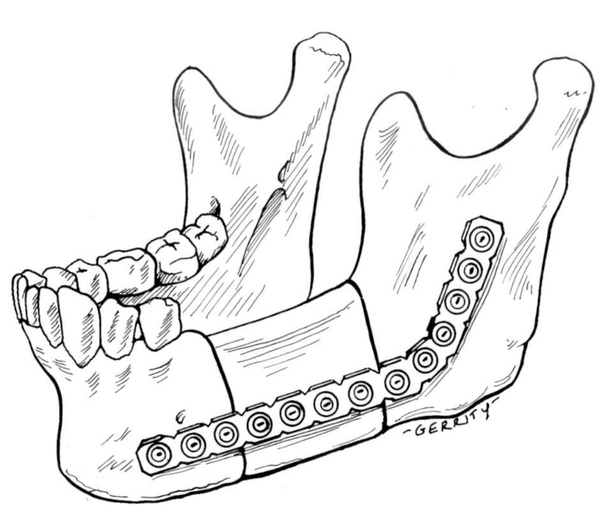

C

FIG. 2C. The bone is trimmed to fit precisely into the defect, and the plate is then fixed into place with the original screws.

struction, the distal fibula is used to provide long donor vessels from the end of the flap (Fig. 6B).

The patient is placed in a supine position, with a roll under the ipsilateral hip, and a tourniquet is placed on the thigh. The fibular head at the knee, the peroneal nerve just below the fibular head, and the lateral malleolus at the ankle are marked. Hash marks are drawn at 10, 15, 20, and 25 cm from the fibular head, and the skin paddle is centered between these marks, taking into account the location of the mandibular defect as already described (Fig. 7). In the anteroposterior plane, the paddle is centered along the posterior border of the fibula. The leg is elevated and the tourniquet inflated.

Because the peroneal artery and vein course along the medial side of the fibula, a lateral approach is used to begin the dissection (Fig. 8A). An anterior incision down through the deep muscle fascia is made; the inclusion of this fascia in the flap is crucial, as is avoidance of the superficial peroneal nerve as it emerges from the anterolateral intermuscular septum (Fig. 8B). The dissection continues posteriorly exposing the peroneal muscles, down to but not through the anterior aspect of the posterolateral intermuscular septum (Fig. 8C). This key structure must be preserved. The anterior aspect of the septum is then followed to the fibula, with the peroneal musculature being retracted anteriorly. Once the lateral border of the fibula is reached, it is exposed by taking down the origins of the peroneal musculature along the entire length of the dissection. Care must be taken to avoid injury to the intermuscular portion of the superficial peroneal nerve during the proximal aspect of this dissection. The dissection then proceeds over the anterior aspect of the fibula, dividing the anterolateral intermuscular septum, the muscles of the anterior compartment, and finally the interosseous membrane (Fig. 8D). During the anterior compartment aspect of this dissection, care must be taken to avoid injury to the anterior tibial neurovascular bundle.

Once the interosseous membrane has been divided, the posterior dissection is started. The posterior skin incision is made down through the deep muscle fascia, and the skin paddle is elevated to the edge of the soleus muscle. A 1-cm-deep incision is made in the soleus muscle approximately 1 cm from its lateral edge (Fig. 8E). No further posterior dissection is done at this time. Next, the bone cuts are made to the required length using an oscillating saw. The proximal cut in the fibula should be made as high as possible without damaging the peroneal nerve. Even if one does not plan to use the proximal fibula, it should be harvested to expose the trifurcation of the leg vessels, thus facilitating the pedicle dissection (Fig. 8F).

Once the fibula is cut, it is retracted laterally, exposing the vessel and medial musculature attachments. The dissection proceeds from distal to proximal and from medial to lateral. The peroneal vessels are located distally, ligated, and divided (Fig. 8F). With the knowledge of their location, the flap dissection continues (medially to laterally) with less risk of injuring the perforating vessels to the skin paddle (Fig. 8G).

After the flap is elevated, the tourniquet is released and any residual bleeding controlled. By this time, the ablative team should have the mandible exposed and ready for resection. Before osteotomies are undertaken, the reconstructive team bends a reconstruction plate over the native mandible, stabilizes the plate with screws posterior to the planned mandibulectomy cuts, and then removes the plate and screws. Thus, the original shape of the mandible will be reestablished and the condyles correctly positioned relative to the neomandible.

The ablative team now completes the resection while the reconstructive team uses the shaped reconstruction plate (as a template) to cut the fibula with closing wedge osteotomies; during this sequence, the fibula is perfused in situ (Fig. 1F,G). The bone fragments are fixed before transfer to limit ischemia time. As soon as the resection is finished and tumor-free margins have been confirmed by frozen-section examination, the pedicle is divided and the flap transferred to the recipient site. First, the skin paddle is inset along the tongue because this is technically easier to do before the bone is in place (Fig. 9A). Next, the bony ends of the fibula/reconstruction plate complex are trimmed for a proper fit, with just a bit of bone compression, and the plate is resecured to the native mandible with the screws previously placed (Fig. 9B).

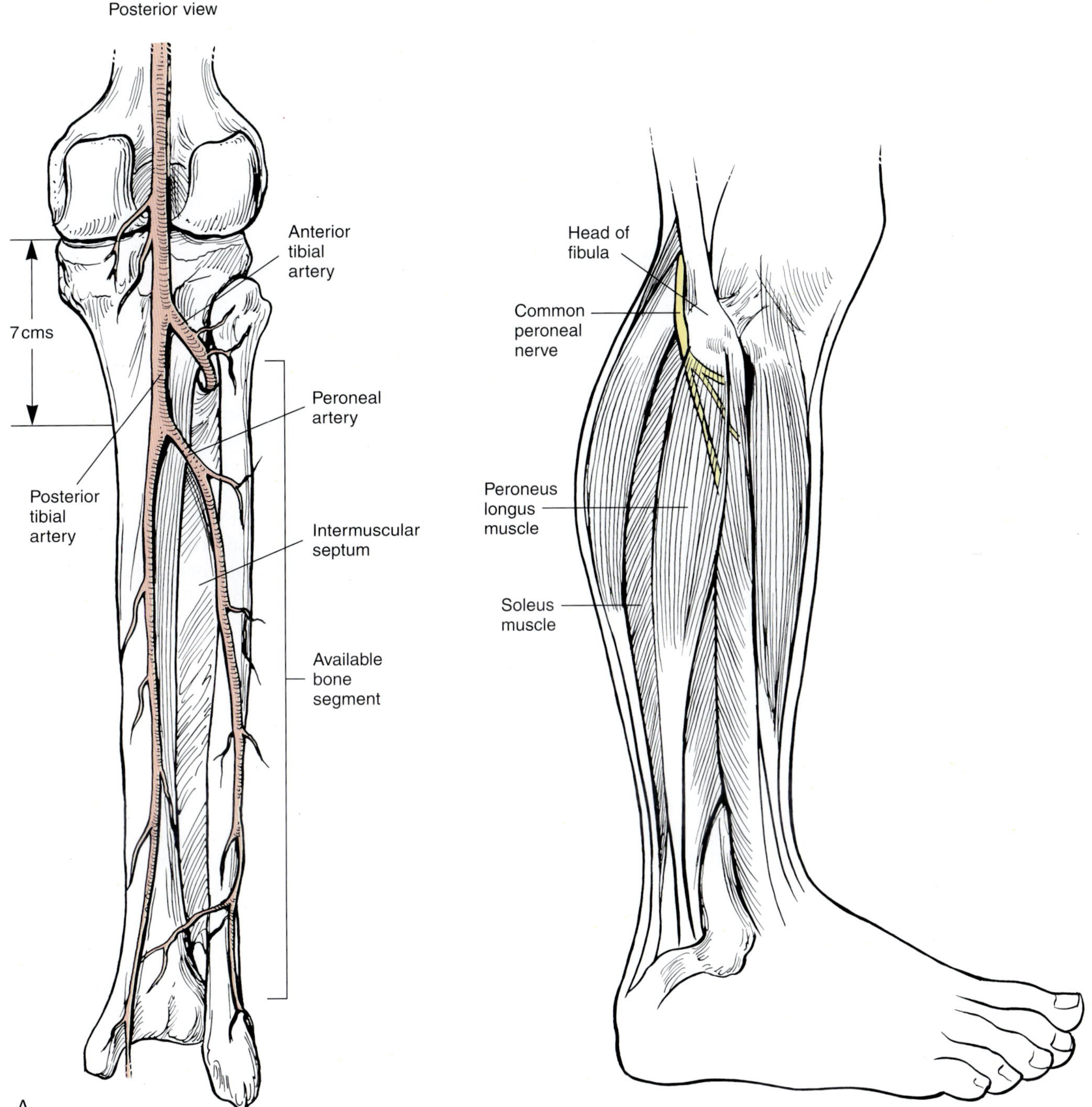

FIG. 3A. The anatomy of the leg vasculature. The peroneal artery branches off the popliteal trunk 7 cm from the knee joint.

FIG. 3B. The common peroneal nerve courses around the fibula head and must be avoided during the dissection.

After inset, the flap is revascularized, preferably using end-to-side anastomoses to the external carotid artery and the internal jugular vein (Fig. 9C). After the anastomoses are completed, the flap is checked for adequate reflow, and the flap inset is completed. The neck is then closed.

The leg donor site is repaired by simply closing the skin over closed-suction drains; no other special closure techniques are needed. If harvest of a large skin paddle precludes primary closure of the skin, a split-thickness skin graft is used for wound closure. The leg is then further dressed with a bulky dressing and posterior splint.

Postoperative care

The patient is transferred to the intensive care unit for recovery and monitoring of the flap. The vascular integrity of the anastomoses must be checked hourly by assessing the color and refill of the skin paddle. Use of the laser Doppler, ultrasonic hand-held Doppler, or implantable 20 MHz Doppler (Swartz) may be used to augment the clinical assessment, but there is no substitute for routine nursing assessment of the flap.

After 72 hours, the patient may be transferred to a regular floor room. On the fifth postoperative day the dressing is changed and the posterior splint removed from the leg. If no skin graft has been used, the patient may be sent to physical therapy for gradual weight bearing and assisted ambulation. If a skin graft has been used to close the donor site, one should wait until the 7th to 10th postoperative day before allowing the patient to put the extremity in a dependent position, and then only when wrapped with an elastic bandage. The drains are removed per routine and the patient is usually ready for discharge on the 10th to 14th postoperative day.

ILIAC CREST/DEEP CIRCUMFLEX ILIAC ARTERY FLAP

Anatomic Considerations

The DCIA arises from the external iliac vessels approximately 1 to 2 cm above the inguinal ligament (Fig. 10A). The DCIA passes beneath the transversalis fascia and under the floor of the inguinal canal, traveling laterally and superiorly toward the anterior superior iliac spine. Approximately 1 cm lateral to the anterior superior iliac spine is the origin of the ascending branch, which can be used as a pedicle for the internal oblique muscle (Fig. 10B). Also at that point, the DCIA is crossed either deeply or superficially by the lateral femoral cutaneous nerve (Fig. 10A). Injury to this nerve must be avoided to prevent paresthesia of the lateral thigh. Once the vessels reach the anterior superior iliac spine, they are located in the fascial fusion of the transversalis and the iliaca fasciae. As the vessels travel underneath the lip of the iliac crest, they give off perforators that traverse all three layers of the abdominal wall and provide the blood supply to the overlying skin (Fig. 10C).

Operative Technique

The patient is placed in the supine position with a rolled sheet or sandbag under the hip. The iliac crest contralateral to the recipient vessels is usually selected. The pubic tubercle and the anterior superior iliac spine are both marked. A line drawn between them indicates the route and location of the inguinal ligament (Fig. 11). An incision is then made parallel to and approximately 1 cm above the inguinal ligament. The spermatic cord or round ligament is then retracted upward and medially to expose the floor of the inguinal canal (Fig. 12A). Care should be taken to avoid injury to the ilioinguinal nerve. The floor of the inguinal canal is then explored medially to expose the iliac vessels and the origin of the deep circumflex iliac vessels. These are then traced from medial to lateral under direct vision. Once the ascending branch is identified, if

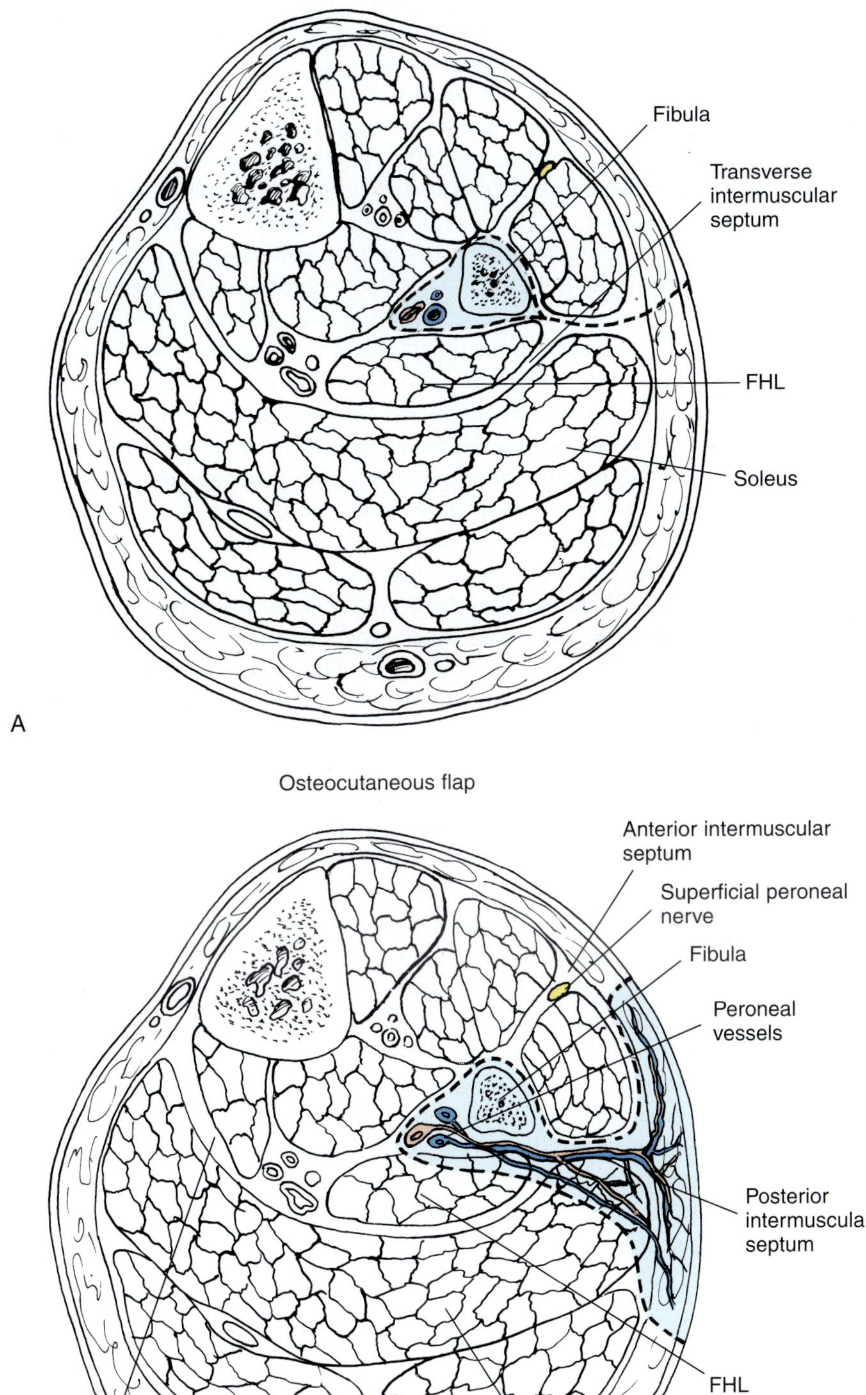

FIG. 4A, B. The peroneal vessels lie in the deep posterior compartment of the leg. Perforators to the skin course along the transverse crural septum, which ends as the posterolateral intermuscular septum. Several of the perforators course through the soleus muscle as well.

a portion of the internal oblique muscle is required for the reconstruction, the artery is preserved, and the internal oblique muscle is dissected along with the flap. If, however, the internal oblique muscle is not required, this vessel is ligated and divided. The lateral femoral cutaneous nerve is then encountered. This nerve can cross either deep or superficial to the DCIA. If it is superficial to the vessels, again care must be taken to avoid injury to the nerve (Fig. 12B). Flap dissection can proceed by mobilizing and freeing this nerve; once the flap is harvested by ligating the DCIA vessels at their origin, these vessels can be brought underneath the lateral femoral cutaneous nerve and the flap transferred without injury to the nerve.

Once the anterior superior iliac spine has been reached, preparation is made for harvest of the bone. If a skin paddle is required, this needs to be incised circumferentially. Care must be taken to mark the skin paddle so that it is located over the lateral aspect of the abdominal wall musculature as it inserts onto the medial aspect of the iliac crest (Fig. 12B). The lateral aspect of the iliac crest is then identified. If a full thickness of iliac crest is to be taken, the lateral muscles must be incised, and the periosteum must be taken off of the lateral aspect of the iliac crest. If, however, only the inner cortex is to be harvested, this maneuver is not necessary. The medial dissection is performed from proximal to distal in such a way that the vessel location is known at all times. The full thickness of the abdominal wall musculature external and internal oblique and transversus abdominis muscles must be incised down to the properitoneal fat, particularly if the skin paddle is to be harvested with the flap. Once the properitoneal fat is identified, the entire inner aspect of the conjoined line between the transversalis and the iliaca fasciae is identified. Then, from proximal to distal, the muscles just below the circumflex iliac vessels are divided, exposing the bone (Fig. 12C). Once the distal aspect of the planned bone harvest is reached, the division of the muscle is carried anteriorly over the top of the iliac crest. An oscillating saw is then used to make the bone cuts. The inner aspect of the cortex is incised proximally and distally. Then, using the saw, an incision is made in the midportion of the top of the crest, into the cancellous bone cavity, thus connecting the proximal and distal osteotomies. The final posterior cut, which is difficult to perform with a saw, can be done with osteotomes inserted into the crest incision, with constant vigilance concerning the location of the DCIA internally (Fig. 12D).

Once the osteotomies are completed, the flap can be shaped in situ and fixed to the reconstruction plate (Fig. 12E). When screws are placed into the bone, care must be taken not to injure the flap vessel, which is on the deep surface of the flap. Donor site closure is accomplished by reapproximating the transversalis abdominis and iliacas fascias (Fig. 13). This must be done meticulously; if necessary, drill holes may be placed in the iliac crest to get a tight, secure closure. If closure is not adequate, use of plastic mesh to reinforce the closure is recommended. The external oblique muscle is then reapproximated, drains are placed in the wound, and the skin is closed in the usual fashion.

SCAPULAR OSTEOCUTANEOUS FLAP

Anatomic Considerations

The scapular flap is based on the cutaneous branches of the circumflex scapular artery. The circumflex scapular artery and thoracodorsal artery are the terminal branches of the subscapular artery. The circumflex scapular artery travels upward and enters the back through the triangular space that is bordered by the teres minor muscle superiorly, the teres major muscle inferiorly, and the long head of the triceps brachii muscle laterally (Fig. 14A). Just prior to reaching the triangular space, however, the circumflex scapular artery gives off numerous branches into the lateral border of the scapula. It is from these branches that the scapula receives its blood supply. In addition, there is an angular artery that arises from the subscapular artery or occa-

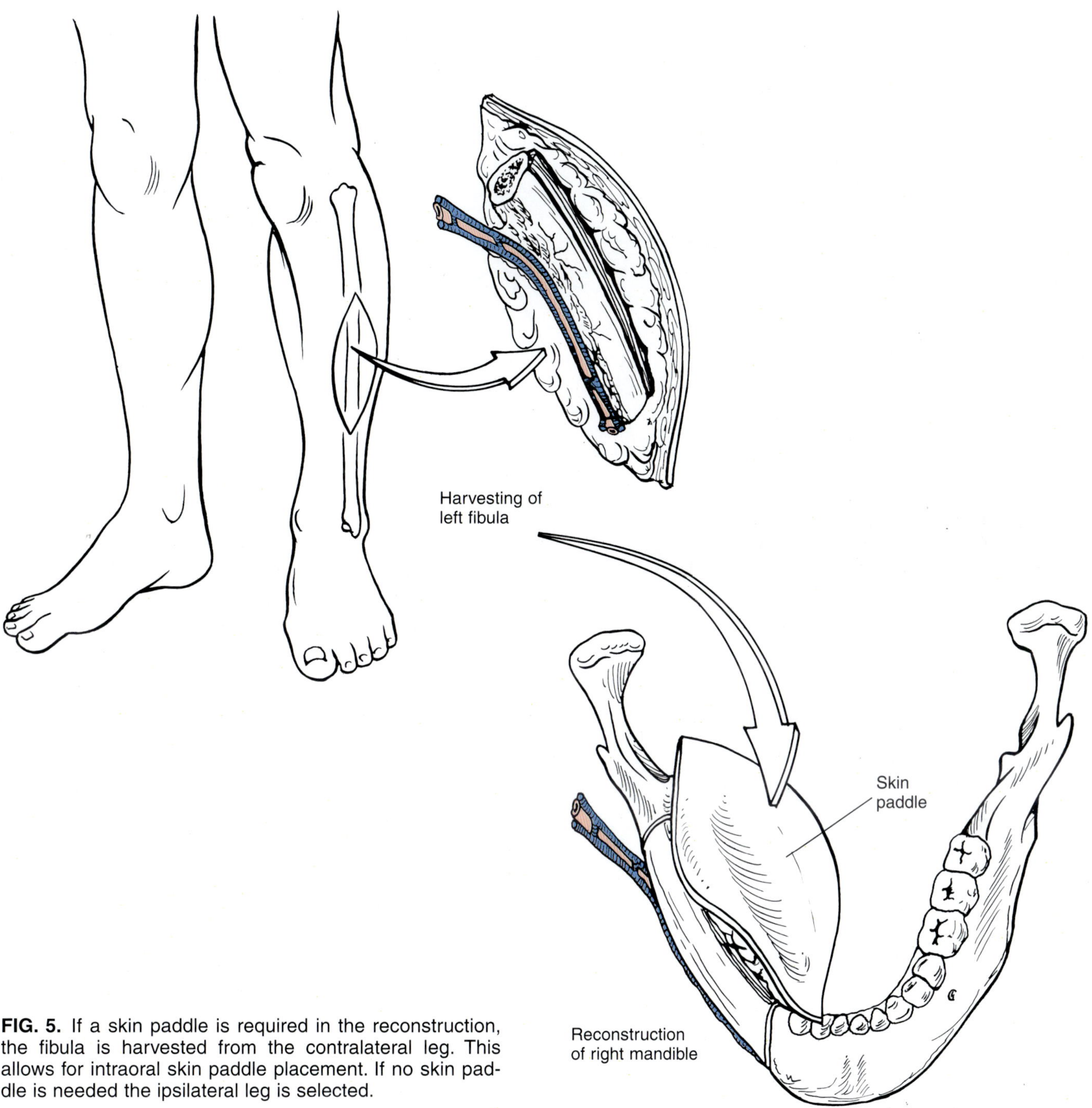

FIG. 5. If a skin paddle is required in the reconstruction, the fibula is harvested from the contralateral leg. This allows for intraoral skin paddle placement. If no skin paddle is needed the ipsilateral leg is selected.

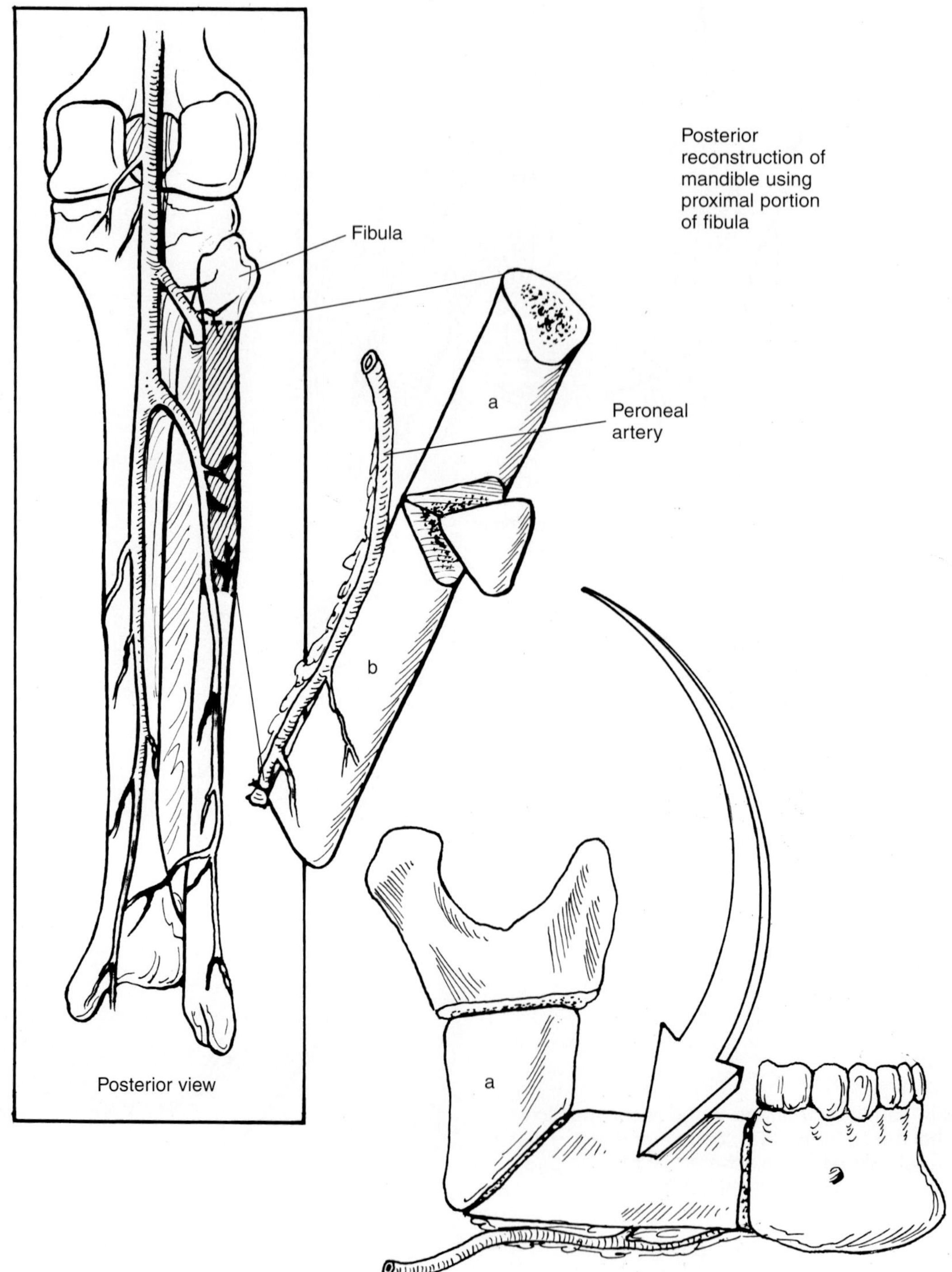

FIG. 6A. If a posterior reconstruction is needed, harvest of the proximal fibula allows for optimal pedicle orientation.

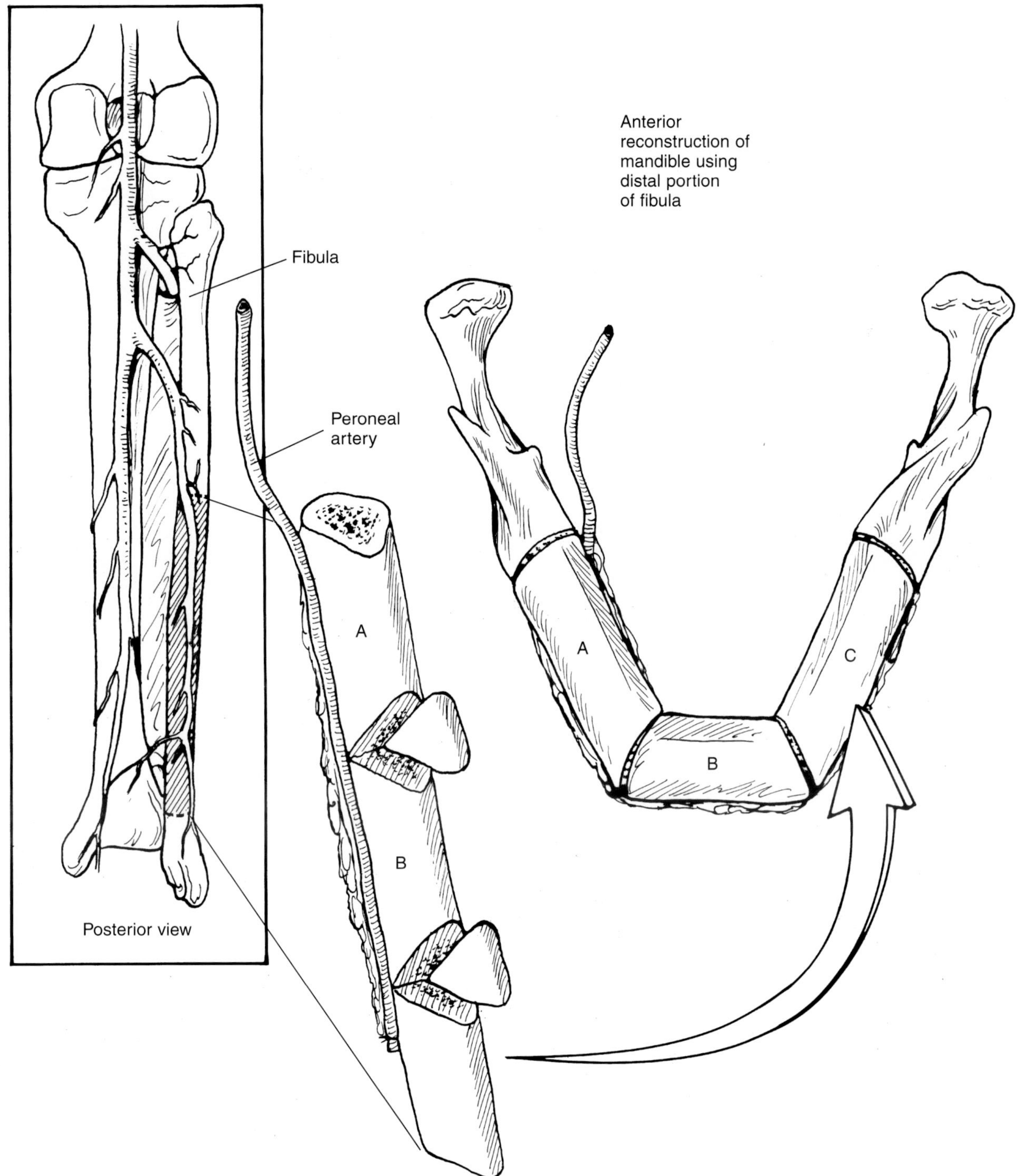

FIG. 6B. Use of the distal fibula is best if anterior reconstruction is required. This configuration gives the longest pedicle, which is often necessary for anterior mandibular reconstructions.

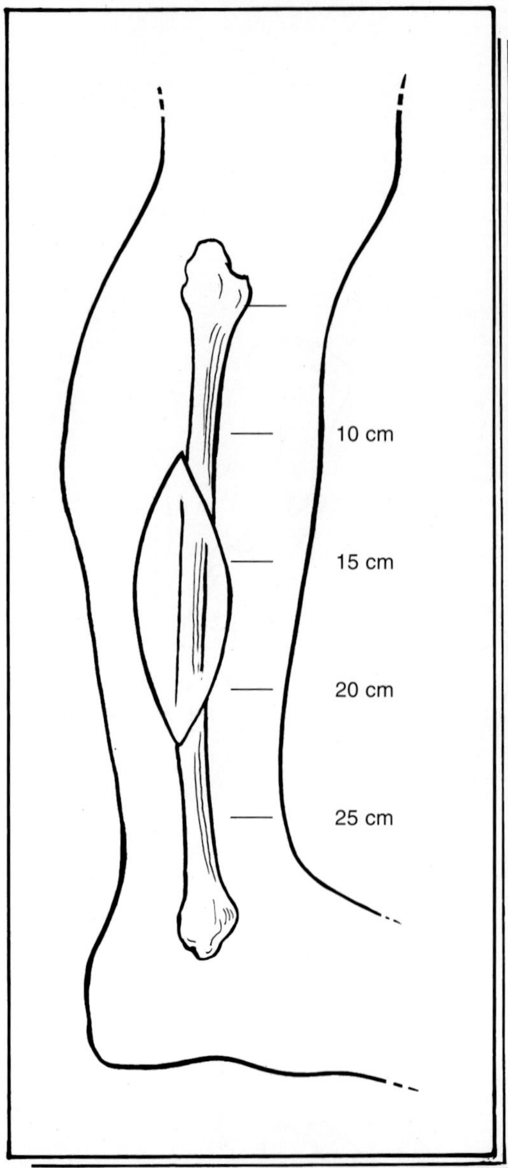

FIG. 7. The skin paddle should be centered over the posterior aspect of the fibula between 150 and 250 cm from the fibular head.

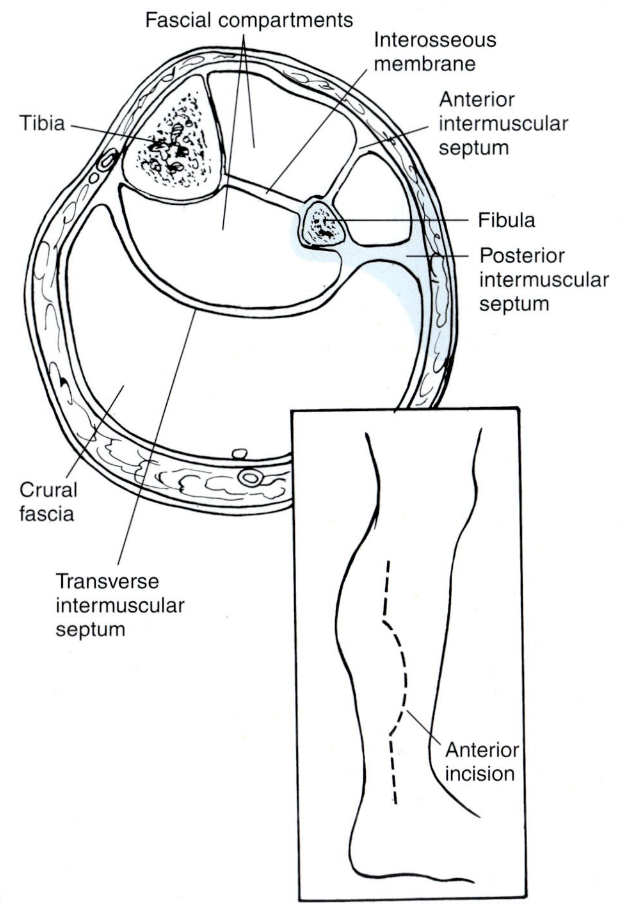

FIG. 8A. The flap harvest is approached from the lateral aspect of the leg.

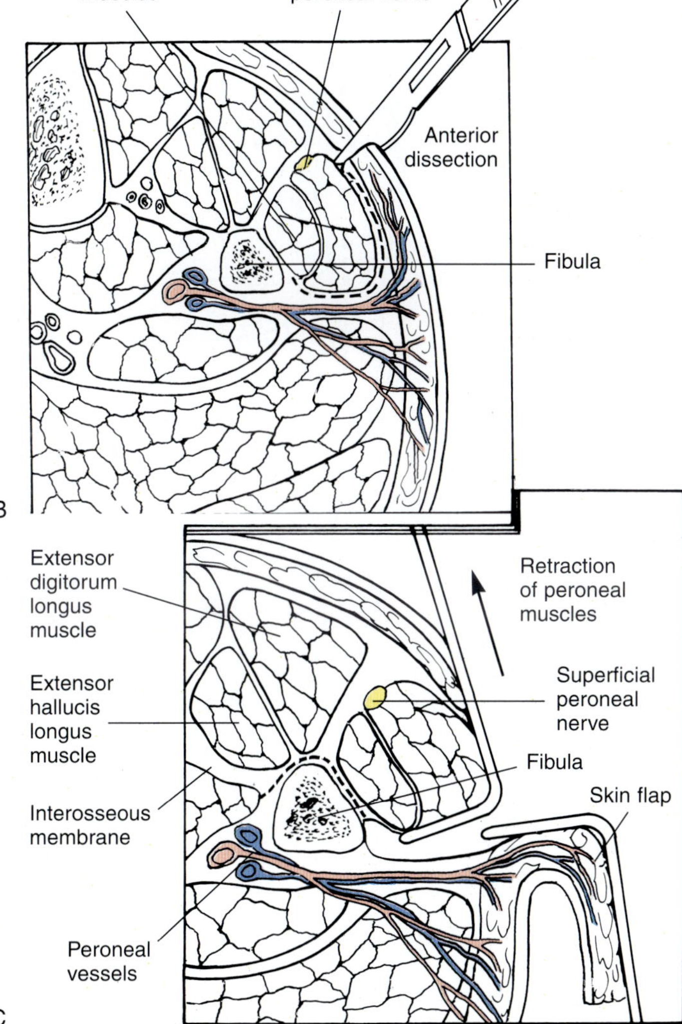

FIG. 8B,C. B: The anterior incision is made over the peroneal musculature, with care taken to avoid injury to the superficial branch of the peroneal nerve. **C:** The incision is made down through the deep muscle fascia and the flap is then elevated toward the posterolateral intermuscular septum, which is preserved, since the skin perforators travel in this fascia.

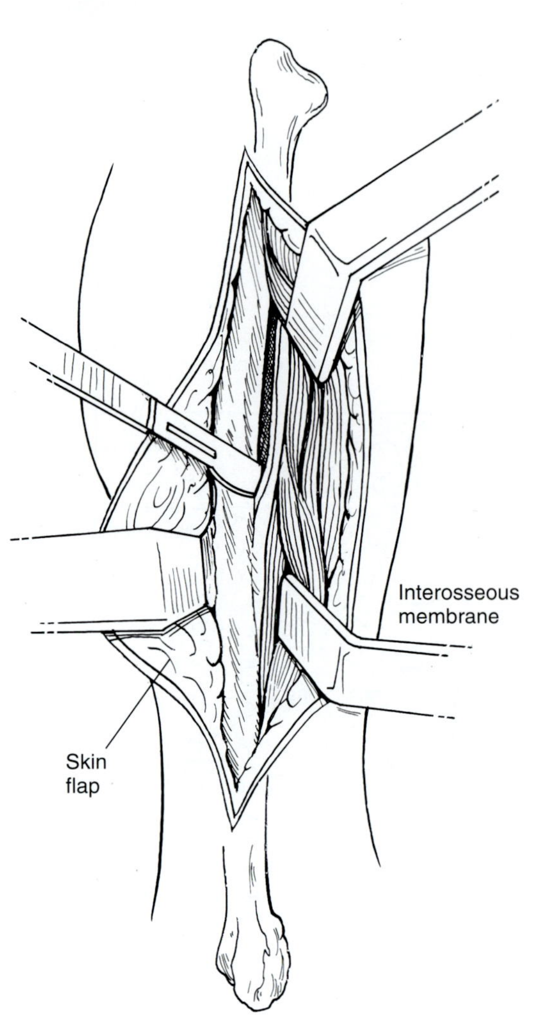

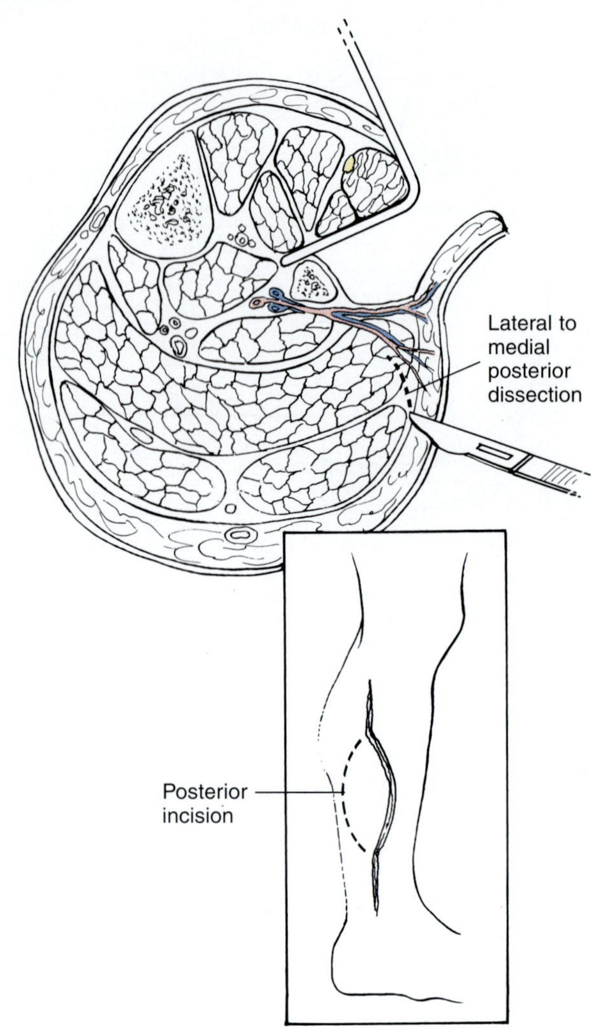

FIG. 8D. The muscles are elevated from the septum up over the top of the fibula, dividing the anterolateral intermuscular septum and the interosseous membrane.

FIG. 8E. After the interosseous membrane has been divided the posterior skin incision is made again including the deep muscle fascia, but the elevation is stopped 1 cm from the edge of the soleus. At that point the soleus muscle is incised for a depth of about 1 cm; then the bone cuts are made.

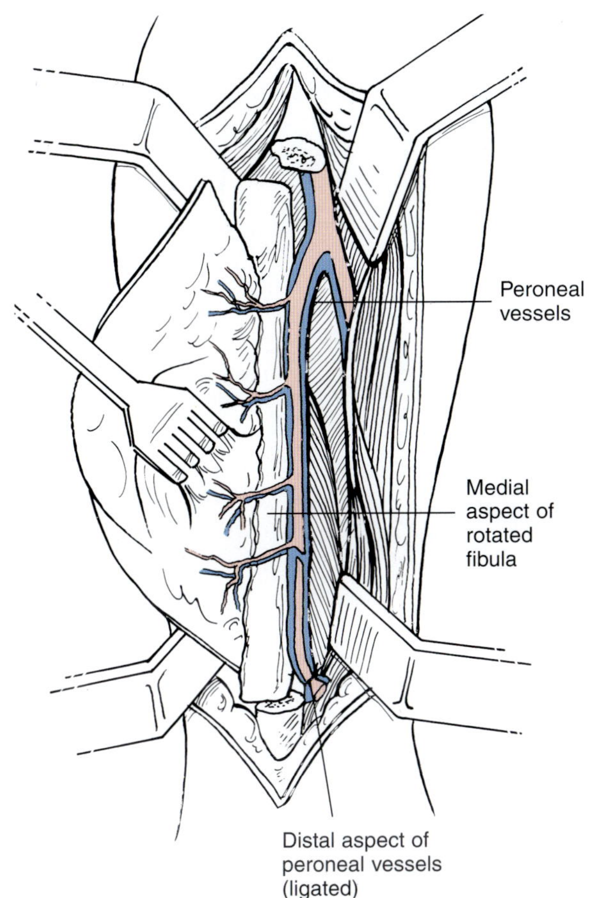

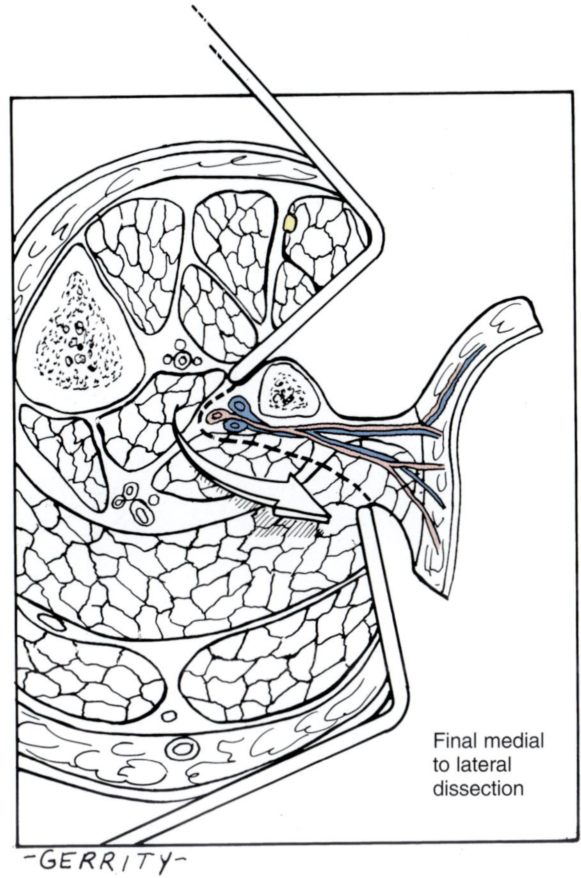

FIG. 8F. The osteotomies are done allowing for traction on the flap, which exposes the deep musculature and helps with the medial dissection. The peroneal vessels are ligated distally, and the musculature is then divided from distal to proximal taking care to avoid injury to the flap vessels.

FIG. 8G. The remainder of the posterior dissection can then be done from medial to lateral, which helps prevent injury to the skin perforators.

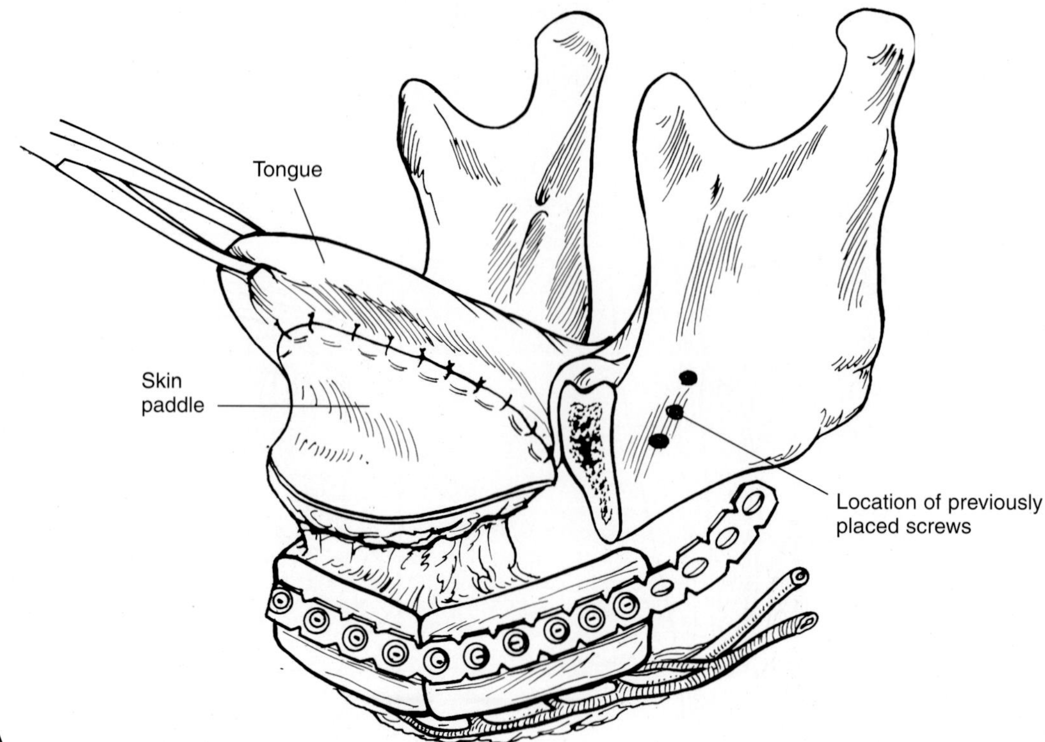

FIG. 9A. Once the bone has been fixed to the plate, the flap/plate unit is transferred to the recipient site, where the skin paddle is inset first.

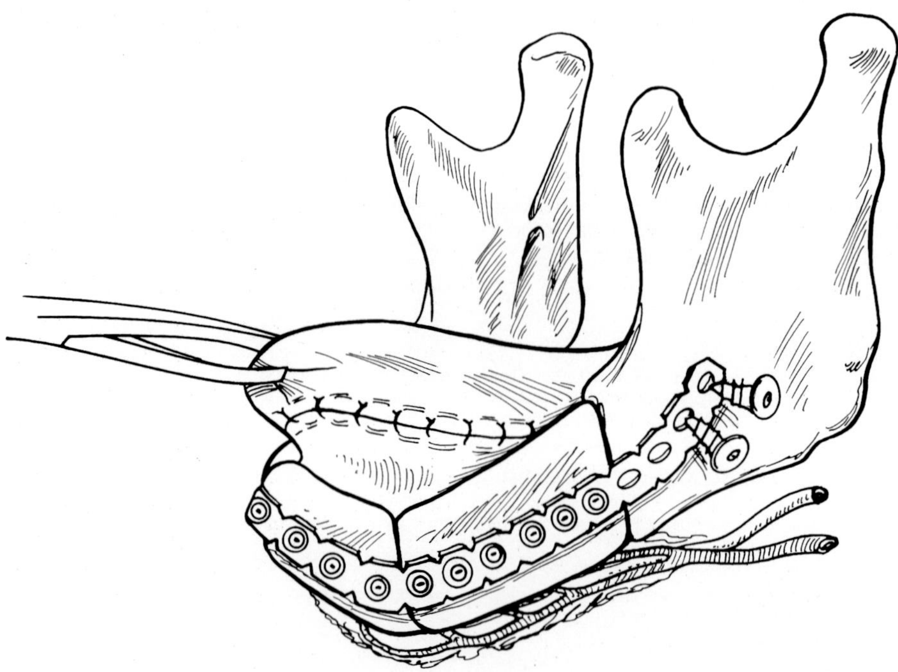

FIG. 9B. The bone is trimmed to size and the plate then refixed into the previously placed screw holes.

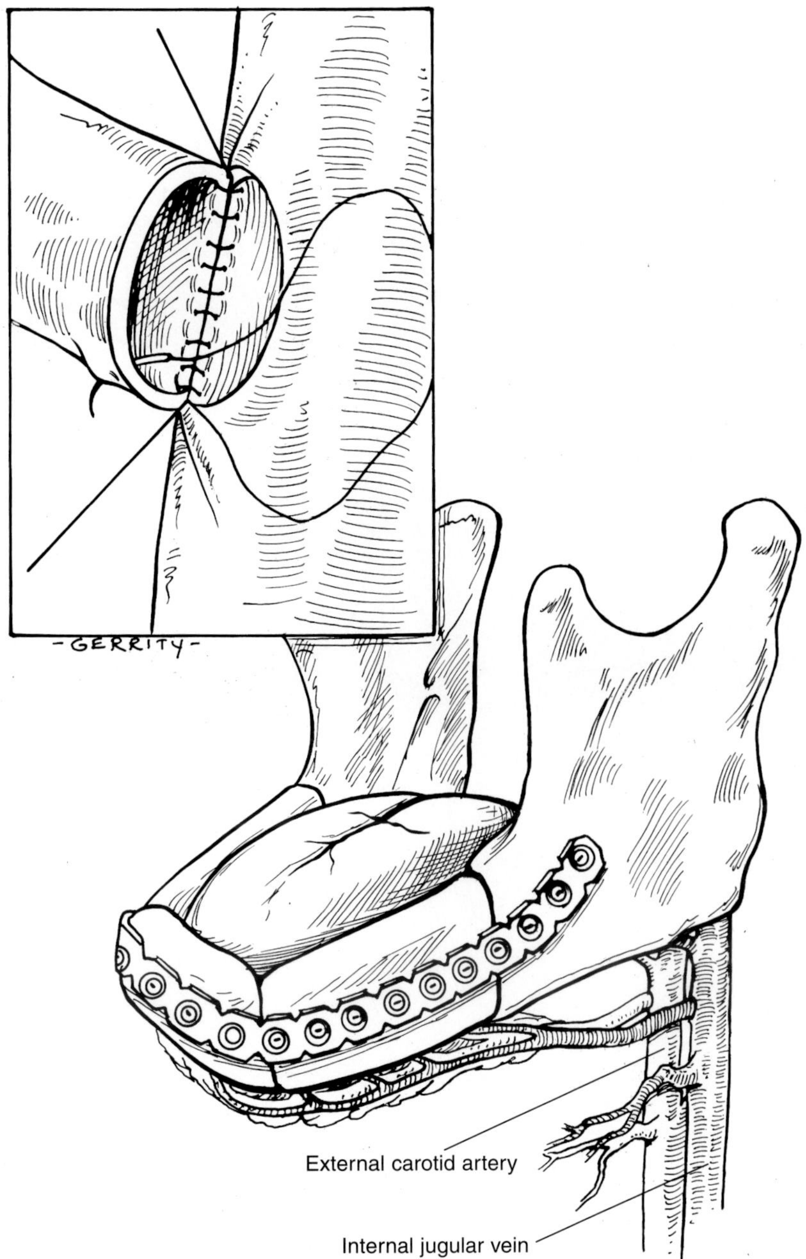

FIG. 9C. Only after inset is the flap revascularized.

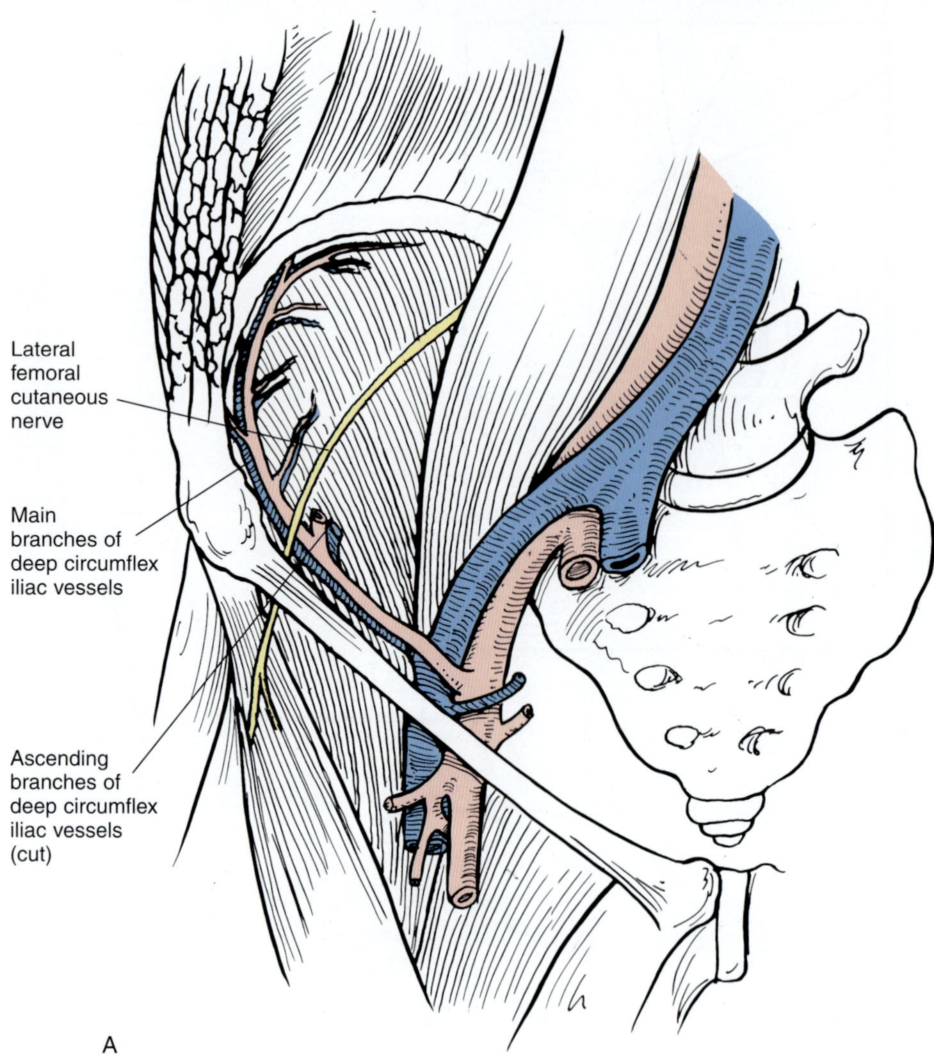

FIG. 10A. The anatomy of the deep circumflex iliac artery (DCIA). Note the origin of the DCI vessels on the external iliac vessels and the course of the DCIA parallel and 2 cm superior to the inguinal ligament. Note also the origin of the ascending branch and the crossing of the DCIA by the lateral femoral cutaneous nerve approximately 1 cm lateral to the anterior superior iliac spine.

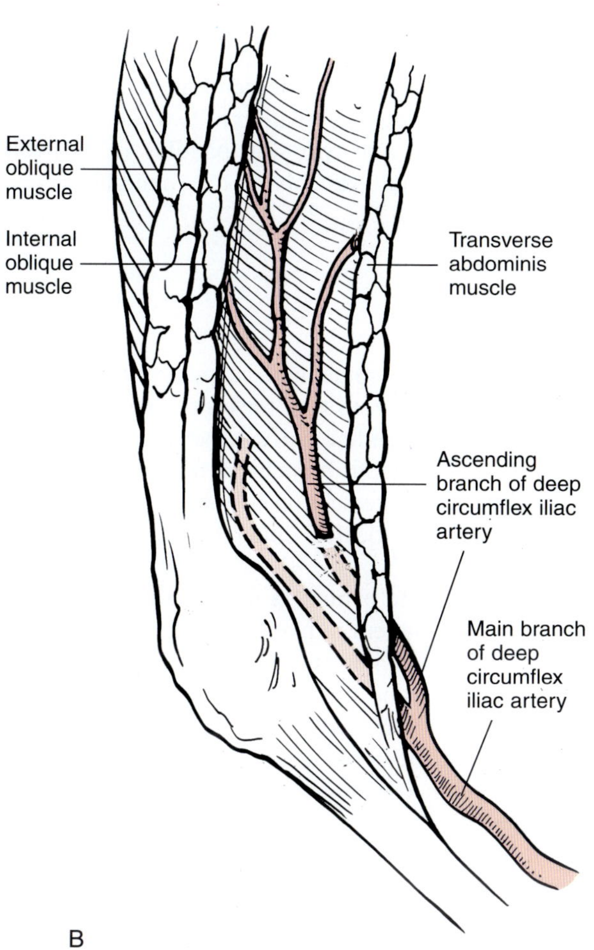

FIG. 10B. The ascending branch of the DCIA is a dominant blood supply to the internal oblique artery; thus, one can use this muscle as part of the flap if necessary.

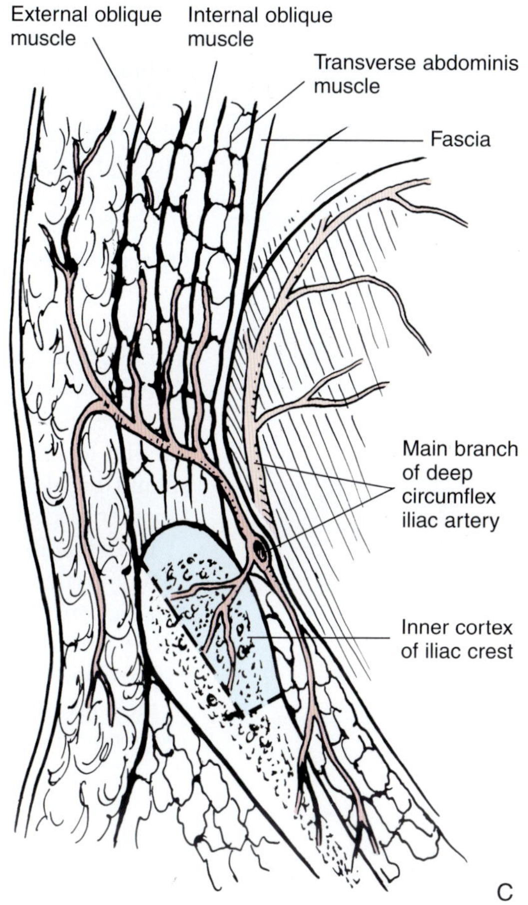

FIG. 10C. The blood supply to the overlying skin is derived from abdominal wall muscle perforators; thus, if a skin paddle is required, one must harvest at least 1 to 2 cm of the entire thickness of the abdominal wall in order to obtain enough perforators to supply the overlying skin.

sionally from the thoracadorsal artery and provides the blood supply to the scapular tip. This vessel can also be harvested to maintain a more reliable blood supply to the tip of the scapula. However, we have not found it necessary to harvest the angular artery in most cases.

After the circumflex scapular artery traverses the triangular space, it splits into two cutaneous branches: a transverse or scapular branch and a descending or parascapular branch (Fig. 14B). These two skin branches allow the creation of two separate skin paddles. The combination of one bone segment and two skin paddles lends itself nicely to the reconstruction of through-and-through defects of the mandible (Figs. 14C and 15A–G).

Operative Technique

Prior to the operative procedure, the scapular spine and scapular tip are both marked, and the outline of the scapula is drawn. The course of the transverse cutaneous branch can be approximated by drawing a transverse line halfway between the scapular spine and the scapular tip. The descending cutaneous branch can be drawn on a line parallel to the lateral border of the scapula. The intersection of theses two branches should be at the triangular space, which can be located either by palpation or by Doppler ultrasound (Fig. 15A).

The mandibular resection is performed with the patient in a supine position (Fig. 15B,C). After completion of the resection, the patient is placed in a lateral position, and the arm is prepared so that it can be manipulated during surgery. The skin paddles are dissected by incising them circumferentially and then elevating them from distal to proximal. These fasciocutaneous flaps should be elevated beneath the deep fascia of the back. As the teres muscles are identified, the dissection should be slowed as one nears the triangular space. Once the main cutaneous branch is identified, the remainder of the cutaneous dissection is completed. The muscles are retracted, and the vessel is traced through the space down to its origin. On the undersurface of the vessel, the dissection should be limited so that injury to the bone branches is avoided. The dissection can be performed circumferentially after the border of the scapula has been passed. The side branches should be ligated and controlled under direct vision and the vessel traced to its origin, where it branches with the thoracodorsal vessel. A decision must be made at this time whether to sacrifice the thoracodorsal vessel to obtain 1 cm of extra length.

Once the vascular dissection has been completed, the bone is harvested. The medial limit of bone harvest is ascertained by palpating the groove between the teres muscles and infraspinatus muscle. This is then incised with a cautery down to the bone, and the teres minor muscle is further elevated laterally to expose the lateral border of the scapula. A periosteal elevator is then used to expose a portion of the bone to perform the osteotomies. The superior extent of this dissection should be just below the glenoid fossa of the scapula. An oscillating saw is used to make the incisions in the bone. The upper aspect of the teres minor muscle needs to be divided to release the vascular pedicle and allow release of the bony segment. The bone flap is then elevated out of the wound, and the underlying musculature is divided with either the cautery or scissors, with care taken not to injure the vascular pedicle (Fig. 15D).

Once the flap has been elevated, it can be allowed to perfuse in situ while the muscular incisions are closed with absorbable suture. The flap vessels are then divided at their origin, and the flap is wrapped in a sterile towel and placed in a basin on ice while the donor site is closed over closed-suction drains. Once closure is completed, the patient is placed again in a supine position and prepared for flap inset and revascularization.

The skin paddle to be used for intraoral lining, usually the transverse skin paddle, is placed first. This allows access to the posterior extent of the soft tissue defect. Once this is done, the bone is fixed into place using either a reconstruction plate or a mini-

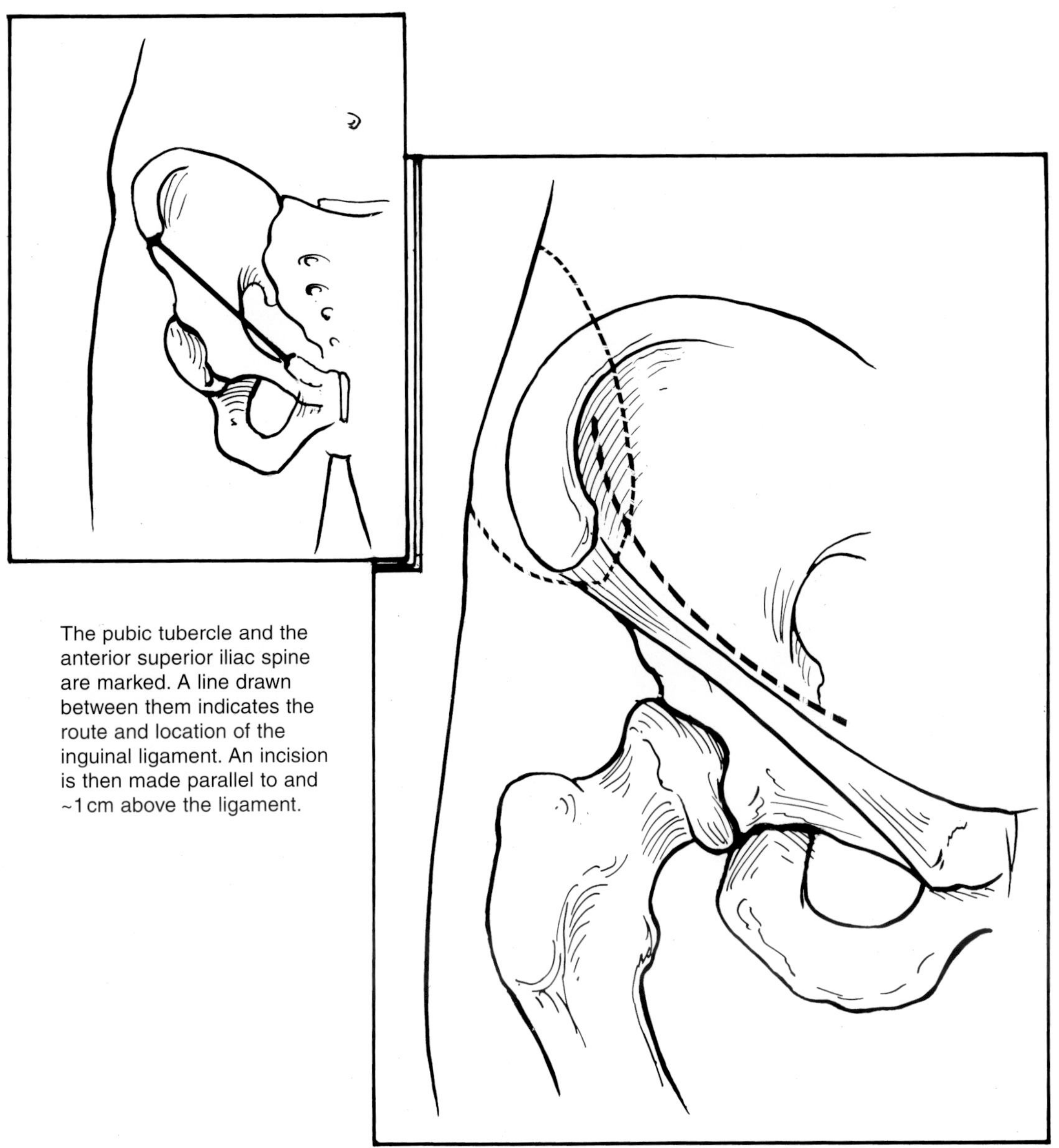

FIG. 11. The landmarks for flap elevation are the anterior superior iliac spine and the pubic tubercle. A line drawn between these two structures denotes the inguinal ligament, and the incision should be made 1 cm above this line.

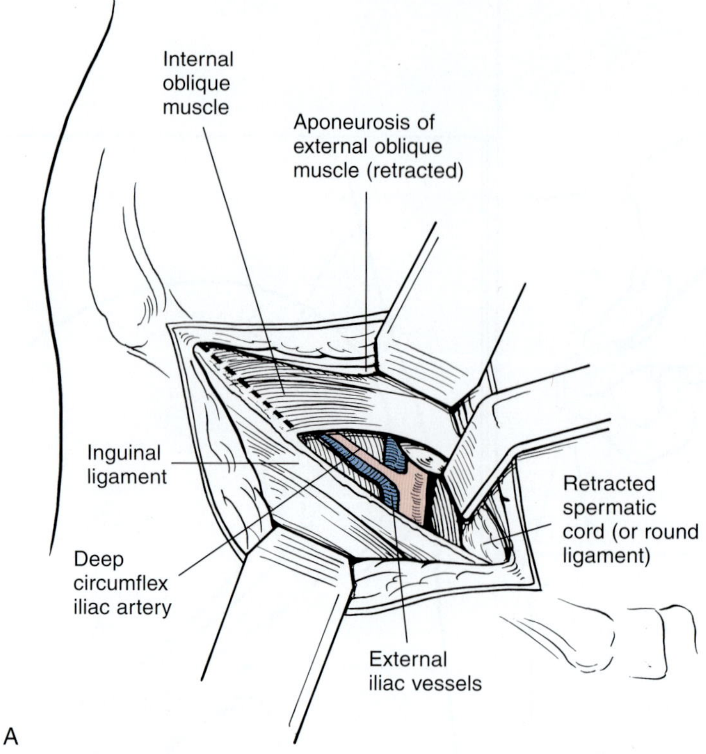

FIG. 12A. Once the incision is made, the spermatic cord or round ligament is mobilized and retracted upward and medially to expose the inguinal floor. After incising the inguinal floor, the origin of the DCI vessels is identified.

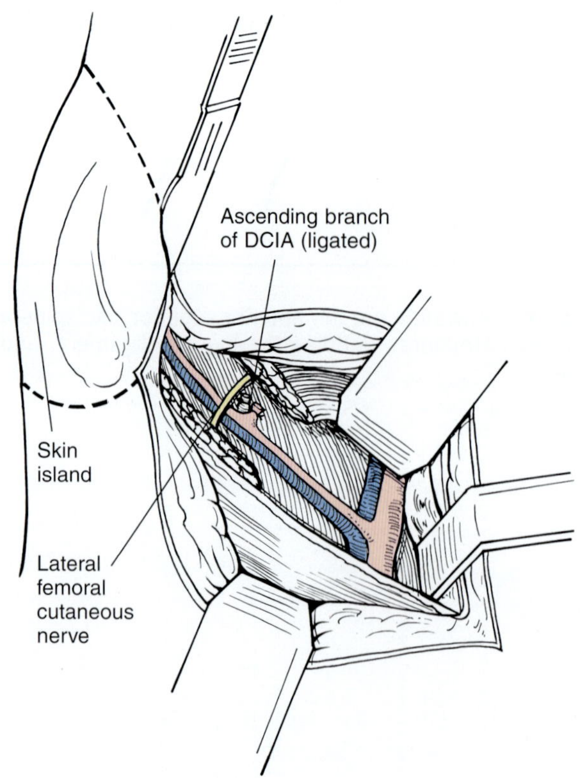

FIG. 12B. The vessels are traced laterally until the area of the origin of the ascending branch, and the crossing of the lateral femoral cutaneous nerve is identified. The ascending branch is divided and ligated if the internal oblique muscle is not needed.

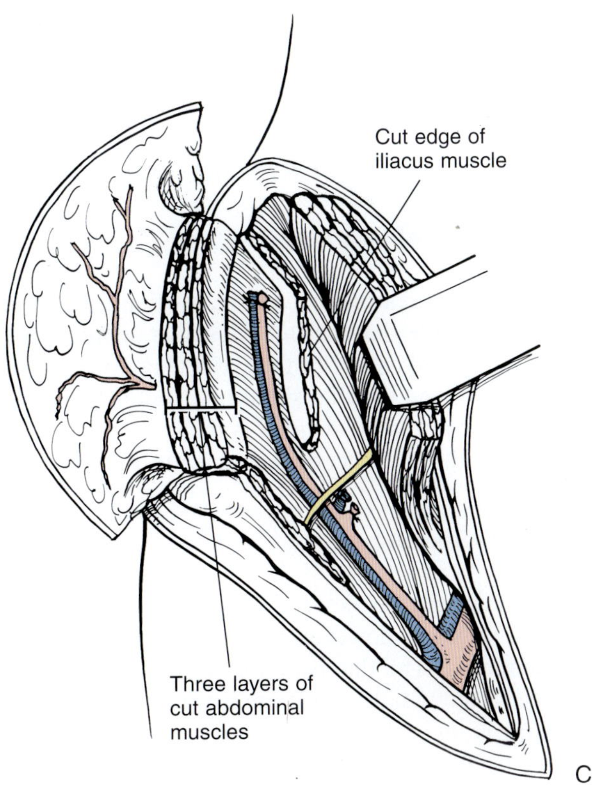

FIG. 12C. The three layers of abdominal wall have been incised to ensure the blood supply to the skin paddle. The iliacus muscle is incised just below the DCI vessels.

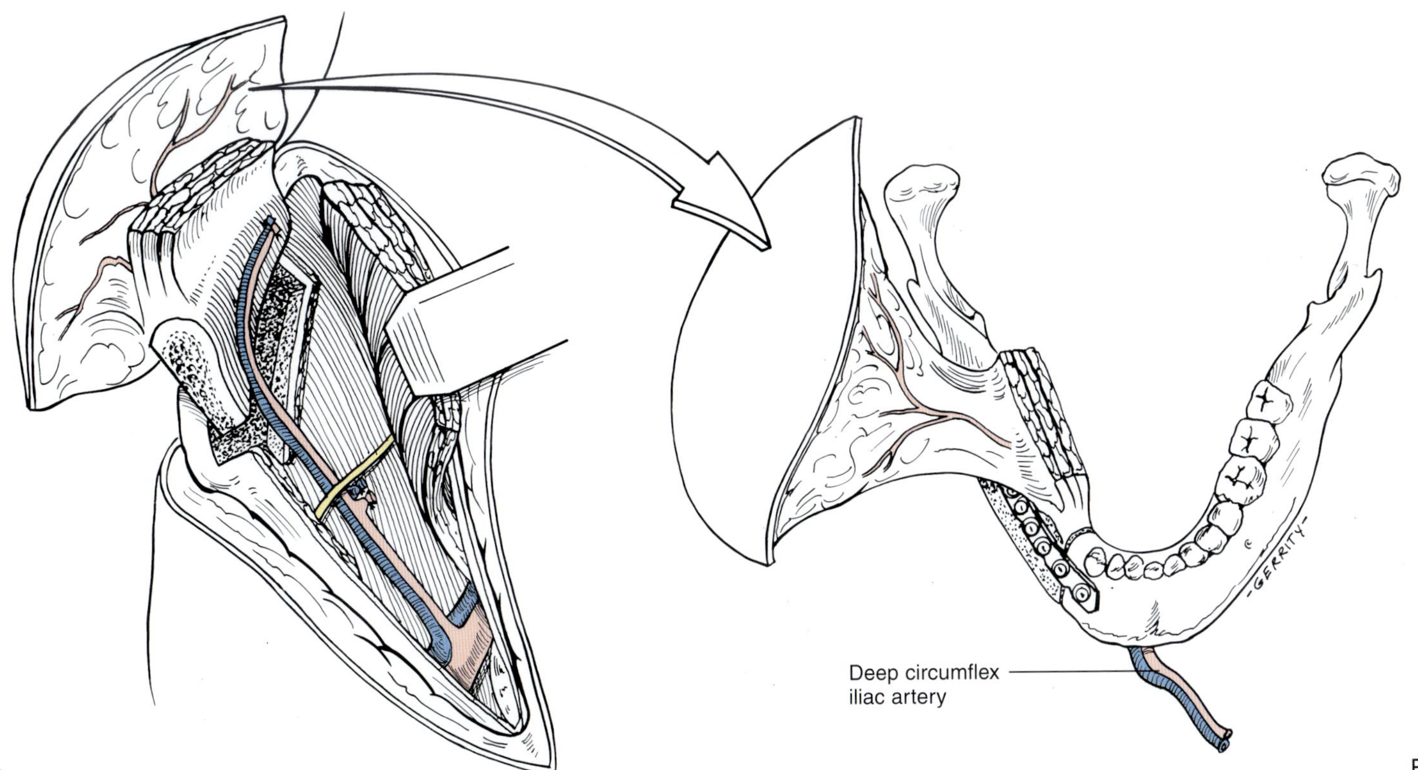

Fig. 12D, E. **D:** Once all the soft tissue has been incised, the bone cuts are made. Note that only the inner cortex is harvested. **E:** The flap is fixed to the reconstruction plate and the whole unit including the skin paddle is transposed to the recipient site. The soft tissue should be inset first if the defect is intraoral.

plate. Usually a single osteotomy will suffice in approximating the native chin prominence (Fig. 15E). After bone fixation, the flap is revascularized. The final step is inset
of the external skin paddle (Fig. 15F,G).

RADIAL FOREARM OSTEOCUTANEOUS FLAP

Anatomic Considerations

The radial forearm osteocutaneous flap is based on the radial vessels, which course
through the anterolateral intermuscular septum, and the cephalic vein, which courses
along the lateral aspect of the wrist (Fig. 16A). These vessels should be marked prior
to elevation, and the flap should be centered over both these vascular axes. The main
neural structure to be avoided is the superficial radial nerve, which is found just adjacent to the distal aspect of the cephalic vein (Fig. 16B).

Operative Technique

This flap may be elevated simultaneously with the ablative surgery. Either forearm
may be selected; however, we attempt to use the arm with the nondominant hand as
the donor site. The flap is incised circumferentially, and the distal ends of the cephalic
veins and the radial vessels are identified, ligated, and divided. The deep fascia of the
forearm is incised and the flap elevated from the periphery toward the anterolateral
intermuscular septum, where the radial vessels reside. Along the lateral aspect of this
dissection, the cephalic vein is elevated with the flap, the side branches are ligated and
divided, and the superficial branch of the radial nerve is identified and dissected free
from the fascia to remain in the donor site. As the lateral aspect of the septum is
encountered, the brachioradialis muscle and tendon are retracted laterally to expose
the lateral aspect of the radius. As the dissection continues along the medial, the flexor
carpi radialis muscle is retracted medially, exposing the flexor digitorum profundus
and pronator quadratus muscles. These muscles are incised to expose the radius, and
then a reciprocating saw is used to harvest the lateral portion of the radius bone. This
cut is made in a curvilinear fashion, which has been shown to minimize strength
deficits at the donor site (Fig. 16C). No more than a third of the diameter of the radius
should be harvested, thus yielding an approximate 1 cm bone segment.

Once this has been done, the remainder of the dissection is completed in the same
manner as for the radial forearm skin flap. The flap is then transferred to the recipient
site and fixed into place. This can be done by means of a reconstruction plate, miniplates, lag screws, or wires. The donor site is closed with a skin graft after the muscles are reapproximated. The forearm is then placed in a cast for a minimum of 6
weeks. If instability of the radius is noted at the time of flap harvest, one may elect to
stabilize the wrist with a plate and repair the defect with an autogenous bone graft harvested from the iliac crest. Again, this flap has limited indications in our opinion, but
in cases in which a small segment of bone is needed and a large soft tissue deficit is
present, the radial forearm osteocutaneous flap may be an excellent choice.

SUMMARY

Free flaps have greatly enhanced our ability to reconstruct the mandible. The free
fibular osteocutaneous flap has found the greatest utility at the University of Texas
M. D. Anderson Cancer Center, but the iliac crest flap is also useful, particularly for
smaller defects. The free scapular osteocutaneous flap is useful for through-and-
through defects of the oral cavity that include the mandible. The free radial forearm
osteocutaneous flap has only limited utility for mandibular reconstruction because of
the limited amount of bone available and the increased donor site morbidity.

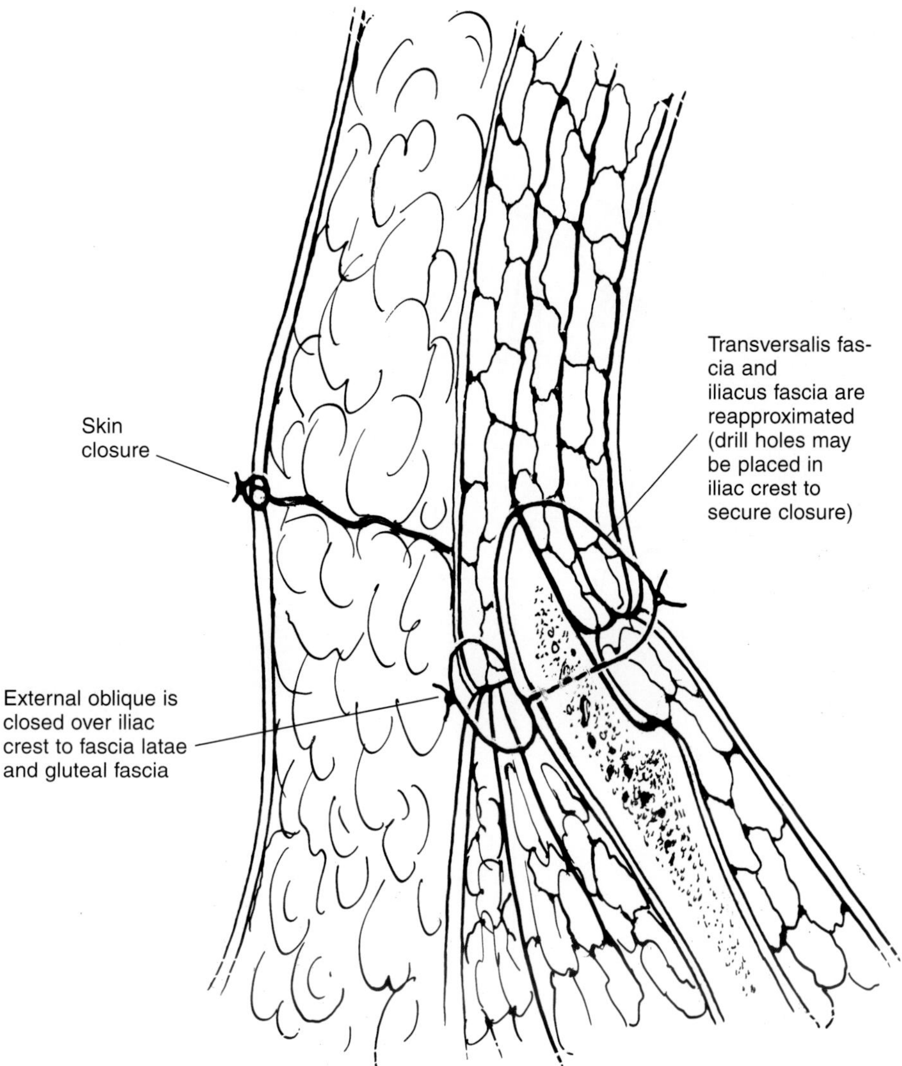

FIG. 13. The closure of the defect is accomplished by suturing the internal oblique and transverse abdominis to the iliacus, and the external oblique to the fascia overlying the remaining crest. Drill holes through the bone are used to further secure and anchor the closure.

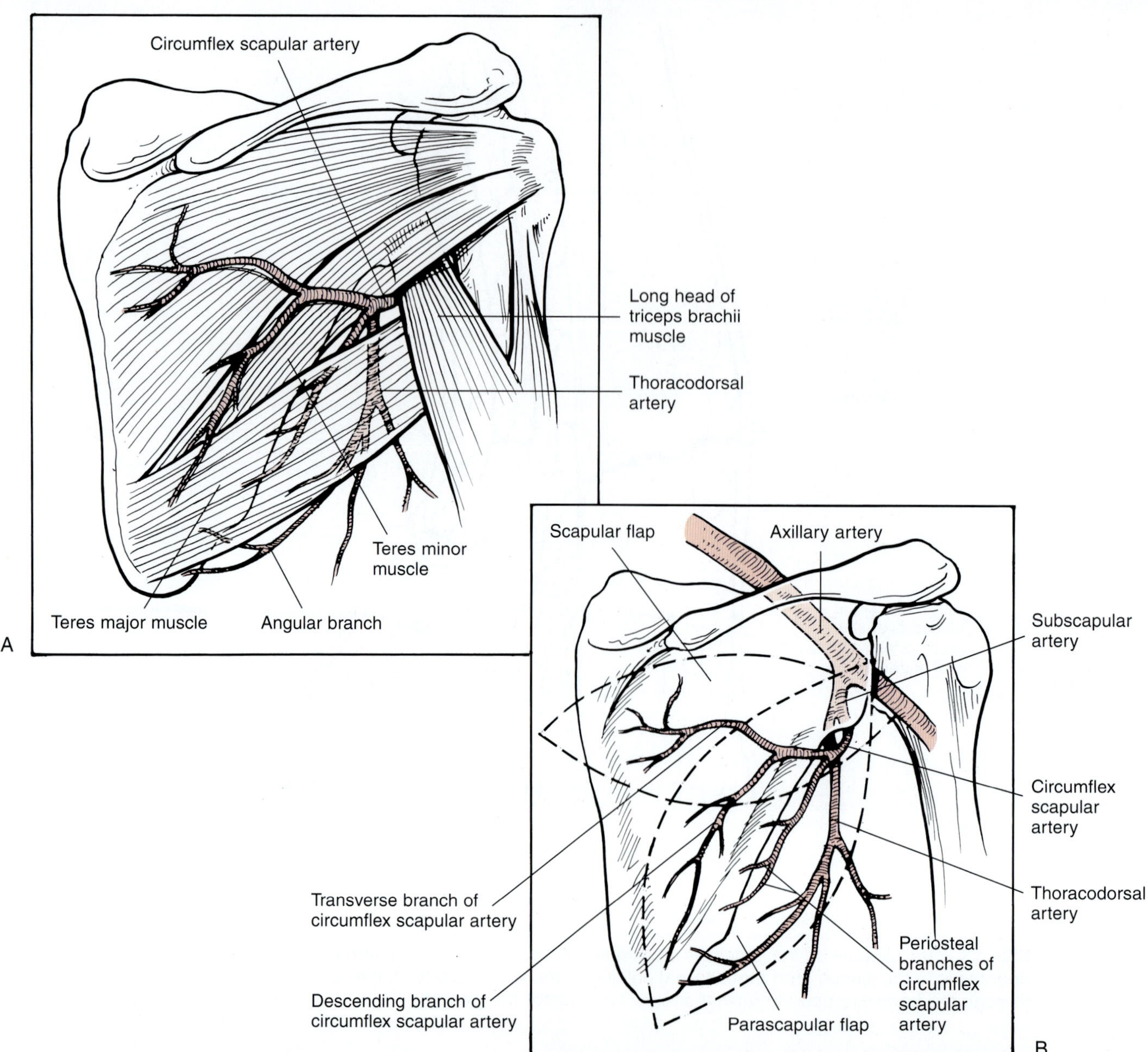

FIG. 14A, B. A: The circumflex scapular artery comes through the triangular space and gives off two skin branches and one bone branch. **B:** The anatomic arrangement allows for the design of one bone paddle and two skin paddles.

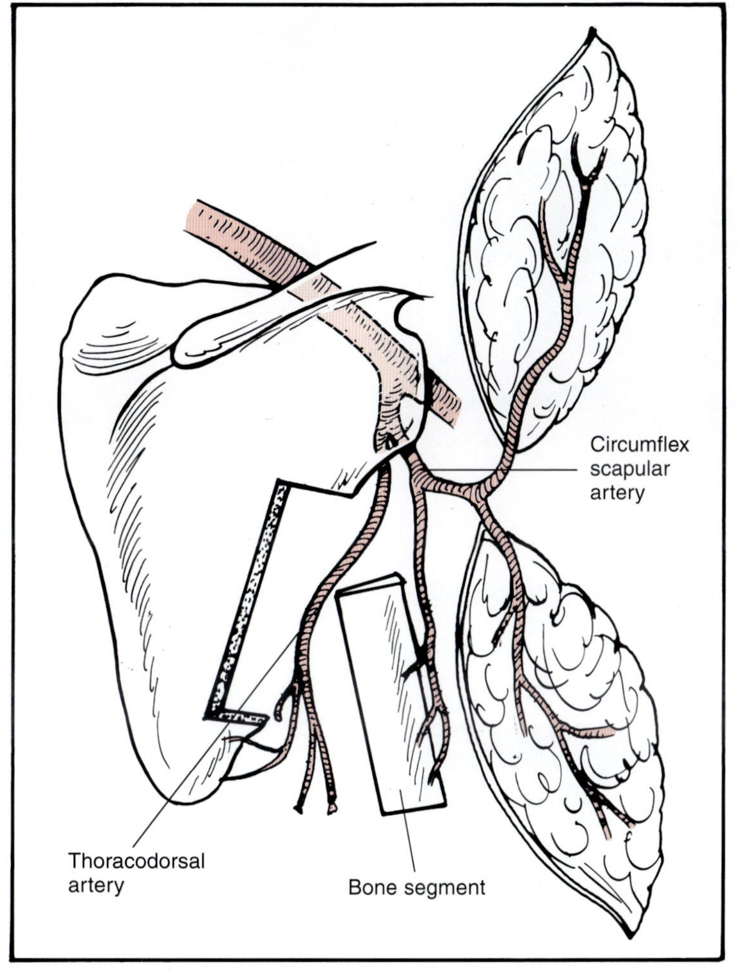

FIG. 14C. Each one of these vascularized units has its own pedicle, thus allowing for greater independent inset of each individual unit.

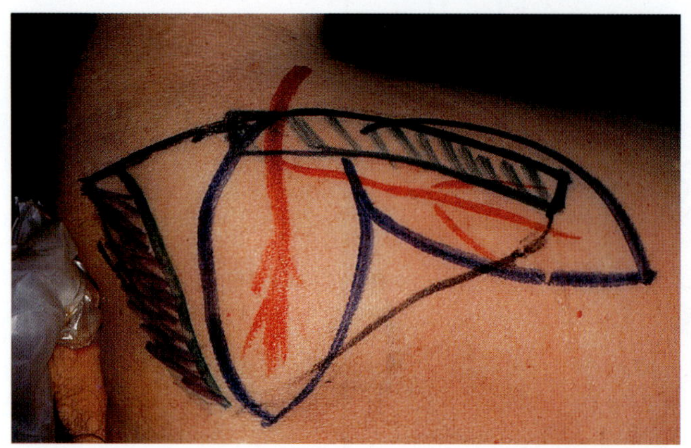

FIG. 15A. The markings for an osteocutaneous bilobed scapular flap.

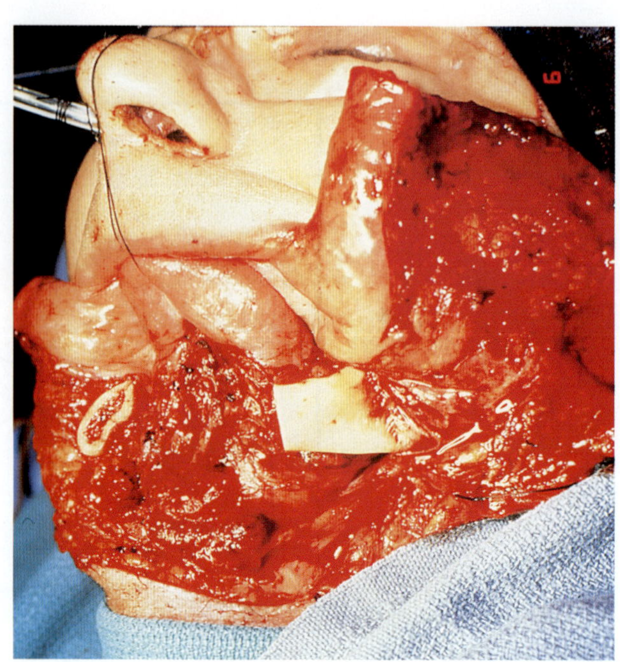

FIG. 15B. The patient after bony resection.

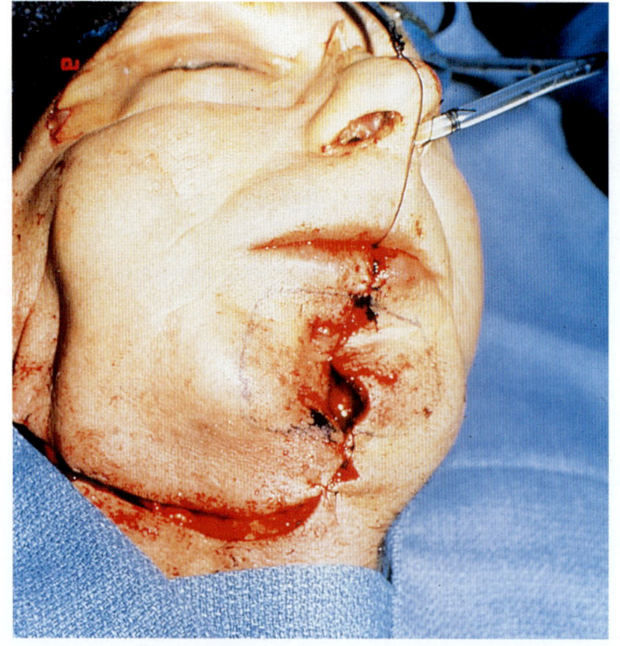

FIG. 15C. An attempt was made to save the chin skin, but the tumor margins dictated further skin sacrifice. The markings for the skin resection are seen in the photograph.

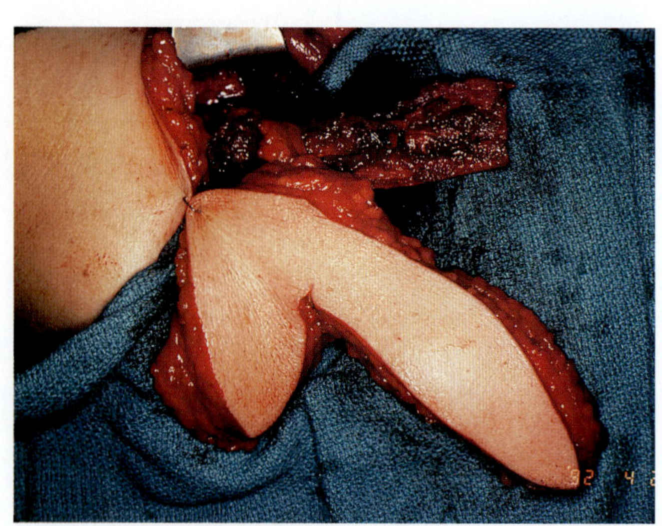

FIG. 15D. The scapular flap after elevation.

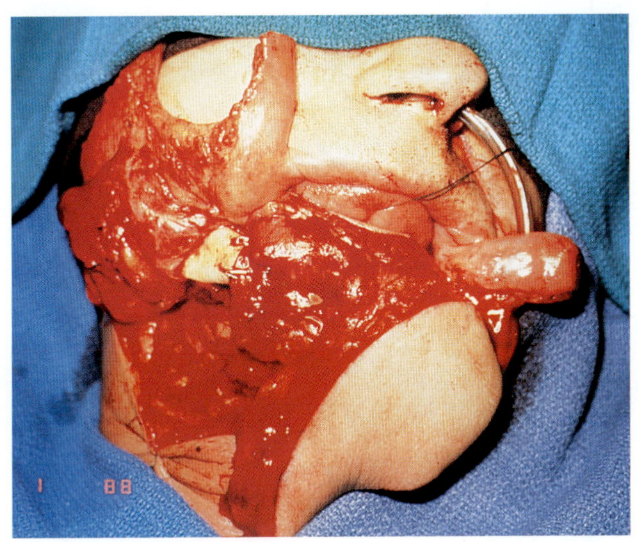

FIG. 15E. The bone and the intraoral skin paddle have been inset. The external paddle is being prepared to be inset as a replacement for the chin skin.

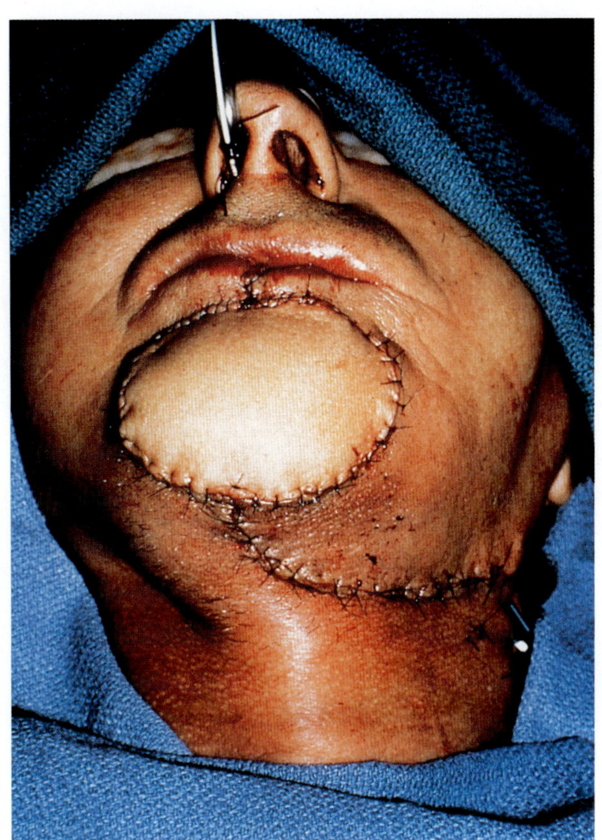

FIG. 15F. The patient after completion of the case.

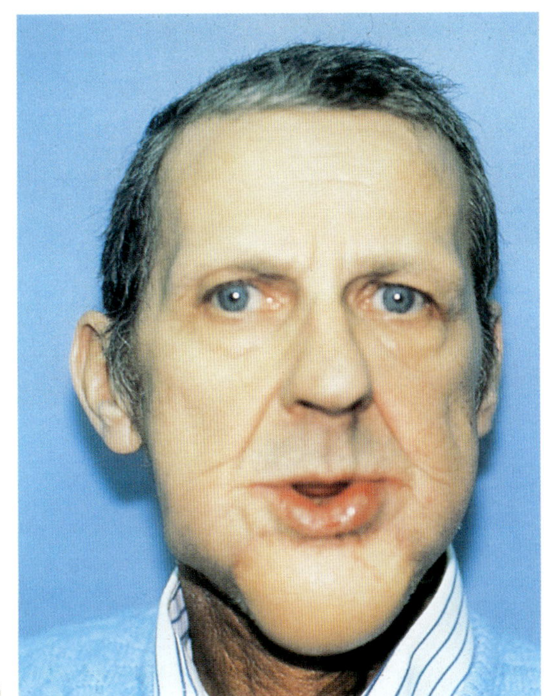

FIG. 15G. Patient appearance after long-term follow-up.

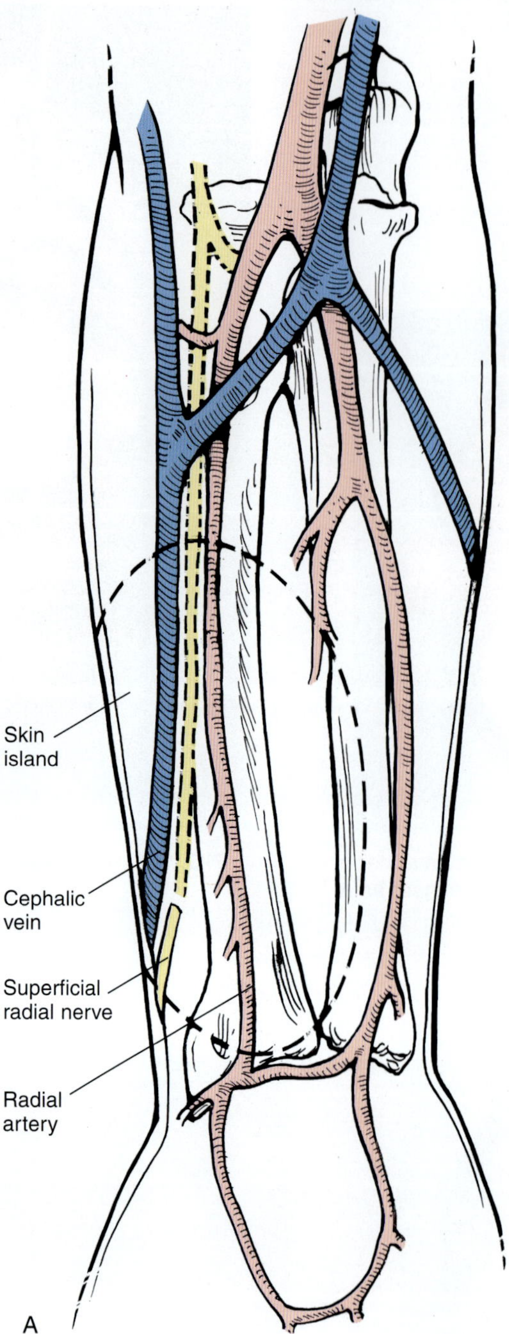

FIG. 16A. The vascular anatomy of the radial forearm flap.

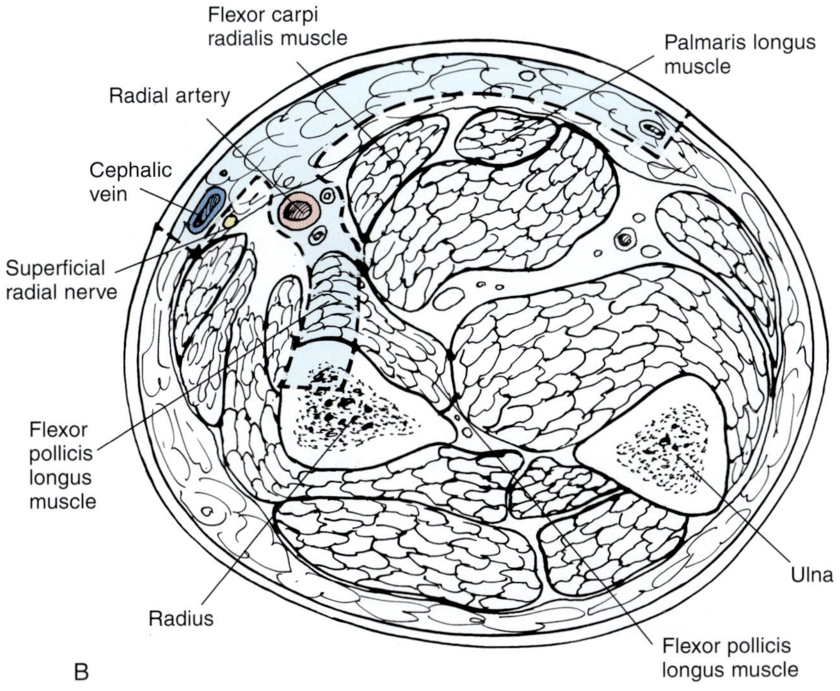

FIG. 16B. A schematic cross section of the flap harvest, which includes a portion of the flexor pollicis longus to provide vascular supply to the bone.

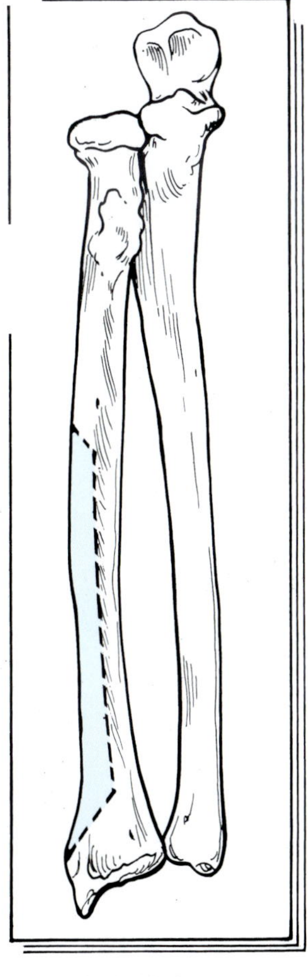

FIG. 16C. The bone is harvested in a curvilinear fashion, which maximizes the strength of the donor site.

SELECTED READINGS

Allison GR, Rappaport I, Salibian AH, McMicken B, Shoup JE, Etchepare TL, et al. Adaptive mechanisms of speech and swallowing after combined jaw and tongue reconstruction in long-term survivors. *Am J Surg* 1987; 154:419–422.

Beppu M, Hanel DP, Johnston GHF, Carmo JM, Tsai T. The osteocutaneous fibula flap: an anatomic study. *J Reconstr Microsurg* 1992;8:215–223.

Boyd JB. The place of the iliac crest in vascularized oromandibular reconstruction. *Microsurgery* 1994;15:250–256.

Boyd JB, Mulholland RS. Fixation of the vascularized bone graft in mandibular reconstruction. *Plast Reconstr Surg* 1993;91:274–282.

Duncan MJ, Manktelow RT, Zuker RM, Rosen IB. Mandibular reconstruction in the radiated patient: the role of osteocutaneous free tissue transfers. *Plast Reconstr Surg* 1985;76:829–840.

Flemming AFS, Brough MD, Evans ND, Grant HR, Harris M, James DR, et al. Mandibular reconstruction using vascularised fibula. *Br J Plast Surg* 1990;43:403–409.

Goodacre TEE, Walker CJ, Jawad AS, Jackson AM, Brough MD. Donor site morbidity following osteocutaneous free fibula transfer. *Br J Plast Surg* 1990;43:410–412.

Hidalgo DA. Fibula free flap: a new method of mandible reconstruction. *Plast Reconstr Surg* 1989;84:71–79.

Hidalgo DA. Aesthetic improvements in free-flap mandible reconstruction. *Plast Reconstr Surg* 1991;88:574–585.

Schusterman MA, Reece GP, Miller MJ, Harris S. The osteocutaneous free fibula flap: is the skin paddle reliable? *Plast Reconstr Surg* 1992;90:787–793.

Shenaq SM, Klebuc MJ. Refinements in the iliac crest microsurgical free flap for oromandibular reconstruction. [Review]. *Microsurgery* 1994;15:825–830.

Soutar DS, Widdowson WP. Immediate reconstruction of the mandible using a vascularized segment of radius. *Head Neck Surg* 1986;8:232–246.

Swartz WM, Banis JC, Newton ED, Ramasastry SS, Jones NF, Acland R. The osteocutaneous scapular flap for mandibular and maxillary reconstruction. *Plast Reconstr Surg* 1986;77:530–545.

Taylor GI, Miller GDH, Ham FJ. The free vascularized bone graft: a clinical extension of microvascular techniques. *Plast Reconstr Surg* 1975;55:533–544.

Taylor GI, Townsend P, Corlett R. Superiority of the deep circumflex iliac vessels as the supply for free groin flaps. Clinical work. *Plast Reconstr Surg* 1979;64:745–759.

Urken ML, Vickery C, Weinberg H, Buchbinder D, Lawson W, Biller HF. The internal oblique-iliac crest osseomyocutaneous free flap in oromandibular reconstruction. Report of 20 cases. *Arch Otolaryngol Head Neck Surg* 1989;115:339–349.

Urken ML, Weinberg H, Vickery C, Buchbinder D, Lawson W, Biller HF. Oromandibular reconstruction using microvascular composite free flaps. *Arch Otolaryngol Head Neck Surg* 1991;117:733–744.

Wei FC, Seah CS, Tsai YC, Liu SJ, Tsai MS. Fibula osteoseptocutaneous flap for reconstruction of composite mandibular defects [see comments]. *Plast Reconstr Surg* 1994;93:294–304; discussion 305.

Weinzweig N, Jones NF, Shestak KC, Moon HK, Davies BW. Oromandibular reconstruction using a keel-shaped modification of the radial forearm osteocutaneous flap. *Ann Plast Surg* 1994;33:359–369; discussion 369–370.

Yoshimura M, Shimada T, Hosokawa M. The vasculature of the peroneal tissue transfer. *Plast Reconstr Surg* 1990;85:917–921.

Microsurgical Reconstruction of the Cancer Patient, edited by M.A. Schusterman.
Lippincott-Raven Publishers, Philadelphia © 1997.

4

Pharyngoesophageal Reconstruction

Gregory P. Reece

Reconstruction of the pharyngoesophagus after resection of locally advanced carcinomas of the larynx and pharynx can be a difficult problem for the reconstructive surgeon. Surgery in this group of patients is often complicated by previous cancer therapy, multiple medical problems, poor nutritional condition, and a history of tobacco and alcohol abuse. Moreover, the long-term survival rate for these patients is usually poor; only 25% to 35% survive 5 years. This fact has led many surgeons to conclude that tumor resection and pharyngoesophageal reconstruction are palliative procedures.

Because these patients have so many factors that predispose them to complications and because they have such a limited life expectancy, the method of pharyngoesophageal reconstruction selected must be a reliable, one-stage procedure with minimal morbidity and mortality, and one that restores swallowing function in the shortest time possible. Although several techniques have been described for total pharyngoesophageal reconstruction, in our opinion free jejunal transfer (FJT) is the most versatile method that best fulfills these requirements. Other techniques, such as the radial forearm free flap (RFFF), are better suited for patients who are not candidates for FJT reconstruction and for patients with partial pharyngoesophageal defects.

PREOPERATIVE CONSIDERATIONS

Prior to surgery, all factors that might interfere with the successful use of an FJT or RFFF for pharyngoesophageal reconstruction must be determined from the patient's history and physical examination, chart review, and radiologic examinations of the

G. P. Reece: Department of Plastic Surgery, The University of Texas, M.D. Anderson Cancer Center, Houston, Texas 77030.

head and neck. For example, the computed tomographic examination of the head and neck may indicate that the tumor extends into the thoracic esophagus; a gastric pull-up may be a better reconstructive option in this situation. Similarly, a RFFF may be a better reconstructive option for patients with a history of ascites or significant liver disease and for patients who have had previous abdominal surgery with dense adhesion formation.

All patients who are to undergo pharyngoesophageal reconstruction with a RFFF require an Allen's test to confirm patency of the palmar arch vessels; an arteriogram is rarely, if ever, indicated for this evaluation. In general, the nondominant arm is the preferred donor site whenever possible. The donor arm of a hirsute patient will require shaving at the time of surgery. Hair growth within the lumen of the tubed flap is seldom a significant problem because most of these patients receive postoperative radiation therapy. Also, because these patients are not able to eat in the immediate postoperative period and because of the possibility of erosion of the flap between the feeding catheter and the tracheostomy tube, we prefer to place a percutaneous endoscopic gastrostomy tube prior to surgery.

PHARYNGOESOPHAGEAL RECONSTRUCTION USING FREE JEJUNAL TRANSFER

Operative Technique

Patients presenting for FJT pharyngoesophageal reconstruction usually do not require a preoperative bowel prep. However, broad-spectrum intravenous antibiotics are administered 1 hour before surgery and for 48 hours postoperatively. The patient is positioned on the operating table in the supine position with a roll placed under the shoulder and with the neck in extension. After a urinary catheter is placed, the patient is sterilely prepared and draped from the midface to the pubis.

To decrease the total operative time, the jejunal flap is preferably harvested at the time of tumor resection through an upper midline abdominal incision. The vascular arcade of the proximal jejunum has the most favorable anatomy for this flap and is best examined by transilluminating the mesentery with the operating room lights turned low.

After selecting a vascular arcade, the length of jejunum required to repair the defect and to provide a monitor flap approximately 1 to 2 cm long is determined. The defect should be measured in order to determine the length required (Fig. 1). In most cases, the FJT should be designed so that the vascular pedicle will be located near the level of the recipient vessels when the flap is placed in the neck.

Flap dissection should begin on both sides of the mesentery at the base of the vascular pedicle to assure suitability of the mesenteric vessels for microvascular anastomoses. The mesenteric veins are fragile and require meticulous dissection under loupe magnification to avoid bleeding or hematoma formation. After these vessels are isolated, dissection continues through the mesentery toward the proximal and distal ends of the flap. The proximal end of the jejunal flap is marked with a silk suture placed in the serosa to maintain the flap in an isoperistaltic orientation. A gastrointestinal anastomotic stapling device is then used to divide each end of the jejunal flap. The vascular pedicle is left intact to perfuse the flap until ready for harvest (Fig. 2A–C).

After the tumor has been removed, the recipient vessels are dissected and isolated.

The jejunal flap is then harvested and the flap transferred to members of the reconstructive team working in the head and neck area. The stumps of the mesenteric vessels must be securely ligated to avoid postoperative bleeding from the donor site. While the flap is being inset and revascularized, jejunal continuity is reestablished at the donor site, jejunostomy and gastrostomy tubes are inserted, and the abdomen is closed.

Using the serosal silk suture as a guide, the jejunal flap is inset in an isoperistaltic fashion. We prefer to perform the pharyngojejunal (proximal enteric) anastomosis before revascularizing the flap. This maneuver allows the jejunal segment to be placed

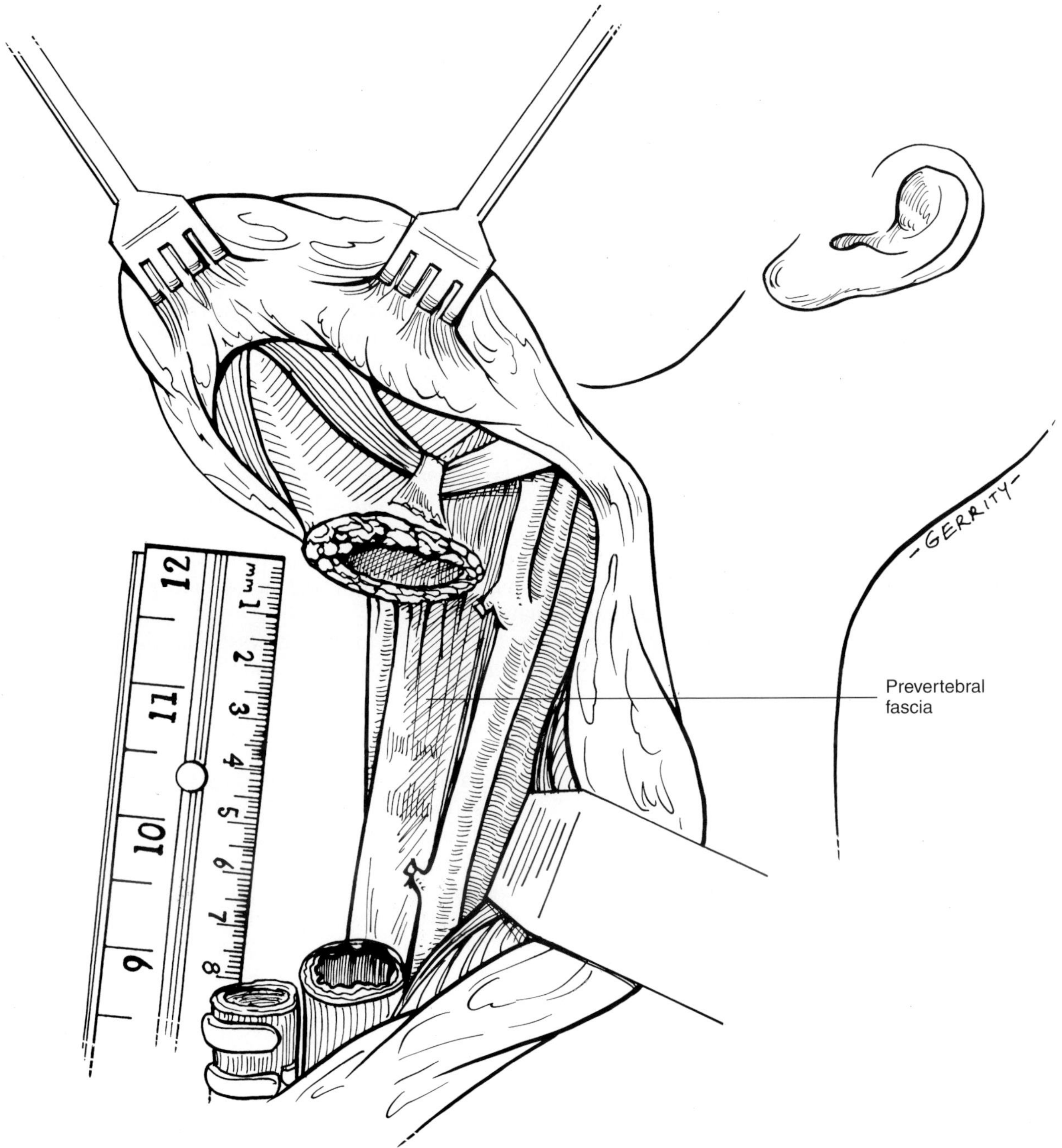

FIG. 1. A typical defect after laryngopharyngectomy. The length of the defect must be measured in its greatest dimension to determine the length of flap required.

in any position necessary to facilitate the bowel anastomosis, prevents disruption of the microvascular anastomoses, and expedites the proximal anastomosis by eliminating the peristalsis, bleeding, and mucus production that occur after revascularization. Although flap ischemia time is increased by 30 to 40 minutes, the additional ischemia is well tolerated by the flap and flap cooling is not required. Because the lumen of the pharyngeal defect is usually larger than that of the jejunum, it is frequently necessary to enlarge the proximal end of the jejunal flap by opening the end of the jejunum along its antimesenteric border for 2 cm or greater.

To avoid fistula formation, the proximal enteric anastomosis is performed in two layers, using interrupted polyglactin and silk sutures for the mucosal and serosal closures, respectively (Fig. 3A–E). The silk sutures are placed in Lembert fashion and should incorporate a portion of the prevertebral fascia posteriorly and a large amount of tongue musculature anteriorly to help support the flap and to take tension off the anastomosis. In our experience, most proximal leaks occur laterally, especially along the mesenteric side of the jejunal flap. Therefore, care must be taken to take a good "bite" of the serosa when placing sutures in this location.

After the proximal enteric anastomosis has been completed, the flap is revascularized (Fig. 4). While the flap is perfusing, the stump of the cervical esophagus is examined. If the esophagus was extensively mobilized, its segmental blood supply may have been interrupted, which may lead to ischemia-induced stricture formation. This situation may be worsened if the cervical esophagus was previously irradiated. For this reason, we usually trim the esophagus to within 1 to 2 cm of intact periesophageal tissue before completing the distal anastomosis.

The neck is flexed to a neutral position to avoid excessive jejunal length, which can lead to a functional dysphagia after surgery. Jejunal redundancy is also avoided by applying slight traction on the jejunum in a caudal direction as the jejunum is marked for the distal anastomosis. The jejunum is then divided at the marked location such that the anterior side is cut longer than the posterior side. The posterior half of the distal enteric anastomosis is then performed using a single layer of interrupted 3-0 absorbable sutures.

To avoid a stricture formation, the distal anastomosis should be enlarged by incising the anterior side of the esophageal stump for 1 to 2 cm before insetting the longer anterior side of the distal jejunal flap into the remaining esophageal defect (Fig. 5A). Placing the sutures for the anterior side of the anastomosis requires great care to avoid "back walling" or bunching the anastomosis. Suture placement is facilitated by passing a 40-Fr Maloney dilator orally, through the jejunum and into the esophagus, and by placing all sutures before they are tied (Fig. 5B). After the distal anastomosis has been completed, a small segment of mesentery or a seromuscular cuff of jejunum can be used to cover the distal anastomosis anteriorly where most distal leaks occur.

The jejunum not required for the interposition flap is used to create the monitor flap. This flap is fashioned by excising the excess jejunum from the mesentery and leaving the last 2 cm of bowel attached to the pedicle (Fig. 6). The monitor is sutured to the neck away from the tracheal stoma and split to expose the mucosa. Because this part of the jejunal flap is still attached to a common vascular pedicle, events occurring in the monitor flap accurately reflect events that are occurring in the FJT. In our experience, this has been the most reliable method for monitoring the FJT. Drain catheters are then placed in the neck away from the bowel and vascular anastomoses and the neck visor flap closed. The exteriorized monitor flap is covered with a petroleum-impregnated gauze to avoid desiccation.

PHARYNGOESOPHAGEAL RECONSTRUCTION WITH THE RADIAL FOREARM FREE FLAP

Operative Technique for Circumferential Defects

The patient is positioned on the operating table in the supine position as described for the FJT. A well-padded tourniquet is placed on the arm proximal to the elbow, and

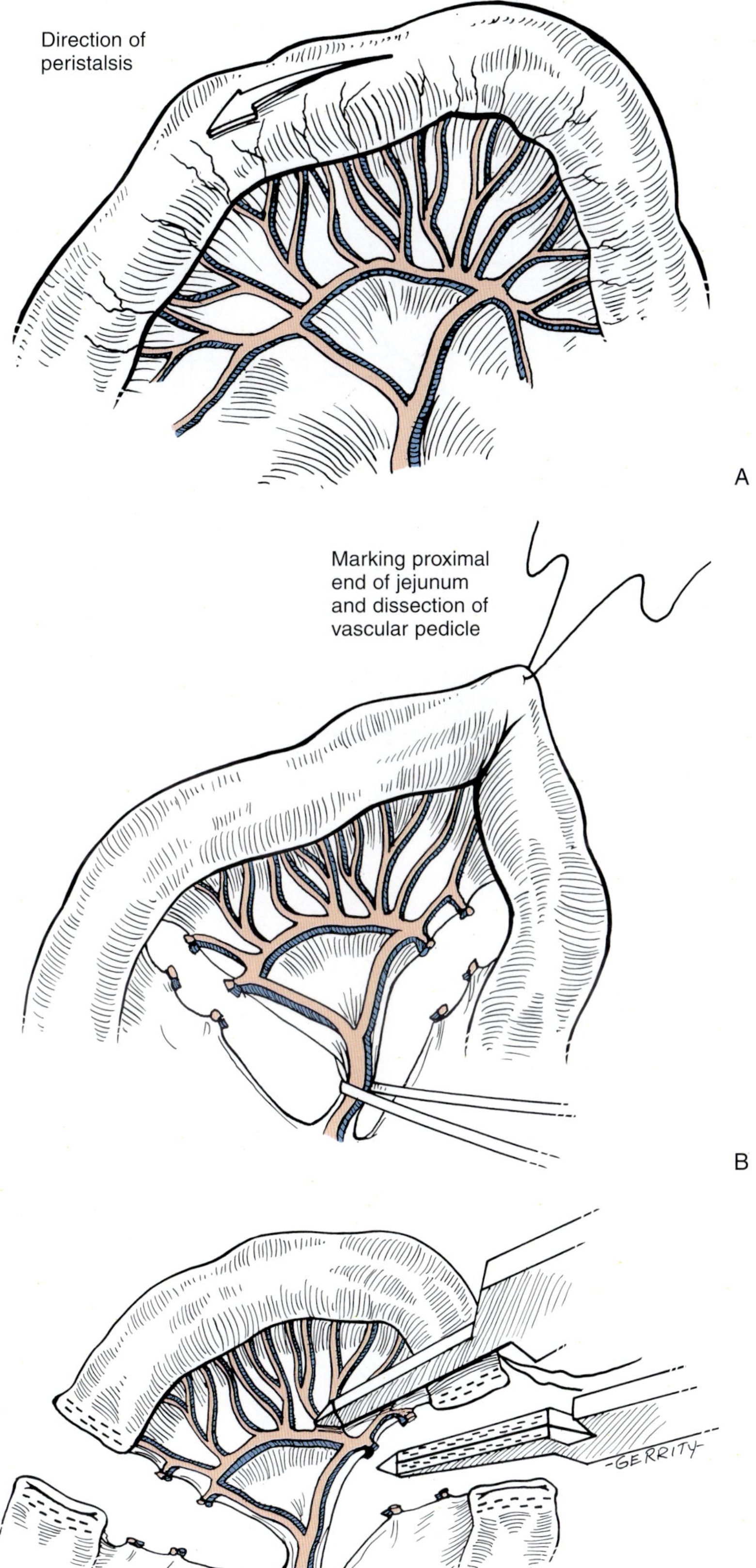

FIG. 2A–C. A suitable segment of jejunum is isolated on its vascular arcade.

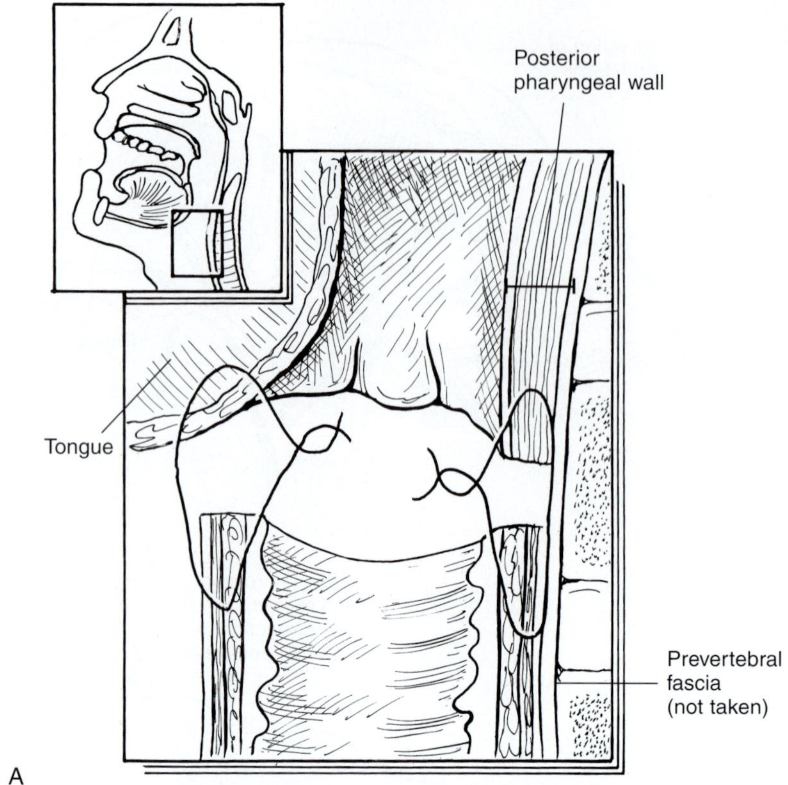

FIG. 3A. Diagram of first layer of inverting absorbable sutures.

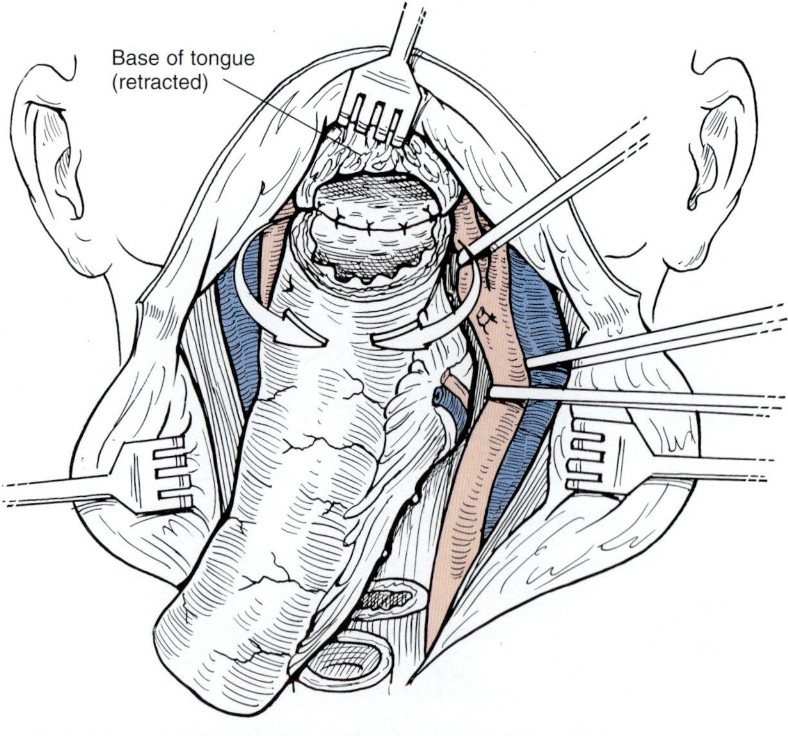

FIG. 3B. The anastomosis is started posteriorly and one works from either side from posterior to anterior until the anastomosis is completed.

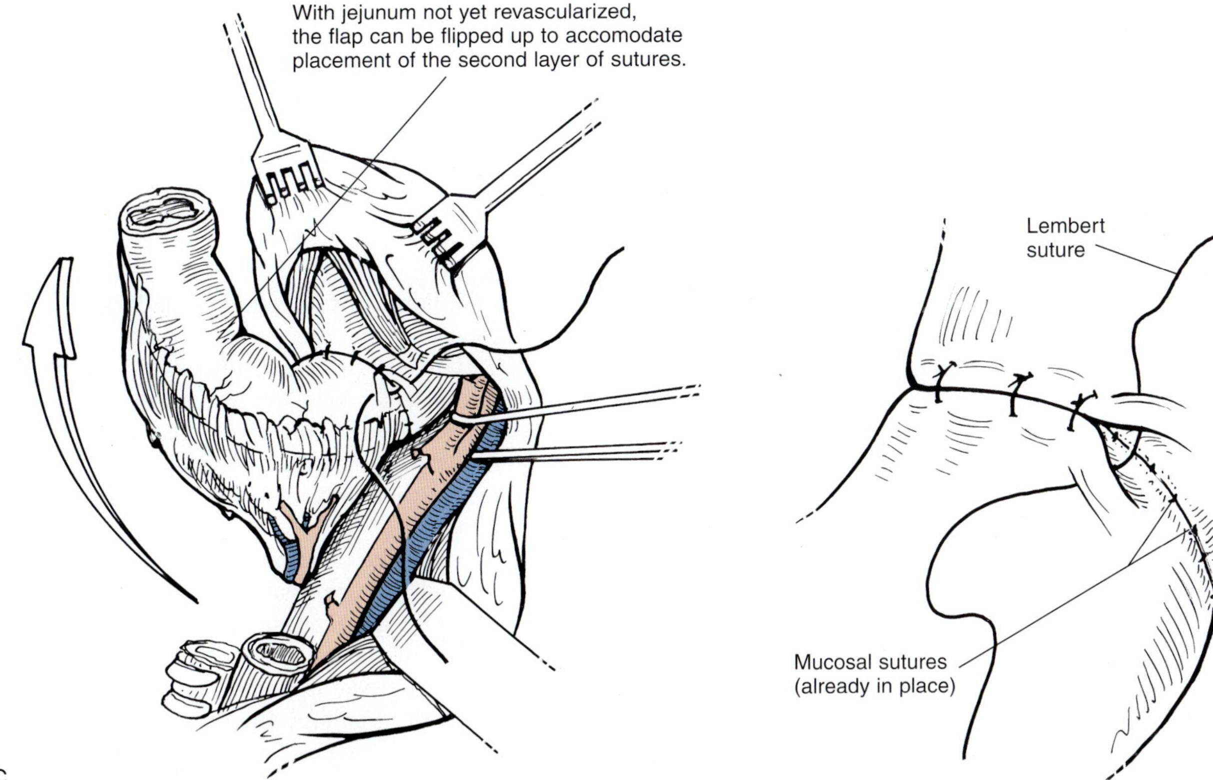

C

FIG. 3C. Once the first layer has been completed, the jejunum is pulled superiorly and the second layer of interrupted silk Lembert sutures are placed.

D

FIG. 3D. Closeup of placement of Lembert sutures.

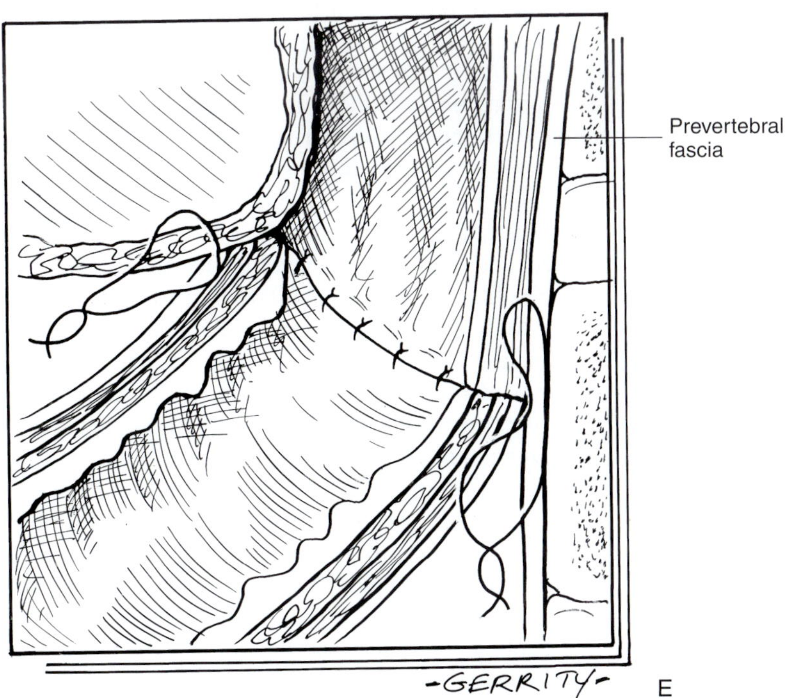

E

FIG. 3E. Cross-sectional diagram of placement of Lembert sutures in the base of tongue and prevertebral fascia.

the arm is placed on an arm board attached to the operating table. The head, neck, donor arm, and skin graft donor site are then sterilely prepared and draped. The skin graft used to cover the donor arm defect is usually obtained from the thigh or hip.

Although the RFFF can be harvested during the tumor resection, we prefer to design and harvest the flap after the tumor has been completely excised and all frozen-section specimens determined to be free of tumor by pathologic examination of the margins of resection. This approach increases the overall operative time by approximately 45 minutes, but allows for a more accurate determination of the defect size and any unusual extensions of the defect prior to designing the flap.

Because of the size discrepancy between the lumina of the pharynx and the cervical esophagus, the RFFF flap must be designed such that one end of the flap is wider than the other end. In most cases, we prefer to use the proximal forearm for the pharyngeal end of the flap because the forearm is wider proximally than distally and because a flap width of 10 to 12 cm is usually required for the pharyngeal anastomosis; a flap width of at least 9 cm is required distally for the esophageal anastomosis (Fig. 7). The length of the flap required for reconstruction varies with the length of the pharyngoesophageal defect.

The flap should be oriented over the long axis of the radial artery and the cephalic vein should be incorporated in the flap design whenever possible to obtain the most optimal perfusion. Because stricture formation at the distal anastomosis is also a problem with a RFFF reconstruction, an extension of the flap is designed along the esophageal end of the flap. Like the FJT, this extra tissue is inset into an incision on the anterior side of the cervical esophageal stump to enlarge the distal anastomosis (Fig. 8A).

After the flap has been designed, the arm is exsanguinated with an Esmarch bandage and the tourniquet inflated to approximately 250 mm Hg. The skin is incised down through the fascia along the planned ulnar and radial margins of the flap. The skin along the distal margin of the flap is also incised through the fascial layer on the ulnar side of the radial artery. To prevent injury to the branches of the superficial radial nerve that are located in the underlying subcutaneous tissue, the skin incision on the radial side of the radial artery extends just to the level of the subcutaneous tissue.

The ulnar side of the flap is dissected first and proceeds in a subfascial plane just over the flexor superficialis tendons toward the radial artery. Care must be taken to leave peritenon over these tendons and to prevent desiccation of these structures by frequent irrigation with sterile saline. Failure to take these precautions can lead to loss of the skin graft used to close the donor site and subsequent tendon exposure. Upon reaching the radial side of the flexor carpi radialis tendon, the deep fascia is incised to reveal the radial artery and its associated venae comitantes. These vessels are clamped, divided, and ligated at the level of the distal margin of the flap (Fig. 8B).

The radial side of the flap is then reflected in a subfascial plane toward the radial artery. After the cephalic vein is identified along the distal flap margin, it is clamped, divided, and ligated before elevating the vein proximally with the rest of the flap. The branches of the superficial branch of the radial nerve are encountered next and the nerve is preserved by dissecting these branches out of the fascia for the length of the flap. Dissection stops at the ulnar margin of the brachioradialis tendon and the deep fascia is incised to reveal the radial vascular pedicle.

The remainder of the flap dissection is performed by completing the skin incision along the planned proximal margin of the flap and elevating the radial vascular pedicle with the flap. This is best done by dissecting under the radial artery and its venae comitantes from distal to proximal. At the proximal end of the flap, the fascia between the flexor carpi radialis and brachioradialis muscles is incised to reveal the rest of the radial vascular pedicle. The cephalic vein in the subcutaneous tissues and radial vascular pedicle are then dissected proximally to the level of the antecubital fossa, ligating all perforating vessels coming off these two vessels proximal to the flap.

The tourniquet is then deflated to let the arm and flap perfuse; hemostasis is then obtained. While perfusing, the flap is tubed on itself by approximating the radial and

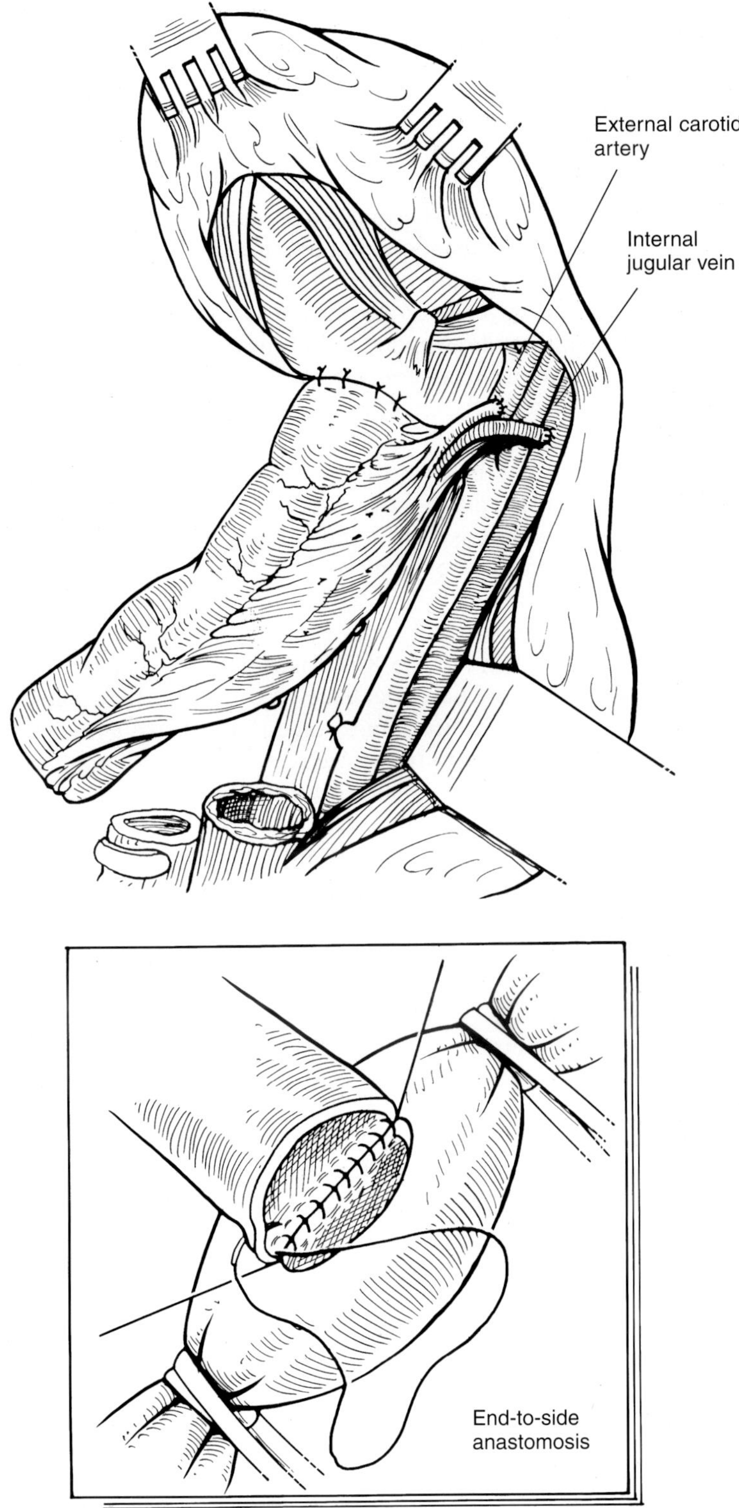

FIG. 4. Flap revascularization with an end-to-side anastomosis into the external carotid artery and internal jugular vein.

ulnar margins of the flap with interrupted 4-0 polygalactin sutures placed in a vertical mattress fashion on the luminal side of the flap (Fig. 8C,D). Care must be taken to approximate the skin edges very carefully to obtain a watertight closure and to avoid postoperative fistulas, which can occur in as many as 67% of patients undergoing reconstruction with this flap. The RFFF is then harvested by ligating the radial vascular pedicle and cephalic vein at the level of the antecubital fossa. The donor arm is covered with a saline-moistened towel until the donor site can be closed.

The proximal anastomosis is performed prior to revascularizing the flap for the same reasons mentioned above for the FJT. This is done using a single layer of 3-0 polygalactin suture placed in an interrupted vertical mattress fashion. As each suture is placed, the edge of the mucosa is carefully approximated to the skin edge of the flap to avoid fistula formation. To relieve tension on the suture line, sutures must include a portion of the anterior spinal ligament posteriorly and deep bites of tongue musculature anteriorly. After the proximal anastomosis has been completed, the flap is revascularized.

The distal (esophageal) anastomosis is performed next. The neck is flexed to a neutral position to avoid tension on the distal anastomosis and the posterior (spinal) side of the anastomosis is completed first using interrupted 3-0 or 4-0 polygalactin sutures placed outside the lumen of the esophagus. To decrease the chance of stricture formation, the lumen of the distal anastomosis is enlarged by incising the anterior (tracheal) side of the cervical esophagus, as is done for the FJT. The flap extension on the esophageal end of the RFFF is inset into the esophageal incision, placing all sutures before they are tied (Fig. 9A,B). As with the proximal anastomosis, care must be taken to achieve a careful skin-to-mucosal approximation.

After all anastomoses are completed, the longitudinal suture line of the flap and the junction of this suture line with the proximal and distal anastomoses may be reinforced by covering these areas with a sternocleidomastoid muscle flap. This is done by dividing the origin of the muscle and tacking the muscle on either side of the suture lines with absorbable sutures. Drains are placed on each side of the neck away from all anastomoses. The vascular pedicle of the flap is inspected for kinking as the neck visor flap is closed. Because flap monitoring is usually achieved with a hand-held Doppler ultrasound unit postoperatively, a suture is placed in the skin of the visor flap over the location of the vascular pedicle of the flap. It is very important to select a portion of the vascular pedicle well away from the great vessels of the neck to obtain an accurate Doppler signal that represents flow through the vascular pedicle.

The RFFF donor site is usually closed by a member of the reconstructive team while the flap is being inset. The proximal incision on the forearm is closed primarily as much as possible and the wound area not amenable to primary closure is closed with a skin graft. The arm and skin graft donor site are dressed with sterile dressings and a splint is applied to the forearm.

Operative Technique for Partial Defects

Partial pharyngoesophageal defects are repaired with the RFFF in much the same manner as for circumferential defects. The only differences are in the size and design of the flap. After the tumor has been resected, a template of the defect is made and the desired location for the radial vascular pedicle is marked on the template. The template is sterilized by soaking it in a 1% Betadine solution (Purdue Frederick, Norwalk, Connecticut) prior to transferring the design to the donor arm. The template is centered over the radial artery on the volar side of the donor arm such that the take off of the pedicle is at the location marked on the template. Every effort is made to incorporate the cephalic vein for better flap drainage. Flap dissection, transfer, inset, and revascularization are exactly the same as for the circumferential defect.

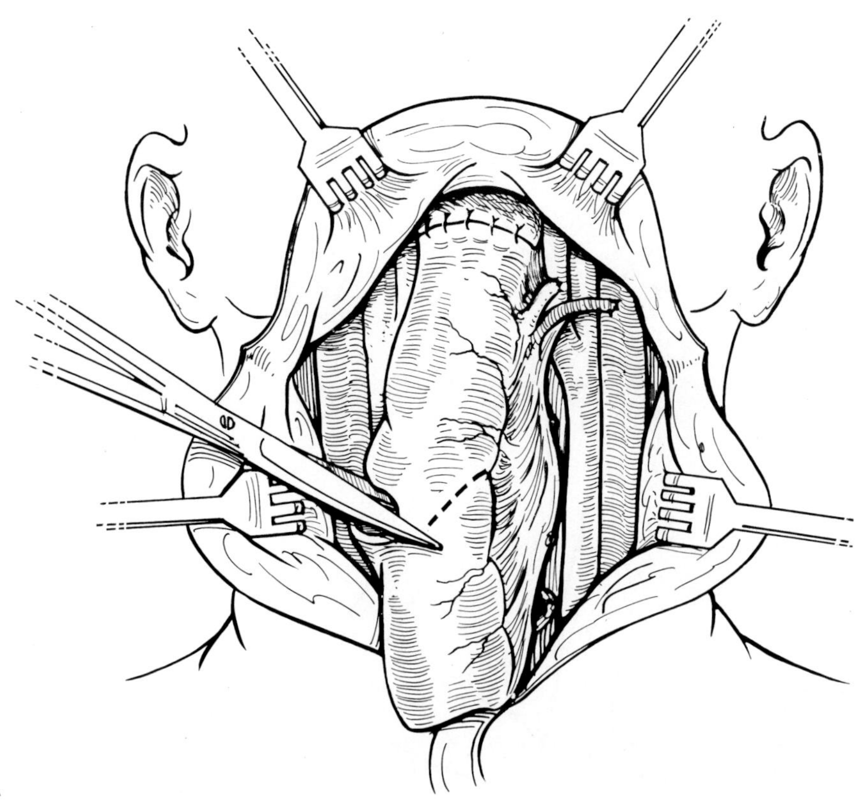

FIG. 5A. Trimming the jejunal flap, leaving the anterior portion longer.

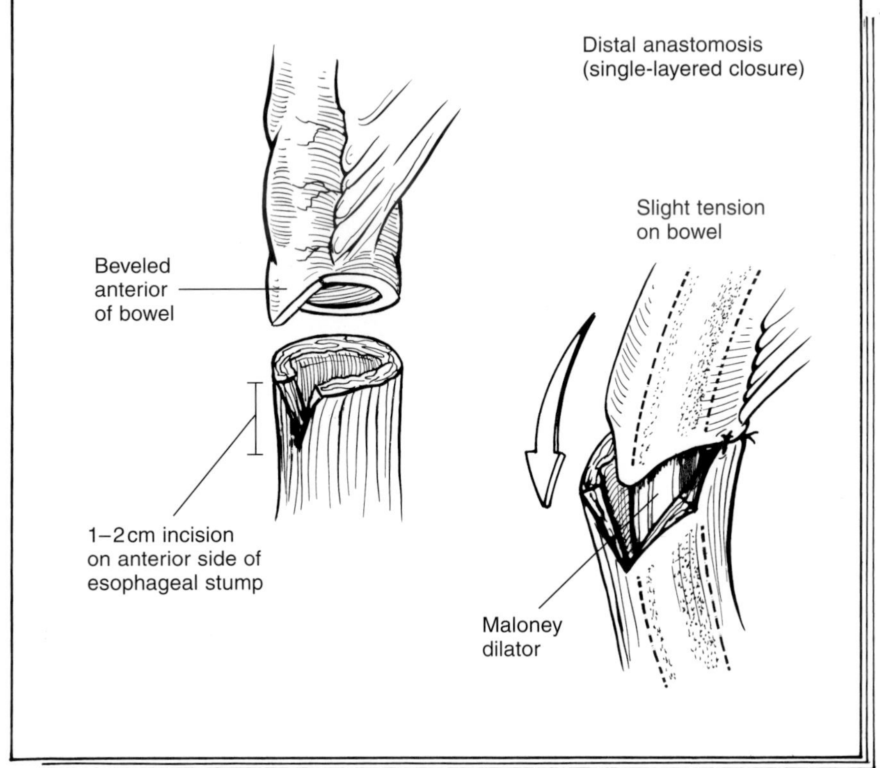

FIG. 5B. This beveled anterior edge is used to break up the circular suture line, which prevents stricture and creates a functionally larger diameter in anastomosis. The anastomosis is completed in one layer.

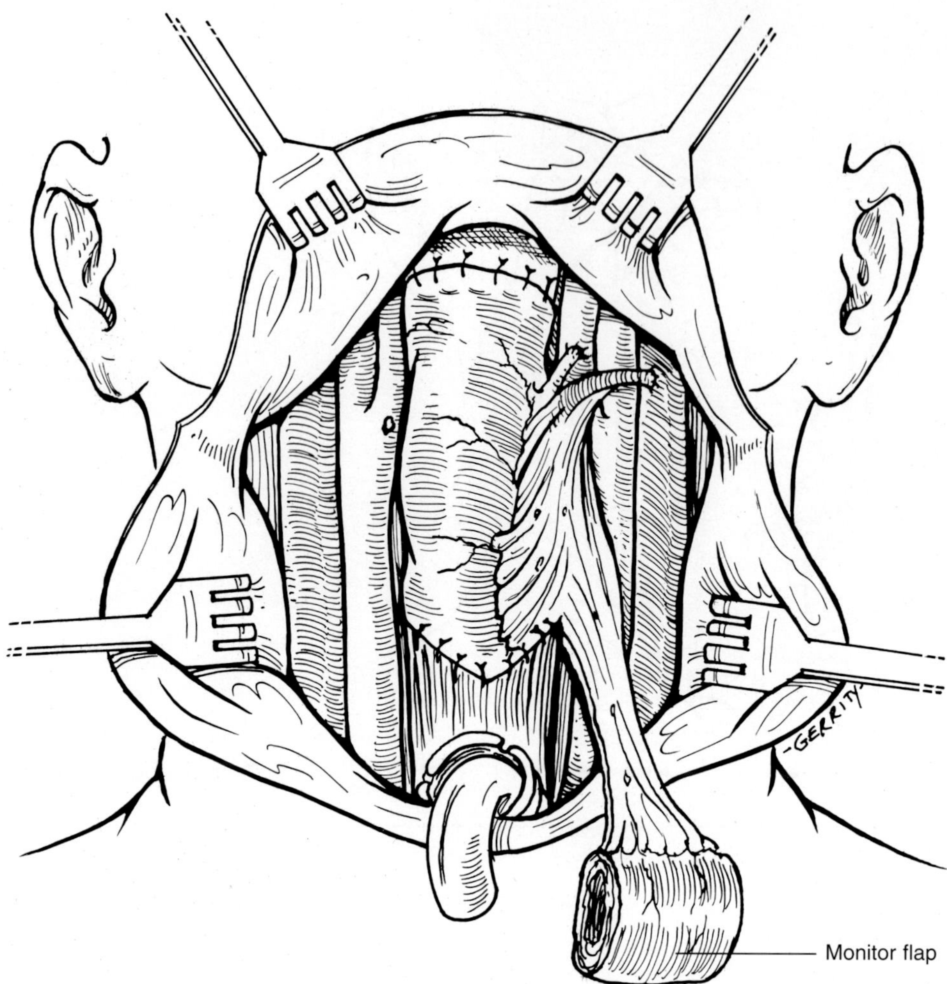

FIG. 6. Schematic of monitor flap used to check for vessel patency postoperatively.

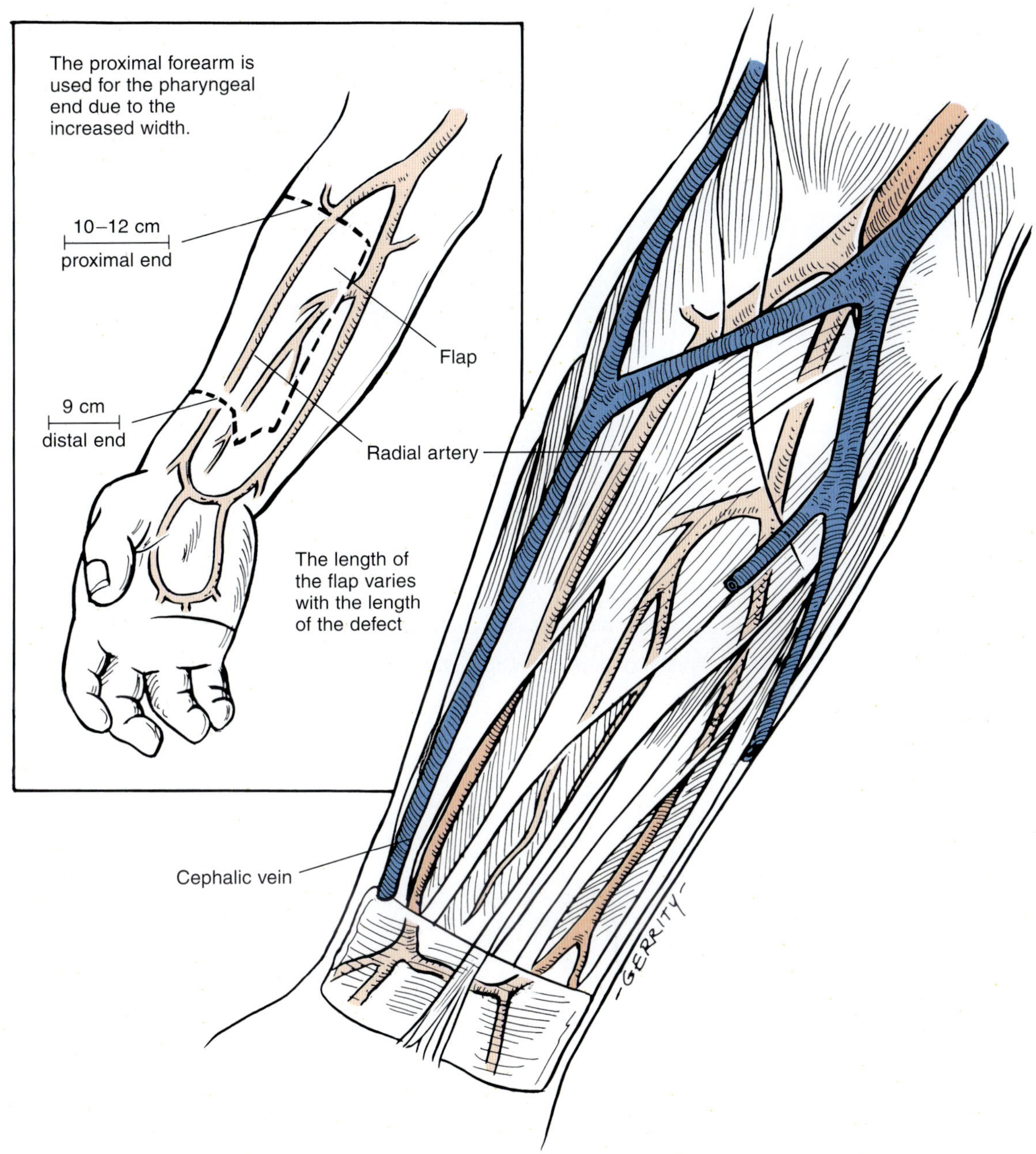

FIG. 7. Diagram of anatomy of the radial forearm flap including design of flap.

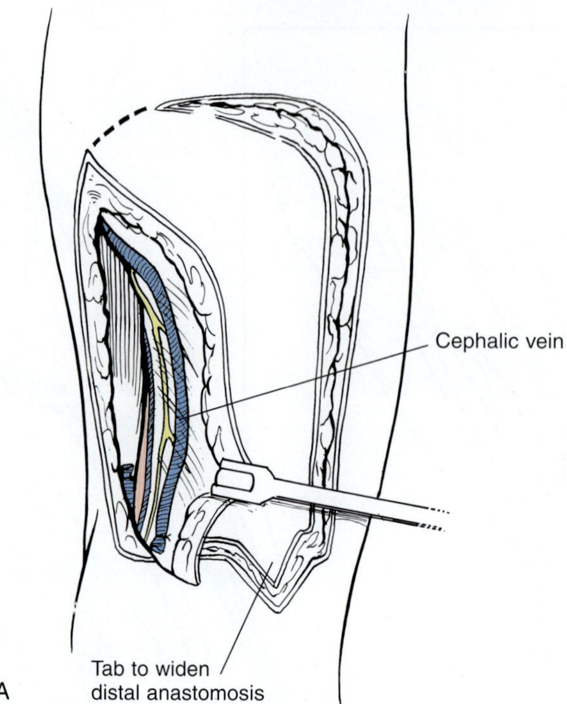

FIG. 8A. Elevation of flap including ligation of cephalic vein.

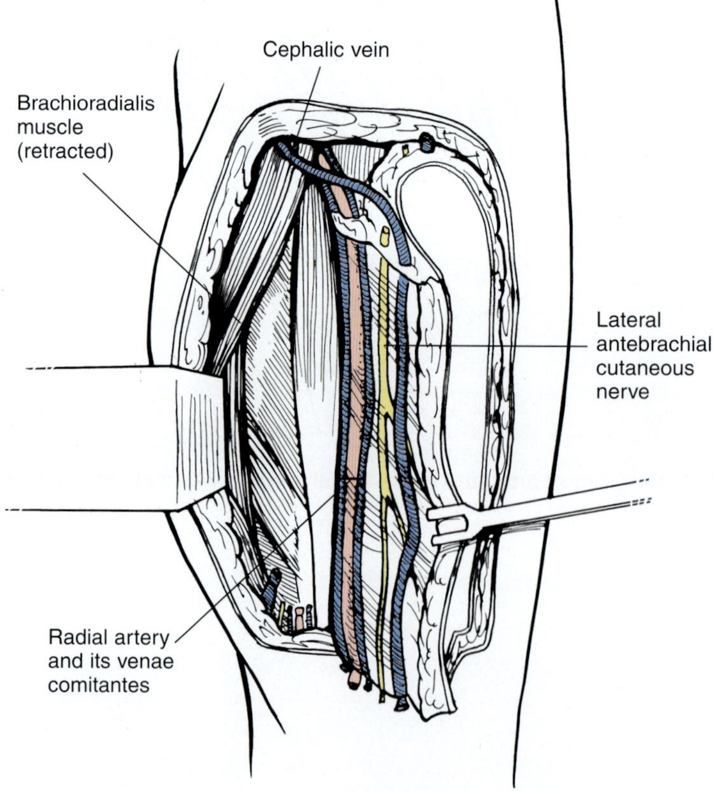

FIG. 8B. Elevation of the radial artery pedicle including retraction of the brachioradialis muscle.

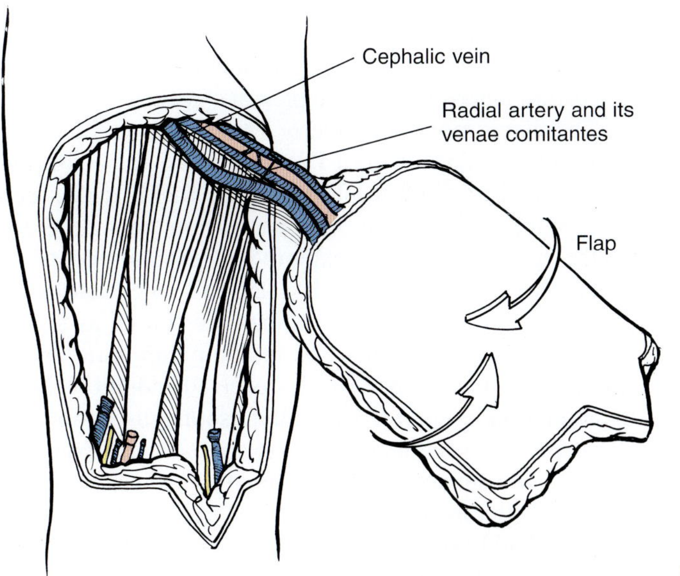

FIG. 8C. Flap after completion of elevation.

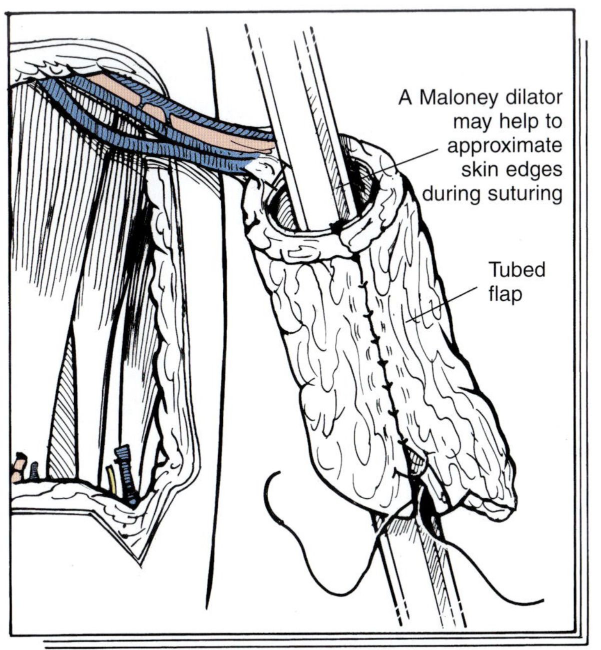

FIG. 8D. Tubing of flap over Maloney dilator.

Postoperative Care

After surgery, patients are transferred to the surgical intensive care unit for overnight observation. The head of the bed is elevated 30° to 40° to decrease venous pressure in the head and neck region. External compression of the vascular pedicle is avoided by suturing the tracheostomy tube to the peristomal skin rather than tying tracheostomy tapes around the patient's neck.

The flap is monitored hourly irrespective of the type of flap used for reconstruction. The monitor flap of the FJT is observed for color and peristalsis and blood flow is determined for both the FJT and the RFFF with a conventional, hand-held Doppler ultrasound device. If any flap parameters change, the patient is immediately returned to the operating room to explore the vascular pedicle.

For patients who have had an FJT, the gastrostomy tube is placed to bedside drainage and jejunal tube feedings are started as soon as bowel activity resumes. On the 7th postoperative day, the monitor flap is removed under local anesthesia and, if the patient has not previously received radiation therapy, a barium cinefluoroscopic examination of the reconstructed esophagus is obtained. If no significant radiologic abnormalities are found on this examination, the patient is allowed to take a liquid diet and the diet advanced as tolerated. In most cases, patients are discharged home on the 10th to 12th postoperative day. Patients who have had previous radiation therapy usually need additional time for healing before stressing the bowel anastomoses and so we prefer to wait until the 12th to 14th postoperative day before obtaining the radiographic examination and beginning an oral diet.

For patients reconstructed with a RFFF, the arm is elevated on several pillows to decrease the edema. The splint is generally removed on the 5th to 7th postoperative day. Nutrition in the early postoperative period is delivered by feeding tube using a protocol similar to the one used for the FJT. A barium cinefluoroscopic examination of the reconstructed esophagus is obtained on the 10th to 12th postoperative day to evaluate the neoesophagus. If the patient has not previously received radiation therapy and if no significant radiologic abnormalities are found on this examination, the patient is allowed to take a liquid diet and the diet is advanced as tolerated. In most cases, patients are discharged home on the 14th postoperative day. As with the FJT reconstruction, patients who have had previous radiation therapy usually need additional time for healing before stressing the suture lines and so we prefer to wait until the 14th postoperative day before obtaining the radiographic examination and beginning an oral diet.

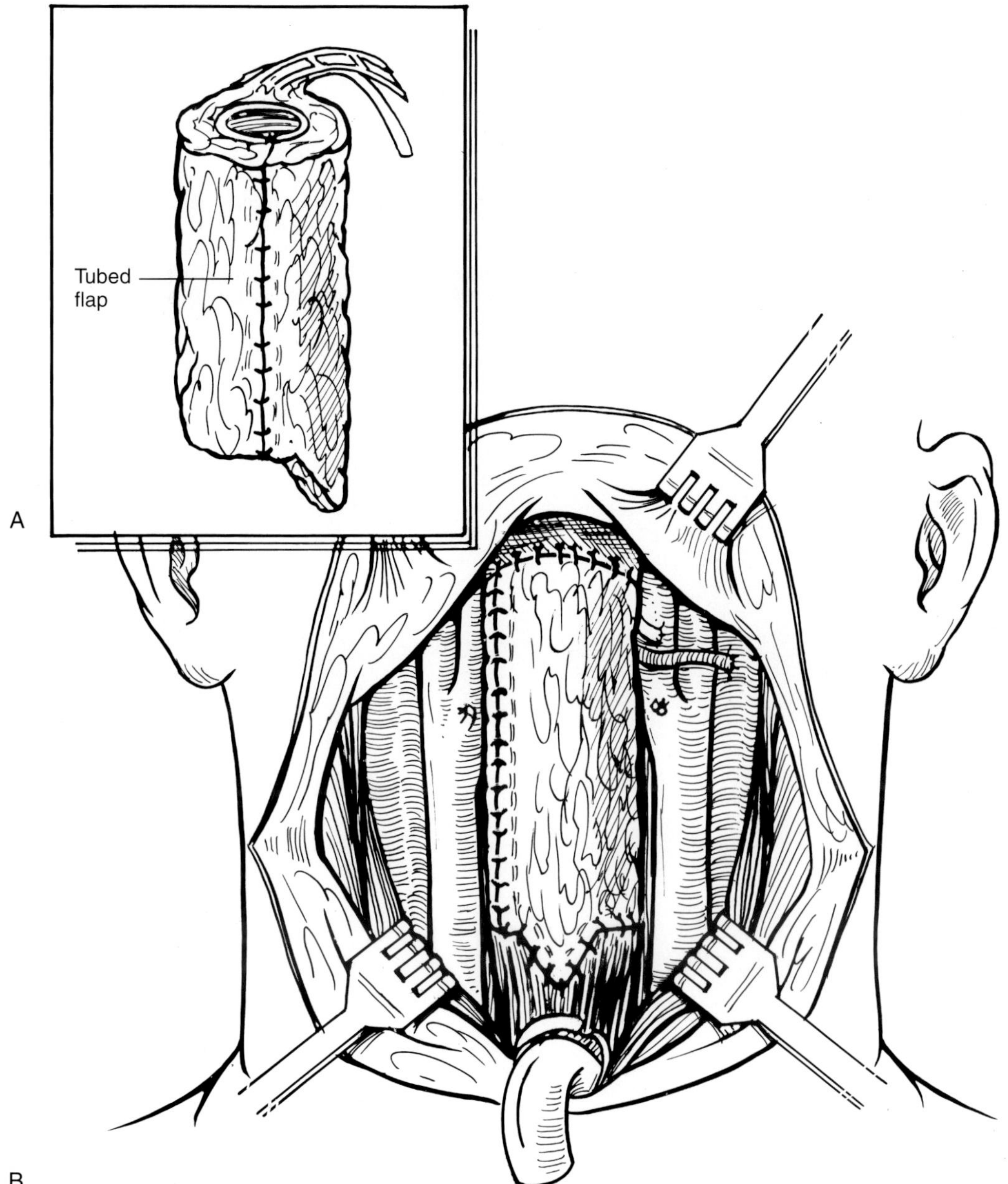

FIG. 9A,B. Inset of flap after the flap is tubed. Note that the tab is off-center to prevent the suture lines all coming together at one point.

SELECTED READINGS

Anthony JP, Singer MI, Deschler DG, et al. Long-term functional results after pharyngoesophageal reconstruction with the radial forearm free flap. *Am J Surg* 1994;168:441.

Anthony JP, Singer MI, Mathes SJ. Pharyngoesophageal reconstruction using the tubed free radial forearm flap. *Clin Plast Surg* 1994;21:137–147.

Coleman JJ III, Searles JM Jr, Hester TR, et al. Ten year experience with free jejunal autograft. Am J Surg 1987; 154:394.

Harii K, Ebihara S, Ono I, et al. Pharyngoesophageal reconstruction using a fabricated forearm free flap. *Plast Reconstr Surg* 1985;75:463.

Kelly KE, Anthony JP, Singer M. Pharyngoesophageal reconstruction using the radial forearm fasciocutaneous free flap: preliminary results. *Otolaryngol Head Neck Surg* 1994;111:16.

Reece GP, Bengston BP, Schusterman MA. Reconstruction of the pharynx and cervical esophagus using free jejunal transfer. *Clin Plast Surg* 1994;21:125.

Reece GP, Schusterman MA, Miller MJ, et al. Morbidity and functional outcome of free jejunal transfer reconstruction for circumferential defects of the pharynx and cervical esophagus. *Plast Reconstr Surg* 1995;96: 1307.

Schusterman MA, Shestak K, deVries EJ, et al. Reconstruction of the cervical esophagus: free jejunal transfer versus gastric pull-up. *Plast Reconstr Surg* 1990;85:16.

Microsurgical Reconstruction of the Cancer Patient, edited by M.A. Schusterman.
Lippincott-Raven Publishers, Philadelphia © 1997.

5

Craniofacial and Midface Reconstruction

Giulio Gherardini, Michael J. Miller, and Mark A. Schusterman

Microvascular reconstruction is particularly useful in the scalp and midface. For large defects, it is difficult to transfer pedicled flaps from the upper chest and back into this area. Even if possible, a rotated flap may have a tenuous blood supply in critical portions and tend to be bulky, causing contour deformities. Often, multistage or delayed procedures may be necessary. For these reasons, microvascular free tissue transfer is usually the most suitable approach for large defects in the scalp and midface. Careful planning and close cooperation between the ablative and the reconstructive surgeons are essential. If maxillofacial prosthetics will be necessary, the patient should be evaluated preoperatively by the prosthodontist so that the tissue reconstruction is planned considering the requirements for a satisfactory prosthesis.

SCALP AND UPPER-THIRD FACIAL RECONSTRUCTION

Defects of the scalp and forehead have similar reconstructive needs. The reconstructive requirements are to protect the brain and cranium with durable tissue of natural-appearing contour and proper color match. For defects involving only the scalp, a split-thickness skin graft applied to vascularized omentum, rectus abdominis, or latissimus dorsi muscle usually provides an effective reconstruction. The rectus abdominis muscle is suitable for smaller areas, the omentum or latissimus dorsi muscle for large defects (>80 cm^2) (Fig. 1A–E). For extreme requirements, the entire thoracodorsal

G. Gherardini, M. J. Miller, and M. A. Schusterman: Department of Plastic Surgery, The University of Texas, M.D. Anderson Cancer Center, Houston, Texas 77030.

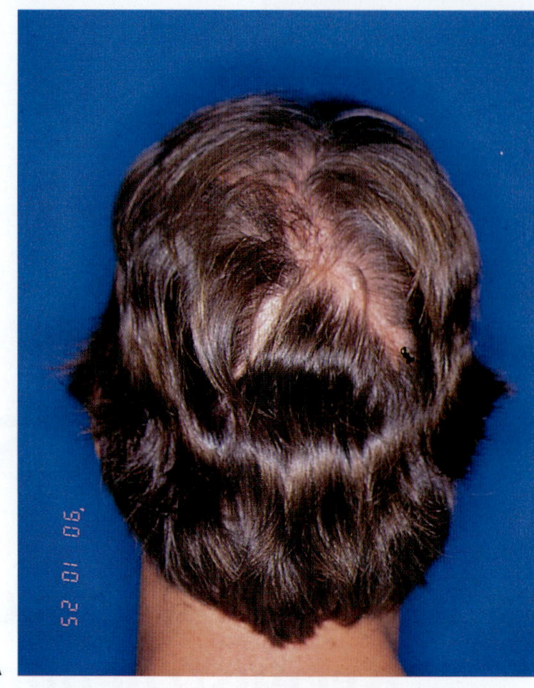

FIG. 1A. Recurrent dermatofibrosarcoma protuberans of the posterior scalp.

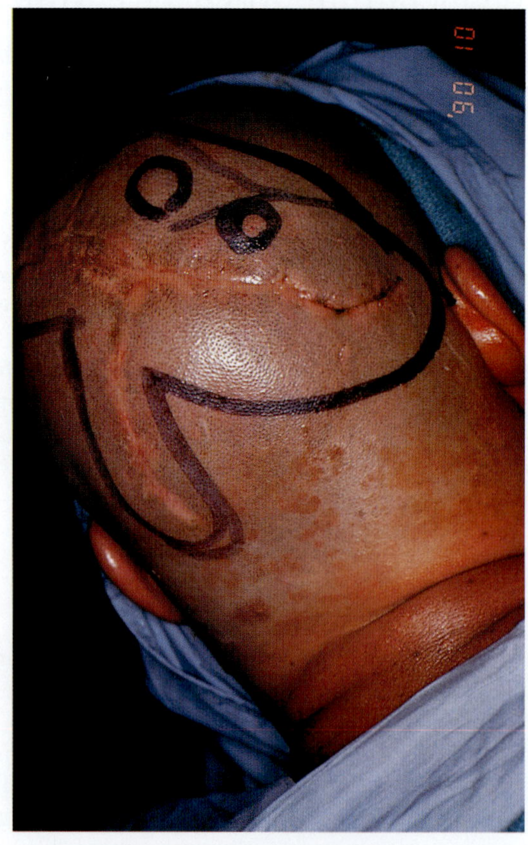

FIG. 1B. Planned resection.

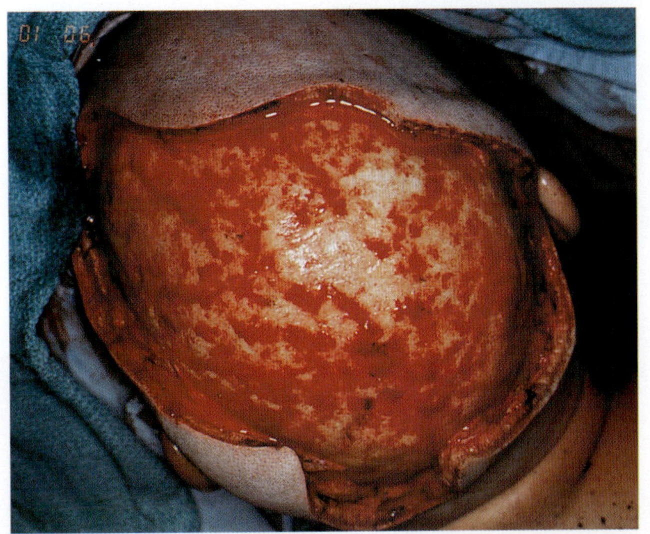

FIG. 1C. Surgical defect includes cranium denuded of periosteum.

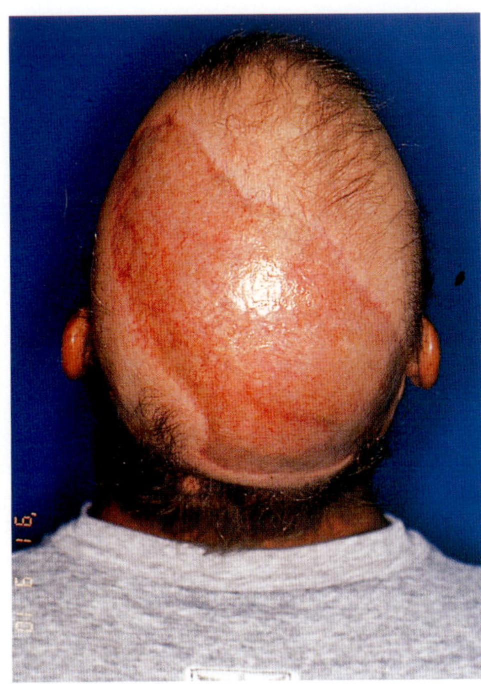

FIG. 1D. Reconstructed with free latissimus dorsi muscle flap. A vein graft was used so that the internal jugular vein and external carotid artery could be utilized as recipient vessels.

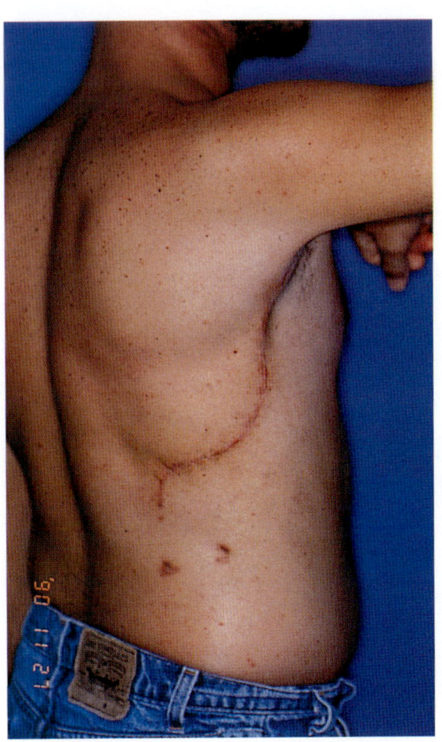

FIG. 1E. Postoperative photo.

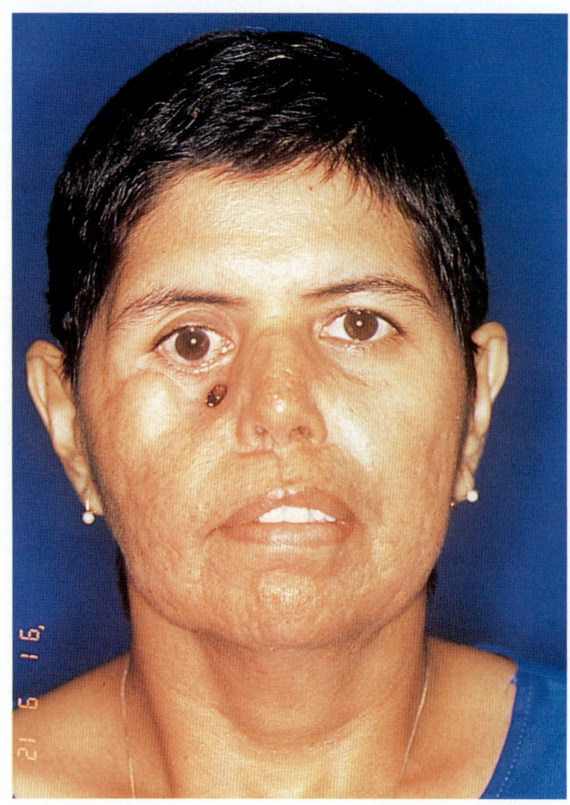

FIG. 2A. Patient with antrocutaneous fistula secondary to maxillectomy that included a portion of orbital rim and floor and was then subsequently treated with radiation therapy.

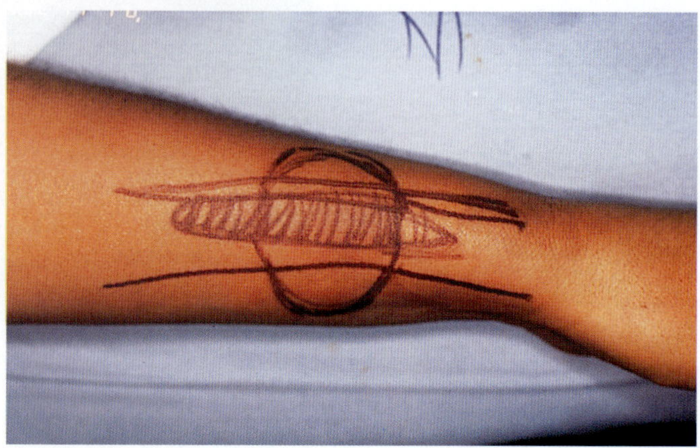

FIG. 2B. Plan was to reconstruct defect with osteocutaneous radial forearm flap.

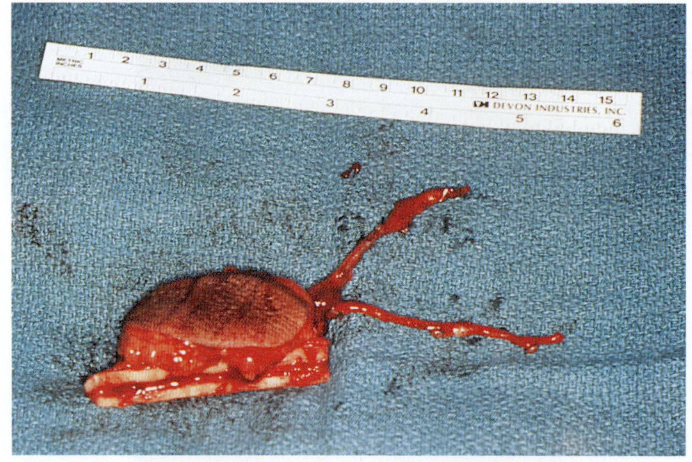

FIG. 2C. Osteocutaneous radial forearm flap after elevation.

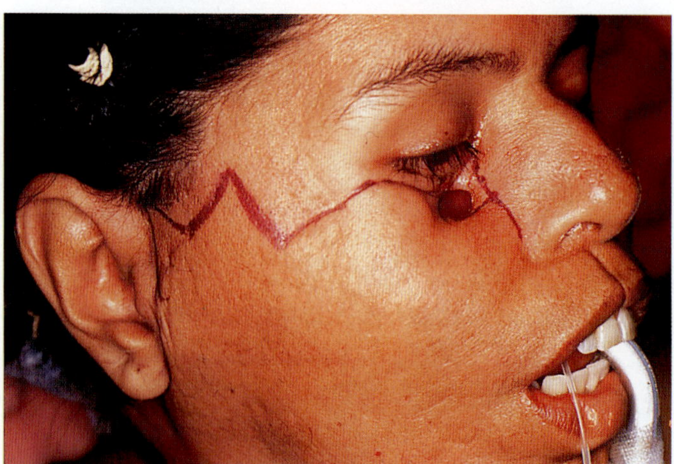

FIG. 2D. Surgical plan for exposure of defect.

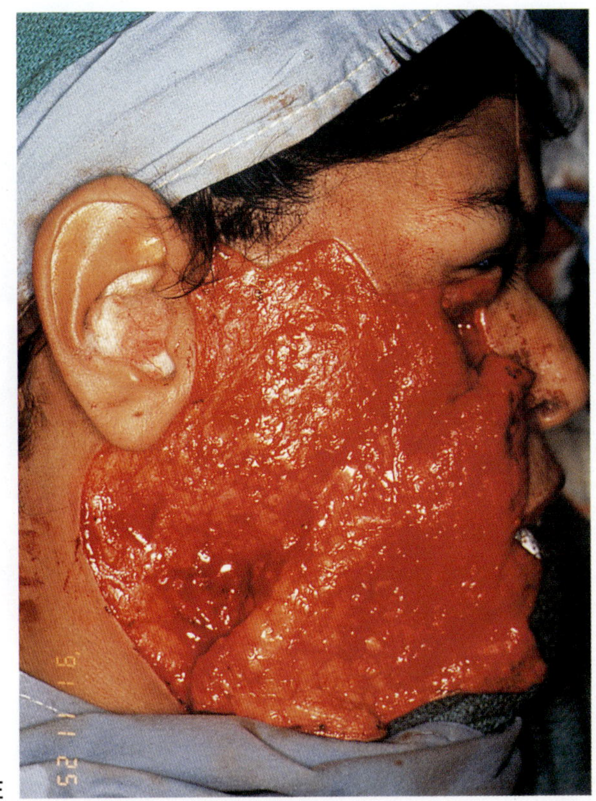

E

FIG. 2E. Elevation of cervicofacial flap allowed access to neck vessels for use as recipient vessels.

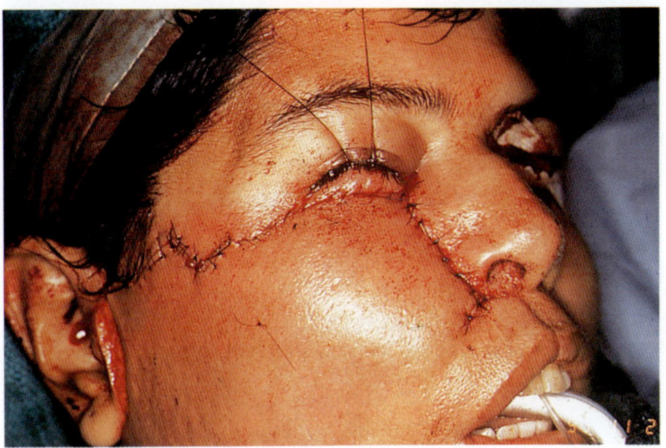

F

FIG. 2F. Result after inset of free flap and wound closure. Note that the skin paddle was used to line the antral cavity, thus protecting the bone from continued contamination, and effectively sealing the fistula. This also allowed for closure of the cheek skin without a patch effect.

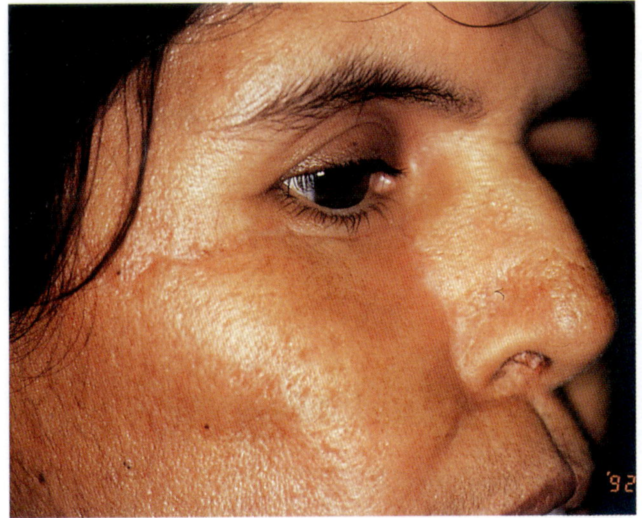

G

FIG. 2G. Late postoperative result.

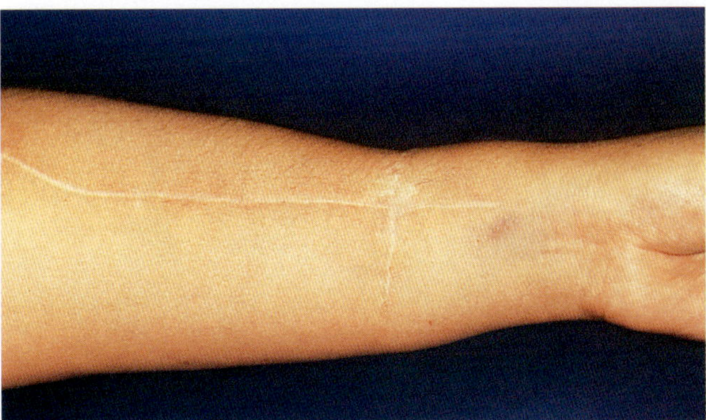

H

FIG. 2H. Donor site result.

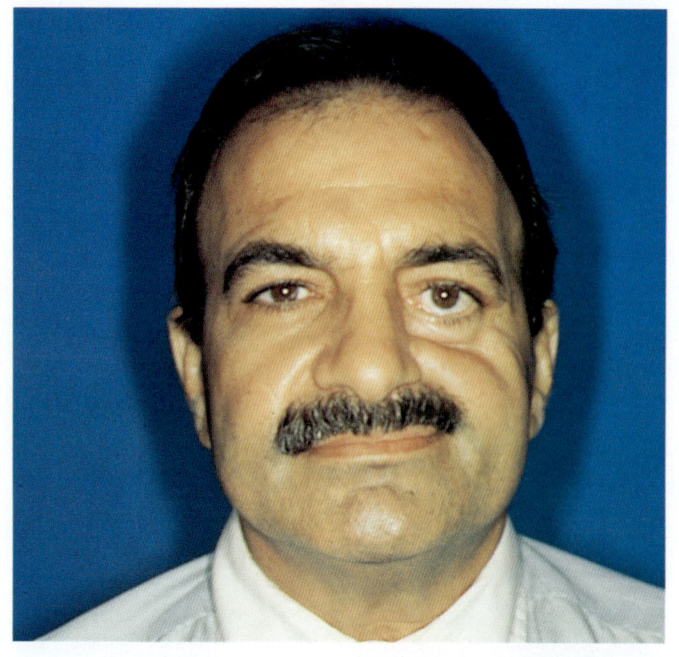

FIG. 3A. Patient after maxillectomy with depressed malar cheek area and inability to retain maxillary prosthesis.

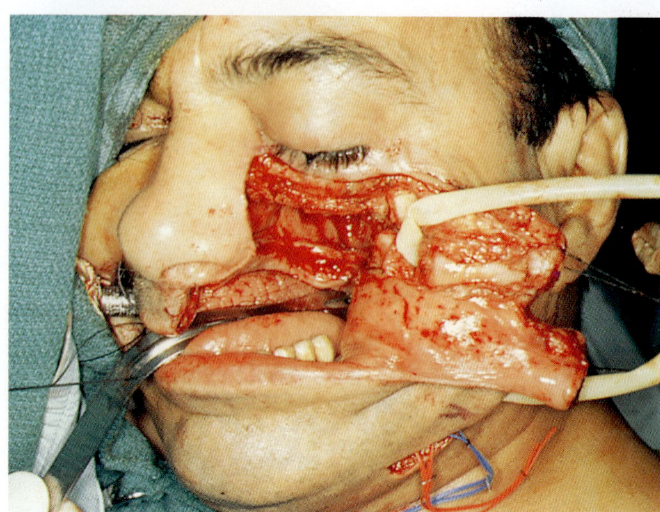

FIG. 3B. Exposure of defect.

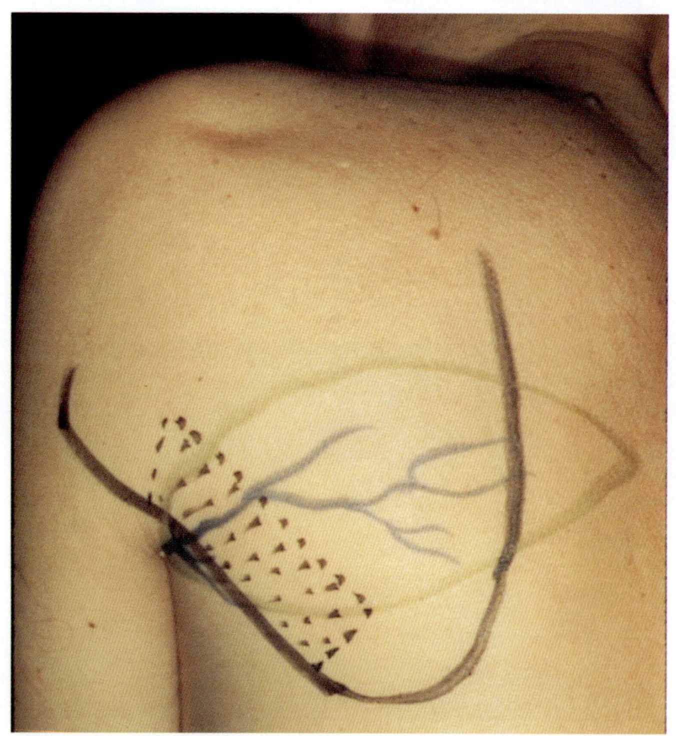

FIG. 3C. Surgical plan for osteocutaneous scapula flap.

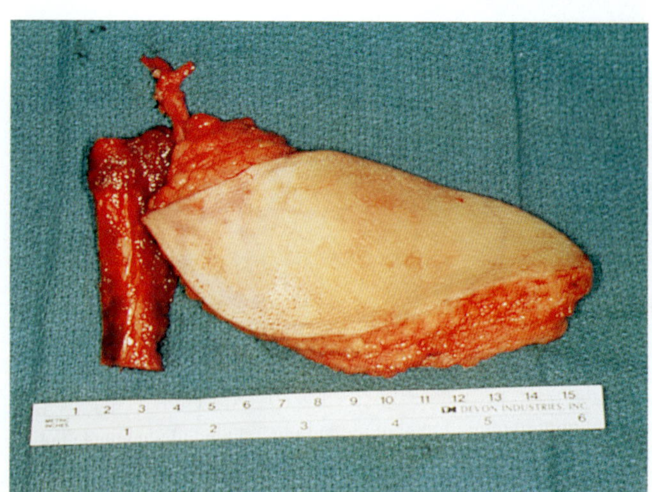

FIG. 3D. Osteocutaneous scapula flap after flap elevation.

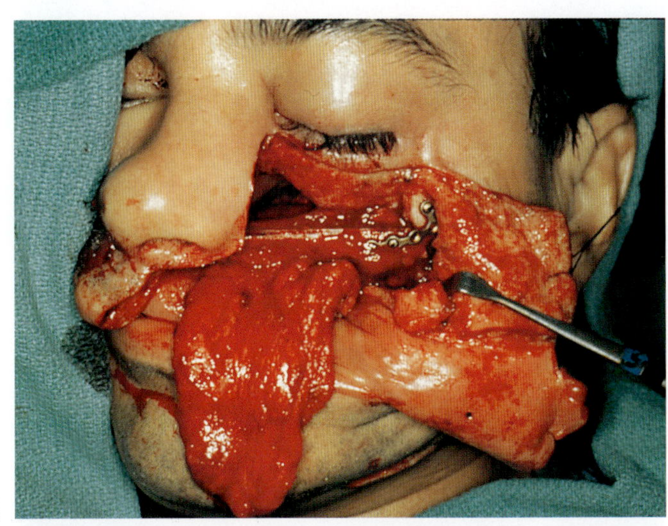

E

FIG. 3E. Flap during inset; note use of skin paddle to obliterate palatal fistula. Skin paddle necrosed and required debridement.

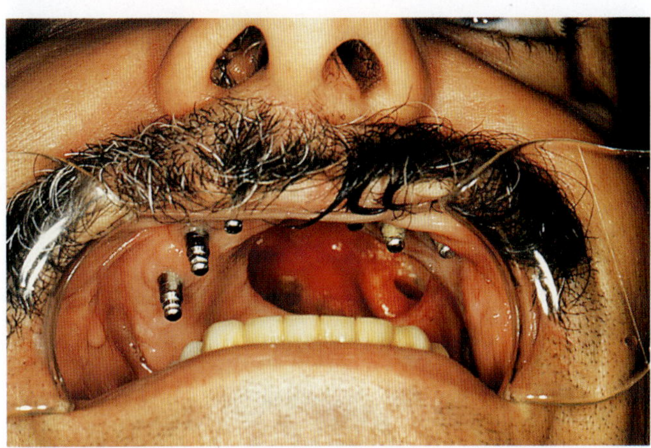

F

FIG. 3F. Despite this complication, osseointegrated implants were placed in the residual scapular bone.

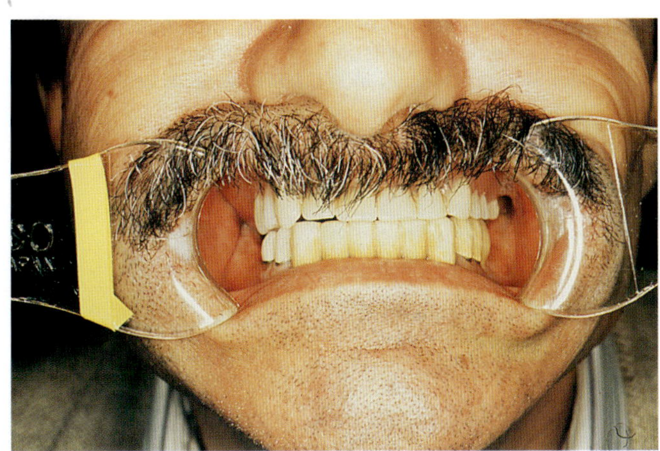

G

FIG. 3G. A palatal prosthesis, and excellent restoration of dentition could then be utilized.

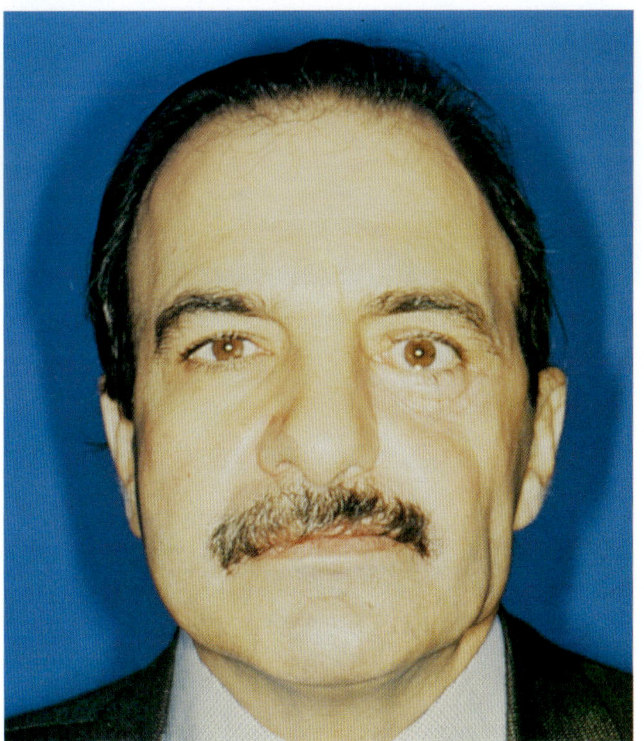

H

FIG. 3H. The bone placement nicely augmented the depressed malar area.

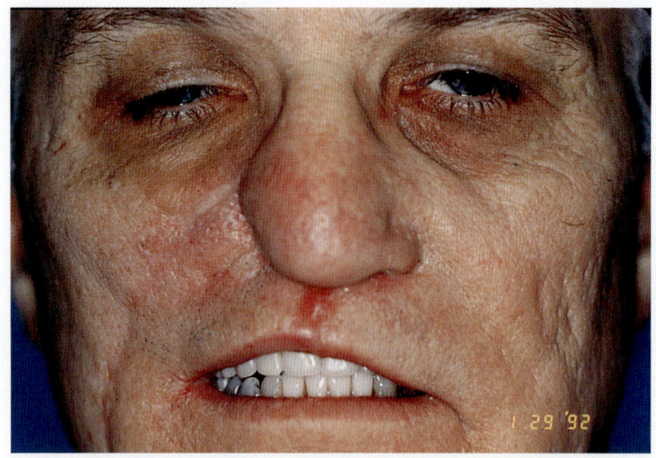

FIG. 4A. Large recurrent basal cell carcinoma of nasolabial fold area.

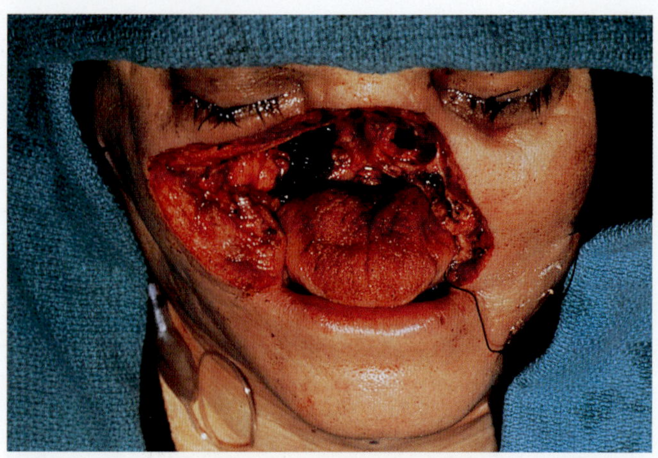

FIG. 4B. Tumor ablation required massive midface resection.

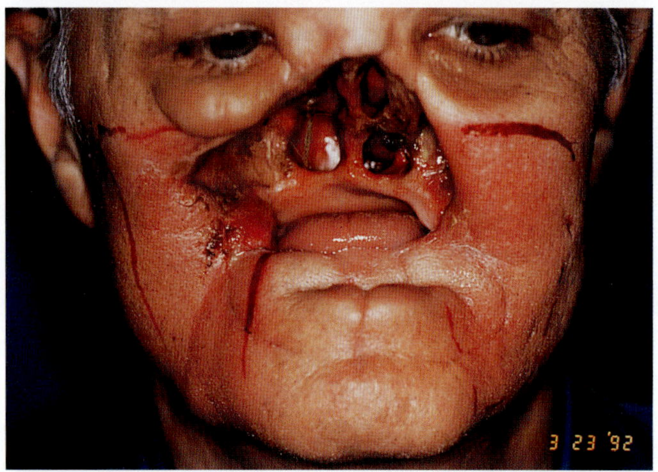

FIG. 4C. This resection was then followed by radiation therapy.

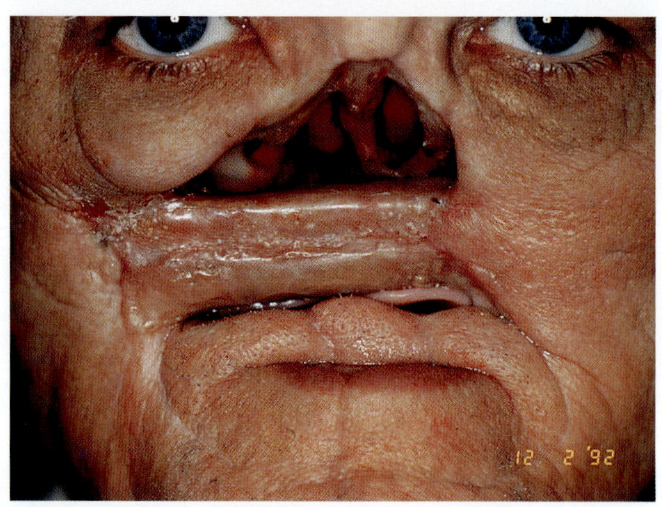

FIG. 4D. Once radiation was done, a free fibula flap was used to augment the midface bony structure. Note that this bone was skin grafted; no skin paddle was utilized.

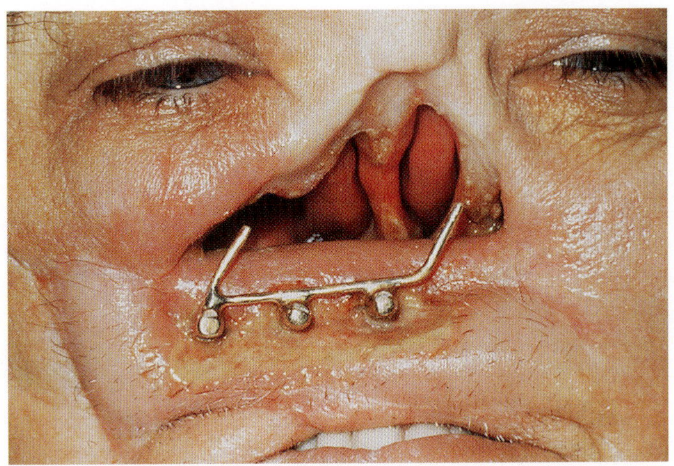

FIG. 4E. Osseointegrated implants were placed.

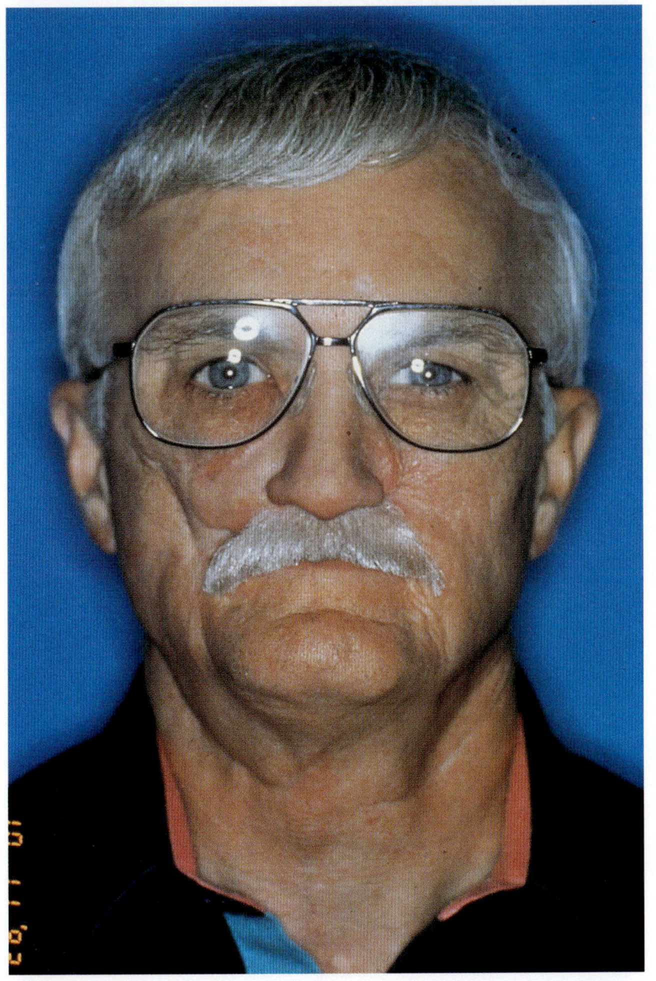

FIG. 4F. The implants allowed fixation of a high-quality facial prosthetic, which was firmly fixed in place.

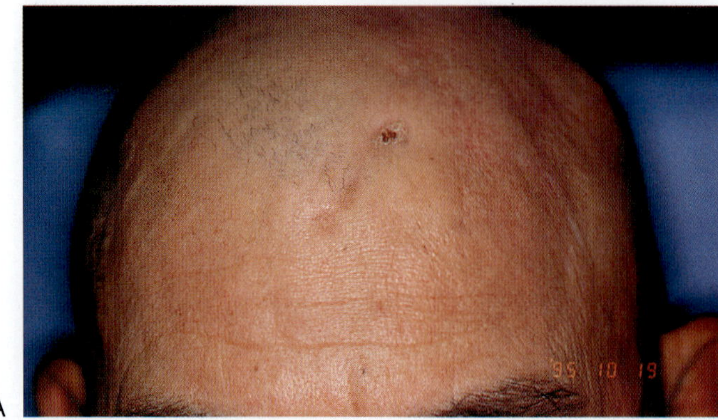

FIG. 5A. Recurrent squamous cell carcinoma after numerous resections and radiation therapy. Local flaps had been used extensively in the past.

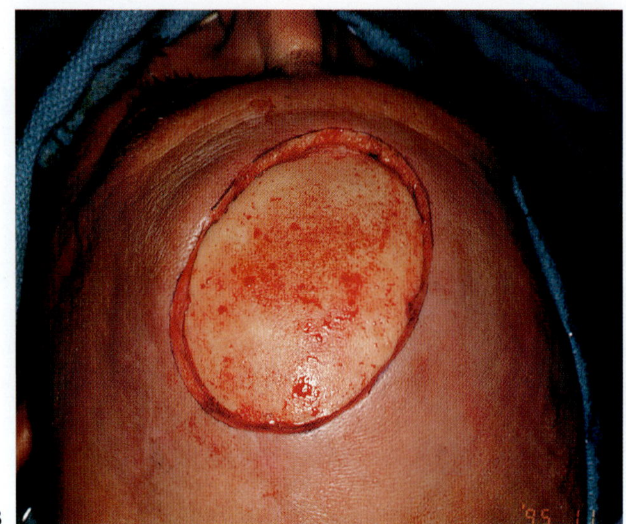

FIG. 5B. Defect after tumor resection.

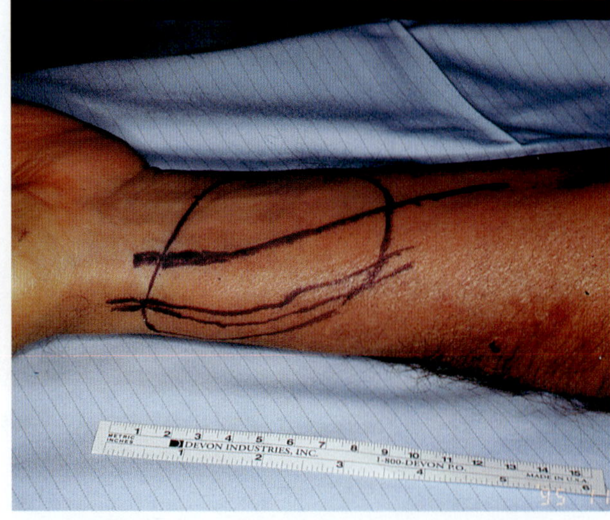

FIG. 5C. Planned use of radial forearm flap.

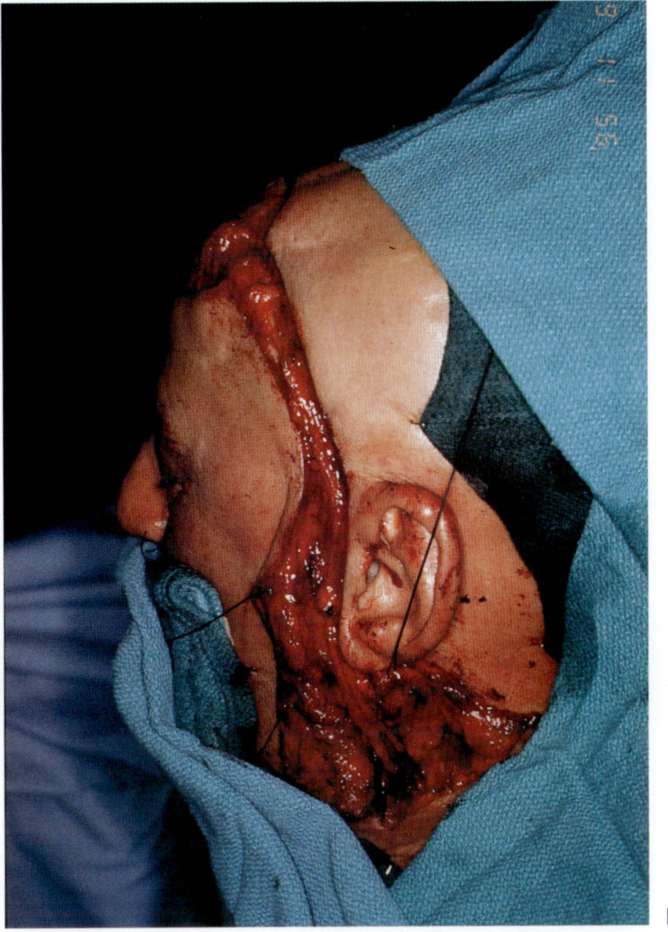

FIG. 5D. Cervicofacial incision used to gain exposure to the great vessel of the neck. A saphenous vein graft was used to span the distance between the neck and the donor vessels in the temporal area.

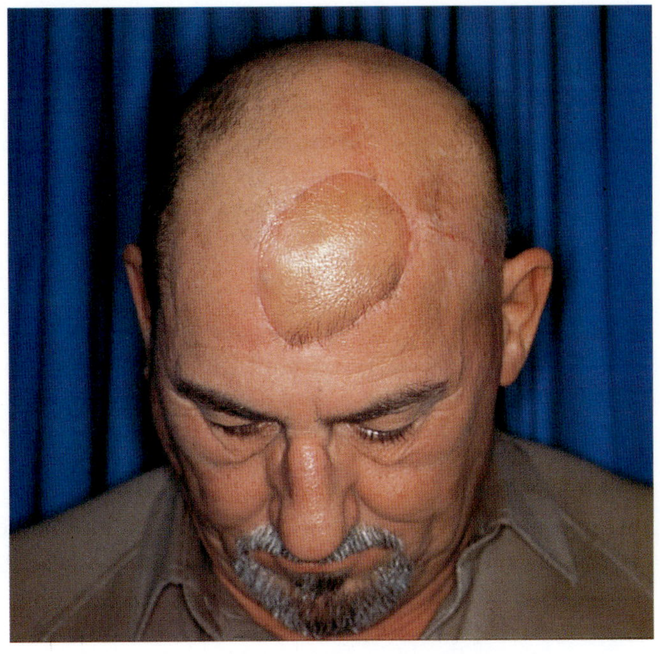

FIG. 5E. Postoperative result.

system (i.e., serratus anterior muscle flap, scapular fasciocutaneous flap) may be harvested. Small associated cranial defects may be repaired with soft tissue alone. Muscle flaps become fibrotic over time and provide some protection and contour preservation. For larger bone defects, an alloplastic cranioplasty or autogenous bone transfer may be necessary. Free tissue transfer will reliably provide the necessary soft tissue coverage. In patients with recurrence following radiotherapy, the bone may have a limited capacity to incorporate conventional grafts and a composite free flap containing bone may be considered.

MIDFACIAL DEFECTS

Reconstructive requirements for the midface vary with the amount of tissue resected and the degree of involvement of specialized facial features (e.g., eyes and nose). The goal is to provide primary wound healing, protect vital structures, allow maxillary dental rehabilitation, and restore facial features. The specific goals are individualized for each patient and depend primarily on whether an immediate or delayed reconstruction is planned. In immediate reconstruction, the primary objective is wound healing and protection of vital structures so that adjuvant therapy is not delayed. It is often also important to avoid totally obscuring the area of resection in order to allow monitoring for tumor recurrence by direct examination. A rectus abdominis musculocutaneous flap, possibly with a split-thickness skin graft to restore multiple surfaces, is often ideal. In delayed reconstruction, more elaborate tissue restoration of the zygoma, orbit, and palate may be considered. A radial forearm osteocutaneous flap offers suitable vascularized tissue for smaller defects involving the palate or orbit (Fig. 2A–H). A scapula or fibula composite flap provides composite tissue best suited for larger defects, such as those involving the maxilla and zygoma (Figs. 3A–H and 4A–F). Usually, a combination of autogenous tissue and maxillofacial prosthetics is required, and the reconstructive surgeon must establish the optimal tissue base for stable prosthetic support. Although some prostheses use adhesives for fixation, osseointegrated implants are now being utilized for fixation of midface prostheses. The final facial contour should be lower than normal to allow the facial prosthesis to re-create normal facial projection.

MICROSURGICAL PROCEDURES

Recipient Vessels

There are three options to revascularize flaps transferred to the scalp or midface: the superficial temporal, the facial, or the cervical vessels. Interposition vein grafts may be required to reach recipients in the neck (Figs. 5A–E and 6A–C).

For scalp reconstructions, the superficial temporal vessels are explored first. An incision is created anterior to the ear from the level of the external auditory meatus upward into the temporal area and the vessels are found in the subcutaneous tissues. If these are unsuitable, then an incision is created in the neck anterior to the sternocleidomastoid muscle and the cervical vessels, usually the external carotid artery (ECA) and internal jugular (IJ) vein are selected. To expose the ECA, the neck is extended and the head rotated to the contralateral side. An incision is made following the anterior margin of the sternocleidomastoid muscle from the mastoid process to the midportion of the muscle. The platysma and the cervical fascia are incised and upper and lower skin flaps are developed. The anterior margin of the sternocleidomastoid is identified, dissected, and retracted exposing the facial vein. The facial vein is also retracted or ligated and divided to expose the carotid sheath. After opening the sheath, the internal jugular vein is identified, isolated, and retracted using vessel loops. The carotid bulb is easily identified and the ECA recognized by the presence of collateral branches. The dissection of the ECA should be performed proximally to identify the hypoglossal nerve. All branches of the ECA are isolated and retracted using vessel loops.

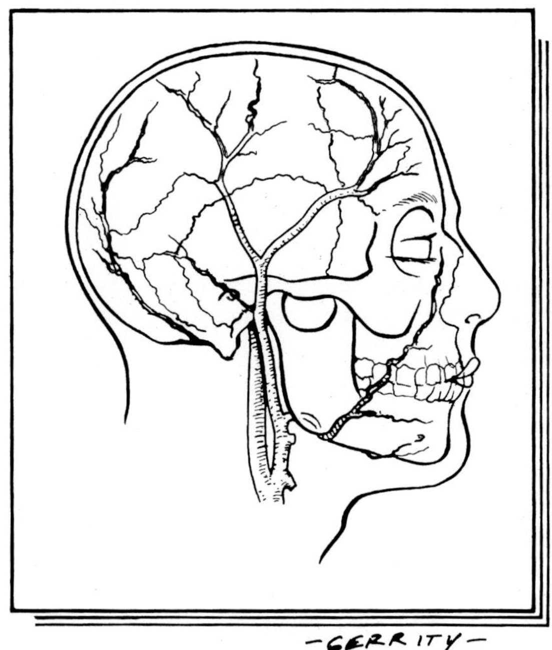

A

FIG. 6A. Vascular architecture of the carotid artery.

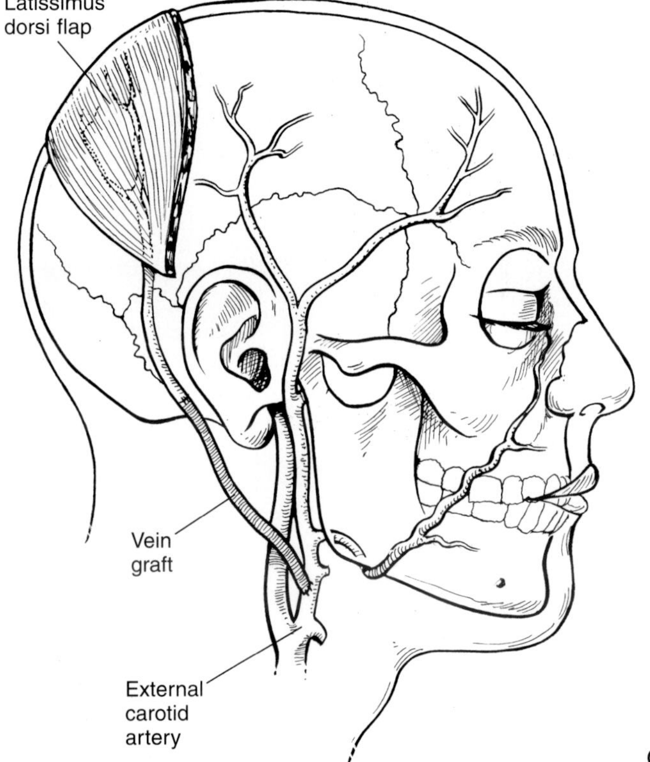

C

FIG. 6C. Use of external carotid artery with interposition vein graft as recipient vessel.

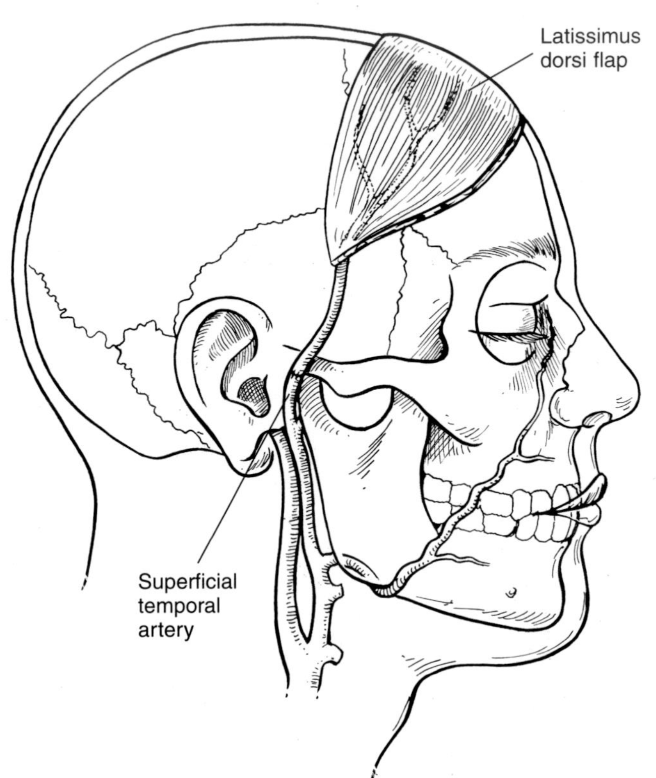

B

FIG. 6B. Use of superficial temporal artery as recipient vessel.

For midface reconstruction, the facial artery and vein are explored through a submandibular incision (Fig. 7). Care is taken to avoid injuring the marginal mandibular nerve. A subcutaneous tunnel is created through the cheek to allow the flap vessels to reach the recipient vessels. If the facial vessels are unsuitable, the next choices are the ECA and the internal jugular vein.

Scapular Flap

When the reconstruction involves the forehead, the scapular flap seems to afford the best color and texture match compared with other fasciocutaneous donor sites. The scapular flap may be harvested with a skin paddle for forehead reconstruction and a fascial extension that may be skin grafted for reconstruction of the hair-bearing scalp. If osseous reconstruction of the cranium is desired, then the lateral border of the scapula may be harvested to provide vascularized bone. The scapular flap system is highly versatile, providing various combinations of skin, fascia, muscle, and bone. Up to 14 cm of corticocancellous bone is available from the lateral border of the scapula and a thin bicortical bone can also be harvested from the body of the scapula to reconstruct specific areas, such as the orbital floor and the maxilla (Fig. 8A–C).

Pertinent Anatomy

The cutaneous territory of the flap extends from the triangular space laterally to the midline of the back. A flap of approximately 20 cm in length and 10 cm in width can be harvested. The vascular anatomy of the scapular flap is dependent on circumflex scapular artery. It arises from the subscapular artery and passes posteriorly through the triangular space, bordered by the teres minor above and the teres major below, and the long head of the triceps. The artery arborizes in several major branches: the infrascapular artery supplying the subscapular muscle, the branches for the teres major and minor muscles, and the descending branch that gives off the cutaneous scapular and the cutaneous parascapular branches.

Technique of Dissection

The scapular landmarks are marked with the patient in the sitting position. Medial and lateral border and tip of the scapula are noted (see Fig. 3). The triangular space is identified by palpation and marked. For flap harvesting the patient is placed in the lateral position and the ipsilateral arm is prepped into the field. The torso is stabilized with a beanbag. There are two ways to elevate the flap, starting from the vascular pedicle (prograde) or raising the skin paddle first (retrograde). We prefer the dissection of the vascular pedicle first. An incision is made on the upper lateral skin marking, and it is deepened to the thoracodorsal fascia, which is just superficial to the deep muscular fascia, and is raised with the flap. The posterior margin of the deltoid is identified and retracted, exposing the teres minor. The dissection proceeds along the surface of the teres minor and the cutaneous branches of the circumflex scapular artery are exposed. At this point the skin incision is prolonged superomedially and inferiorly and the flap elevation is performed in the space between the thoracodorsal fascia and the muscle fascia. If the skin marking is oriented horizontally, the parascapular artery is ligated and divided, or if a larger skin extension is needed, this branch is conserved to supply the inferior part of the flap. Once the entire flap has been freed from the chest wall, the long head of the triceps, the teres major, and the minor are retracted to facilitate further the exposure of the vascular pedicle. The vascular branches directed to the teres major and minor and the infrascapular branch are ligated and divided, allowing 6 cm of pedicle. At this point the recipient vessel are inspected, the circumflex scapular pedicle is ligated and divided, and the flap is transferred to the surgical defect and

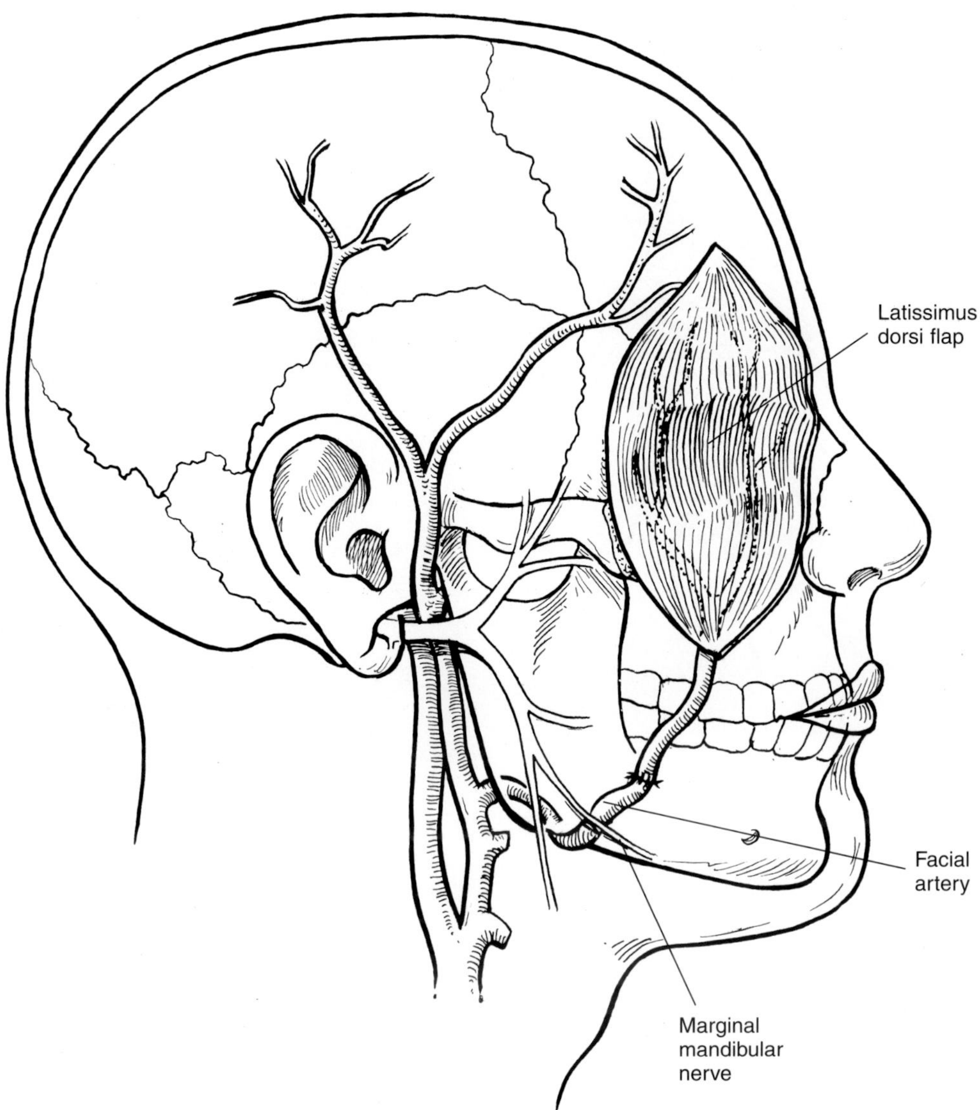

FIG. 7. Use of facial artery as recipient vessel.

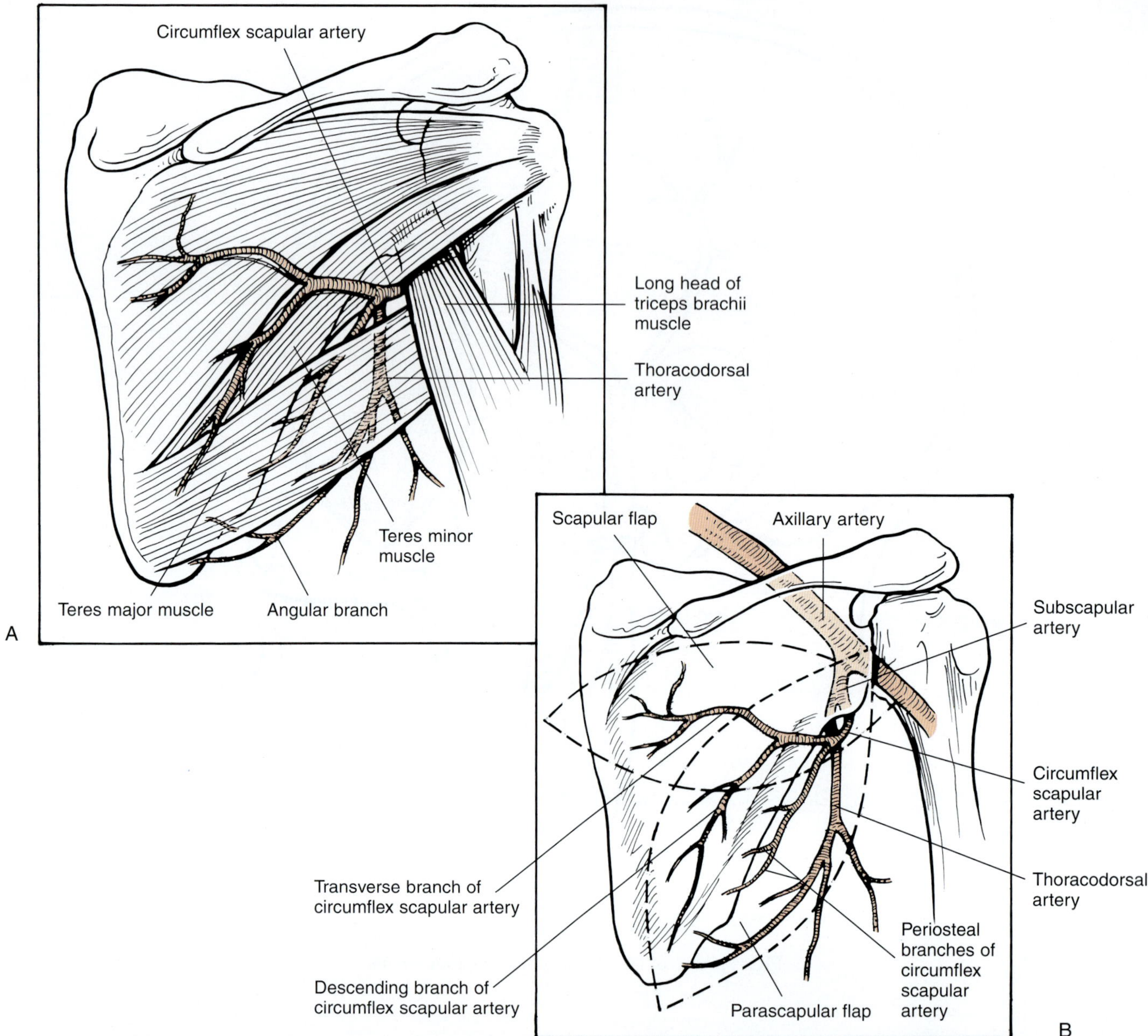

FIG. 8A,B. A: The circumflex scapular artery comes through the triangular space and gives off two skin branches and one bone branch. **B:** The anatomic arrangement allows for design of one bone paddle and two skin paddles.

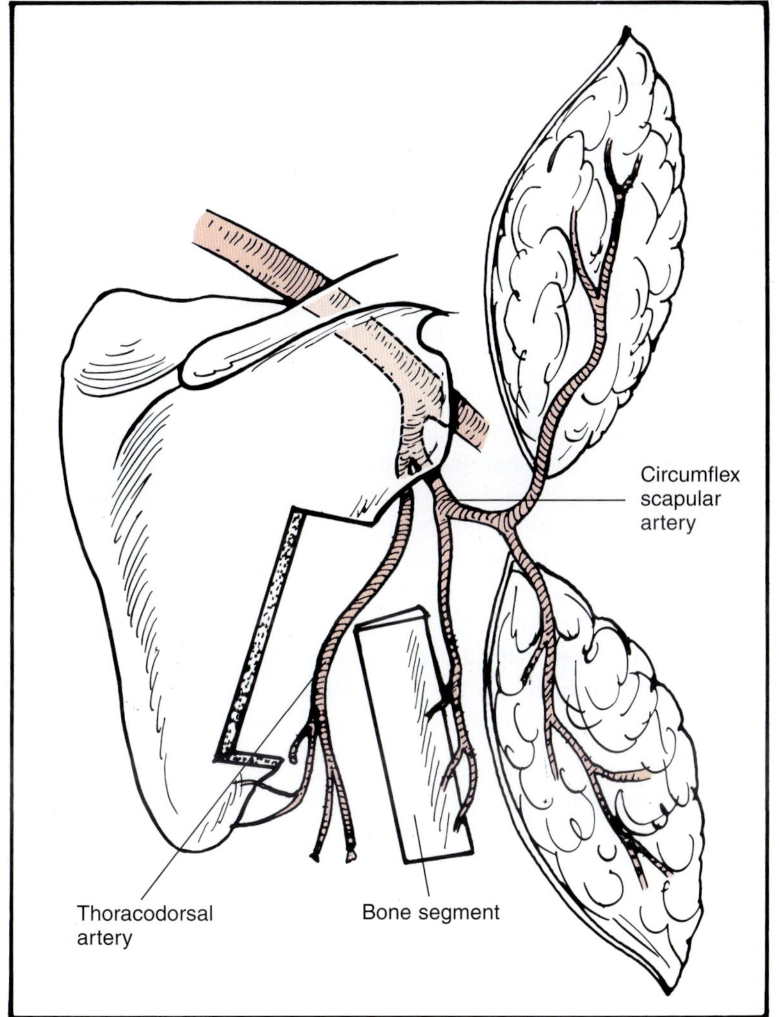

FIG. 8C. Each one of these vascularized units has its own pedicle, thus allowing for greater independent inset of each individual unit.

partially inset. A microvascular anastomosis of the vein is performed first using standard microsurgical techniques. The occluding clamps are released after the vein anastomosis and the presence of a back flow is noted. The anastomosis of the artery is performed next. The blood flow in the vessels is then assessed using an ultrasonic Doppler. Often a pulsation is felt on palpating the artery. The inset of the flap is then completed and one or two drains are left in place. The donor site is closed primarily with interrupted absorbable sutures and with staples.

Flap Inset

The flap is oriented to fill the defect and allow perfect approximation of the vascular pedicle and the recipient vessels. If bone is included in the flap, it is fit into the defect first (see Fig. 3). The surfaces are shaped with a powered saw or bur, and the bone is fixed using microplates and screws. Next, the soft tissue of the flap is partially inset using absorbable sutures. The flap is revascularized, then attention is turned to completing the inset. When resurfacing the forehead, the most important consideration is location of the eyebrows. It is also desirable to design the flap to restore cosmetic units with suture lines placed in a similar location as for a direct brow lift. In most cases, the eyebrow below the reconstruction will be adynamic and prone to ptosis. Tension of the forehead should be adjusted to establish proper elevation and durable support of the eyebrows. These considerations are less significant for reconstructions involving primarily the scalp. Nevertheless, in lateral scalp reconstruction, it is important to adjust flap tension to assure that the ear is in a natural position. Again, it is usually advisable to place closed suction drainage catheters beneath the flap. Care is taken to avoid excessive tension on the skin margins of the flap as it is secured over the unyielding cranium. The blood flow of the flap is then again assessed using capillary refill and perhaps a percutaneous ultrasonic Doppler. A reliable point for obtaining a Doppler signal on the skin of the flap may be marked using a absorbable suture. A dressing is usually not applied, and again, a compressive dressing must be avoided.

Fibula Flap

Anatomic Considerations

The fibular flap is based on the peroneal vein and artery, which is one of three terminal branches of the popliteal artery. As the popliteal artery enters the leg, it gives rise to the anterior tibial artery and, then bifurcates into the posterior tibial and peroneal arteries approximately 7 cm below the knee joint (Fig. 9A,B). The peroneal artery then courses along the medial aspect of the fibula. The fibula itself lies in the deep posterior compartment along the lateral aspect of the leg. It is bordered laterally by the peroneal muscles, anteriorly by the extensor digitorum longus muscle, laterally by the posterior tibialis muscle and inferiorly by the flexor hallucis longus muscle. The blood supply to the skin arises from the inferolateral intermuscular septum and consists of septocutaneous branches as well as musculocutaneous branches arising from the flexor hallucis longus and the soleus muscles (Fig. 10).

At the superior aspect of the fibula, the peroneal nerve crosses just below the head, and care must be taken to avoid injury to this nerve during the dissection. Inferiorly, the fibula is an important contributor to the ankle joint; thus, to preserve ankle joint integrity, the inferior 8 cm of the fibula must not be damaged or sacrificed.

Preoperative assessment of the vascular supply to the lower extremities is essential prior to utilizing the free fibular flap. Although preoperative angiography is not mandatory, it should be considered if there is clinical evidence of vascular compromise such as diminished pulses or atrophy of the skin. Using these clinical criteria for assessment of the lower extremity, we have not had any complications due to vascular compromise of the foot or lower leg.

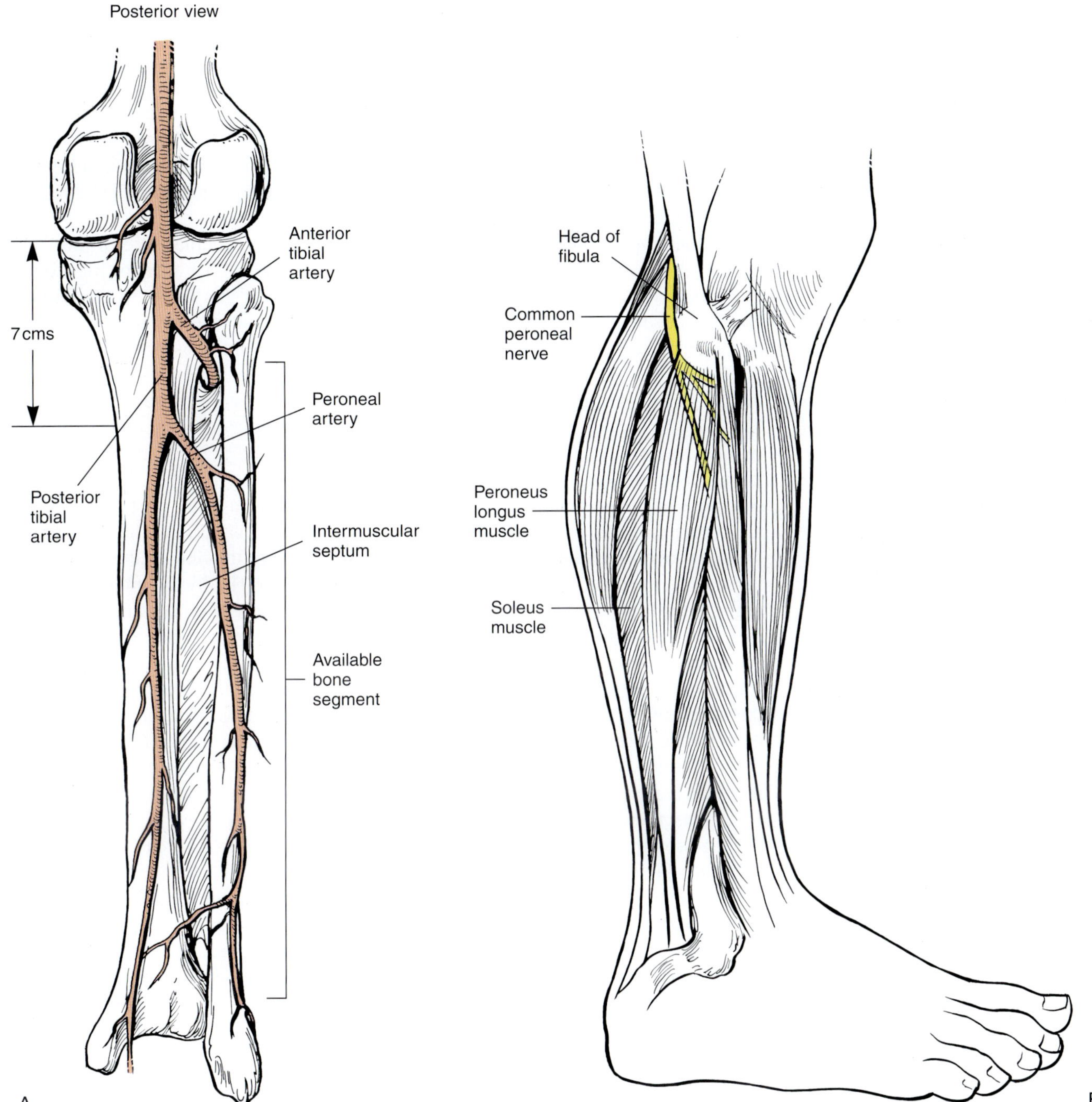

FIG. 9A. The anatomy of the leg vasculature. The peroneal artery branches off the popliteal trunk 7 cm from the knee joint.

FIG. 9B. The common peroneal nerve courses around the fibula head and must be avoided during the dissection.

Operative Technique

The patient is placed in a supine position, with a roll under the ipsilateral hip and a tourniquet is placed on the thigh. The fibular head at the knee, the peroneal nerve just below the fibular head, and the lateral malleolus at the ankle are marked. If a skin paddle is needed, hash marks are drawn at 10, 15, 20, and 25 cm from the fibular head, and the skin paddle is centered between these marks (Fig. 11). In the anteroposterior plane, the paddle is centered along the posterior border of the fibula. The leg is elevated and the tourniquet inflated.

Because the peroneal artery and vein course along the medial side of the fibula, a lateral approach is used to begin the dissection (Fig. 12A). An anterior incision down through the deep muscle fascia is made; the inclusion of this fascia in the flap is crucial, as is avoidance of the superficial peroneal nerve as it emerges from the anterolateral intermuscular septum (Fig. 12B). The dissection continues posteriorly exposing the peroneal muscles, down to but not through the anterior aspect of the posterolateral intermuscular septum (Fig. 12C). This key structure must be preserved. The anterior aspect of the septum is then followed to the fibula, with the peroneal musculature being retracted anteriorly. Once the lateral border of the fibula is reached, it is exposed by taking down the origins of the peroneal musculature along the entire length of the dissection. Care must be taken to avoid injury to the intermuscular portion of the superficial peroneal nerve during the proximal aspect of this dissection. The dissection then proceeds over the anterior aspect of the fibula, dividing the anterolateral intermuscular septum, the muscles of the anterior compartment, and finally the interosseous membrane (Fig. 12D). During the anterior compartment aspect of this dissection, care must be taken to avoid injury to the anterior tibial neurovascular bundle.

Once the interosseous membrane has been divided, the posterior dissection is started. The posterior skin incision is made down through the deep muscle fascia, and the skin paddle is elevated to the edge of the soleus muscle. A 1-cm-deep incision is made in the soleus muscle approximately 1 cm from its lateral edge (Fig. 12E). No further posterior dissection is done at this time. Next, the bone cuts are made to the required length using an oscillating saw. The proximal cut in the fibula should be made as high as possible without damaging the peroneal nerve. Even if one does not plan to use the proximal fibula, it should be harvested to expose the trifurcation of the leg vessels, thus facilitating the pedicle dissection.

Once the fibula is cut, it is retracted laterally, exposing the vessel and medial musculature attachments. The dissection proceeds from distal to proximal and from medial to lateral. The peroneal vessels are located distally, ligated, and divided (Fig. 12F). With the knowledge of their location, the flap dissection continues (medially to laterally) with less risk of injuring the perforating vessels to the skin paddle (Fig. 12G).

After the flap is elevated, the tourniquet is released and any residual bleeding controlled. The bone is usually inset first then the skin paddle. Wires or miniplates can be used to fix the bone to one of the remaining midface buttresses. After inset, the flap is revascularized, preferably using end-to-side anastomoses to the external carotid artery and the internal jugular vein. After the anastomoses are completed, the flap is checked for adequate reflow, and the flap inset is completed. The neck is then closed.

The leg donor site is repaired by simply closing the skin over closed-suction drains; no other special closure techniques are needed. If harvest of a large skin paddle precludes primary closure of the skin, a split-thickness skin graft is used for wound closure. The leg is then further dressed with a bulky dressing and posterior splint.

Postoperative Care

The patient is transferred to the intensive care unit for recovery and monitoring of the flap. The vascular integrity of the anastomoses must be checked hourly by assessing the color and refill of the skin paddle. The laser Doppler, ultrasonic hand-held

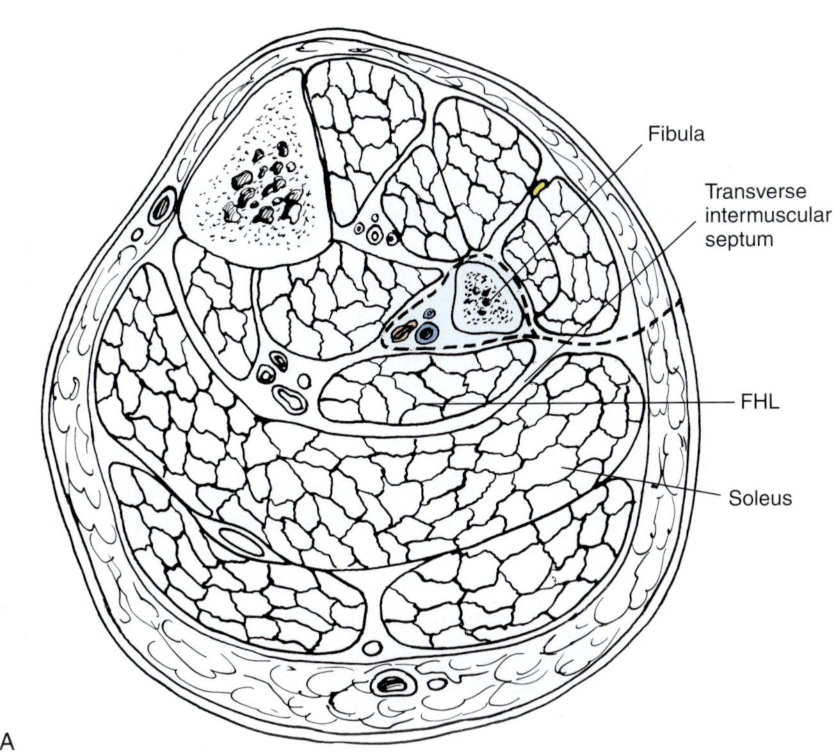

FIG. 10A,B. The peroneal vessels lie in the deep posterior compartment of the leg. Perforators to the skin course along the transverse crural septum, which ends as the posterolateral intermuscular septum. Several of the perforators course through the soleus muscle as well.

Doppler, or implantable 20 MHz Doppler (Swartz) may be used to augment the clinical assessment, but there is no substitute for routine nursing assessment of the flap.

After 72 hours, the patient may be transferred to the floor. On the fifth postoperative day the dressing is changed and the posterior splint removed from the leg. If no skin graft has been used, the patient may be sent to physical therapy for gradual weight bearing and assisted ambulation. If a skin graft has been used to close the donor site, one should wait until the seventh to tenth postoperative day before allowing the patient to put the extremity in a dependent position, and then only when wrapped with an elastic bandage. The drains are removed per routine and the patient is usually ready for discharge on the tenth to fourteenth postoperative day.

Rectus Abdominis Muscle Flap

The rectus abdominis flap can provide a large amount of tissue with a long vascular pedicle with good-sized vessels. The flap is suitable for filling of deep defects and for covering large surfaces and even the entire scalp. The major advantage is that the patient's position for flap harvesting does not require altering, and there is enough space for two surgical teams to work simultaneously. Reconstruction of the orbit after exenteration is often performed by using the rectus abdominis free flap. The skin paddle can be used to provide external coverage or internal lining, if necessary. The flap can be folded double and provide bulk for missing maxillary bone. The vascular pedicle is usually long and reaches the vessel of the neck easily. Sometimes for deep skull base reconstructions a vein graft may be required.

Pertinent Anatomy

The rectus abdominis muscle originates from the symphysis pubis and pubic crest and inserts in the fifth, sixth, and seventh costal cartilages. It measures about 30 cm in length and 6 cm in width (Fig. 13). The blood supply is provided by the superior and inferior epigastric arteries. The superior epigastric artery originates from the internal mammary artery at the level of the six intercostal space, where it gives off the musculophrenic artery. This vessel is generally accompanied by two venae comitantes and communicates with the inferior epigastric artery at the level of the umbilicus. It pierces the sheath of the rectus abdominis lying behind the muscle. Several perforators are provided to the muscle and skin. The inferior epigastric artery is the vascular pedicle used in the free rectus flap. It arises from the external iliac artery, immediately above the inguinal ligament, then directs superiorly and medially penetrating the transversalis fascia in front of the arcuate line. It reaches the posterior aspect of the muscle where it divides in two or three branches below the level of the umbilicus. These arteries communicate with branches of the superior epigastric artery. The length of the inferior epigastric artery is about 10.7 cm, and its diameter ranges between 2 and 2.7 mm. Segmental branches of the deep epigastric system anastomose with branches of the intercostal arteries and deep circumflex iliac artery, and the system provides several perforating arteries emerging through the anterior rectus sheath. These branches are placed in two parallel rows on each rectus muscle and reach their highest concentration in the periumbilical area.

Technique of Dissection

The patient is placed supine and the skin marking is performed. If the skin flap is required, this may be outlined vertically or horizontally (Figs. 13 and 14). Usually, the vertical component is used. But, in some cases the horizontal orientation (i.e., transverse rectus abdominis myocutaneous [TRAM]) is most appropriate. The superior and inferior extensions of the marking may cover the entire length of the muscle, but gen-

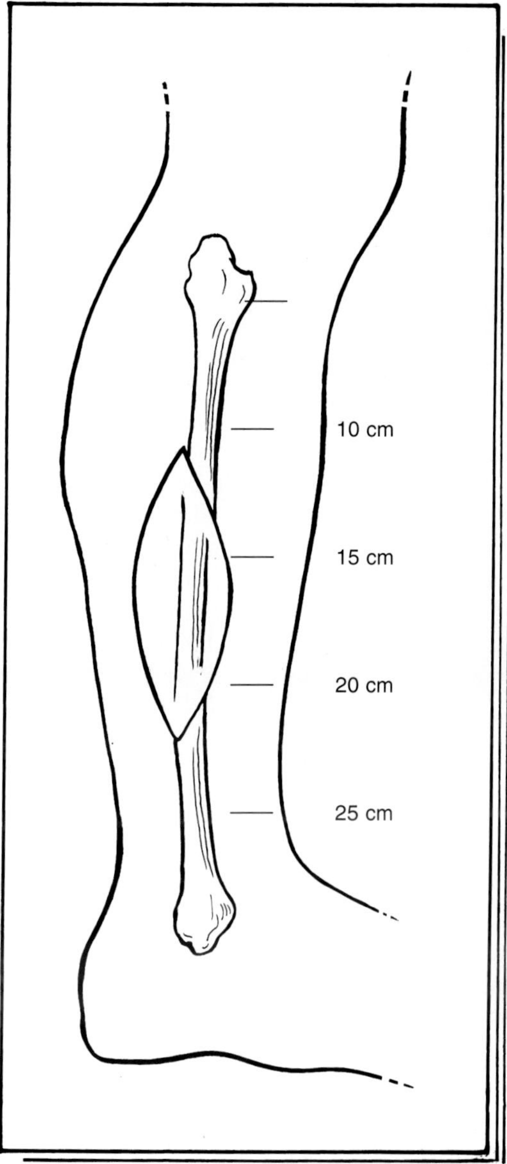

Skin paddle is centered in the anteroposterior
plane along the posterior border of the fibula

FIG. 11. The skin paddle should be centered over the posterior aspect of the fibula between 150 and 250 cm from the fibular head.

erally the proximal marking is placed at the level of the ninth rib, and the distal inferior to the paraumbilical area. The skin incision is performed with the knife, but the dissection is carried on with the electrocautery to minimize blood loss. The anterior rectus fascia is visualized laterally and medially and the flap is then elevated to visualize the medial and lateral rows of perforators (Figs. 15A–C and 16A–D). The fascia is incised with the cautery a few millimeters lateral to the lateral perforators and then reflected laterally to expose the underlying rectus muscle. The lateral border of the muscle and the inferior epigastric artery must be identified. The same procedure is performed on the medial side of the muscle. If no skin paddle is needed the fascia is approached through the skin incision, incised vertically, and reflected laterally and medially. The muscle is then divided superiorly and reflected inferiorly. At this point the dissection of the vascular pedicle is completed to reach the external iliac vessels by using blunt dissection and coagulating with the bipolar cautery all small branches of the vessel. Larger branches require ligatures or clips. Attention is then directed to the recipient vessels that have been already dissected. The vascular pedicle of the flap is ligated and divided, and the flap is transferred to the reconstruction area. The fascia in the donor defect is closed with large nonabsorbable sutures. Care is taken to include all layers in the closure in order to prevent later development of an abdominal bulge or hernia. A mesh prosthesis may be used as an onlay to reinforce the fascial closure in patients with attenuated tissues or in those who demonstrate a tendency for the sutures to tear through when being placed. Drains are usually not necessary unless the skin and subcutaneous tissues were significantly undermined during flap harvest.

Flap Inset

The muscle is positioned to cover the defect and oriented so that the vascular pedicle and the recipient vessels easily approximated without tension. Absorbable sutures may be used to secure the perimeter of the flap to the surrounding tissue. After partial insetting, the flap is revascularized by anastomosis of the vein followed by the artery using standard microsurgical techniques. The inset of the flap is then completed. It may be folded to fill contour depressions, but care must be taken to avoid compression at the fold and thus to prevent ischemia of the folded tissue. Again, closed suction drainage catheters may be placed beneath the flap. Most often, the muscle is used alone and requires a split-thickness skin graft. (Fig. 17A–F). This skin graft is then dressed lightly (e.g., Xeroform [Sherwood Medical, St. Louis, Missouri] or Adaptic [Johnson and Johnson, Harlington, Texas] and antibiotic ointment) to prevent desiccation, but no compressive dressing is used that may cause compromise to the blood supply of the flap. The blood flow of the flap is then again assessed using an ultrasonic Doppler, and a reliable point for Doppler reading on the skin graft is marked using a nonabsorbable suture.

Latissimus Dorsi Muscle Flap

The latissimus dorsi muscle and musculocutaneous flap can provide a large skin flap, sufficient to cover a total scalp. It also can be transferred together with the serratus anterior and/or scapular flap, using the common vascular pedicle comprising the subscapular-thoracodorsal and/or circumflex scapular vessel system.

Pertinent Anatomy

The muscle originates from a broad front, extending from the iliac crest and the surface of the external oblique muscle inferiorly to the thoracolumbar fascia and the spines of the lower six vertebrae posteriorly (Fig. 18). Superiorly it is densely adherent to the surface of the teres major muscle. The latissimus dorsi inserts into the lesser tubercle and the intertubercular groove in front of the proximal humerus. It is flat,

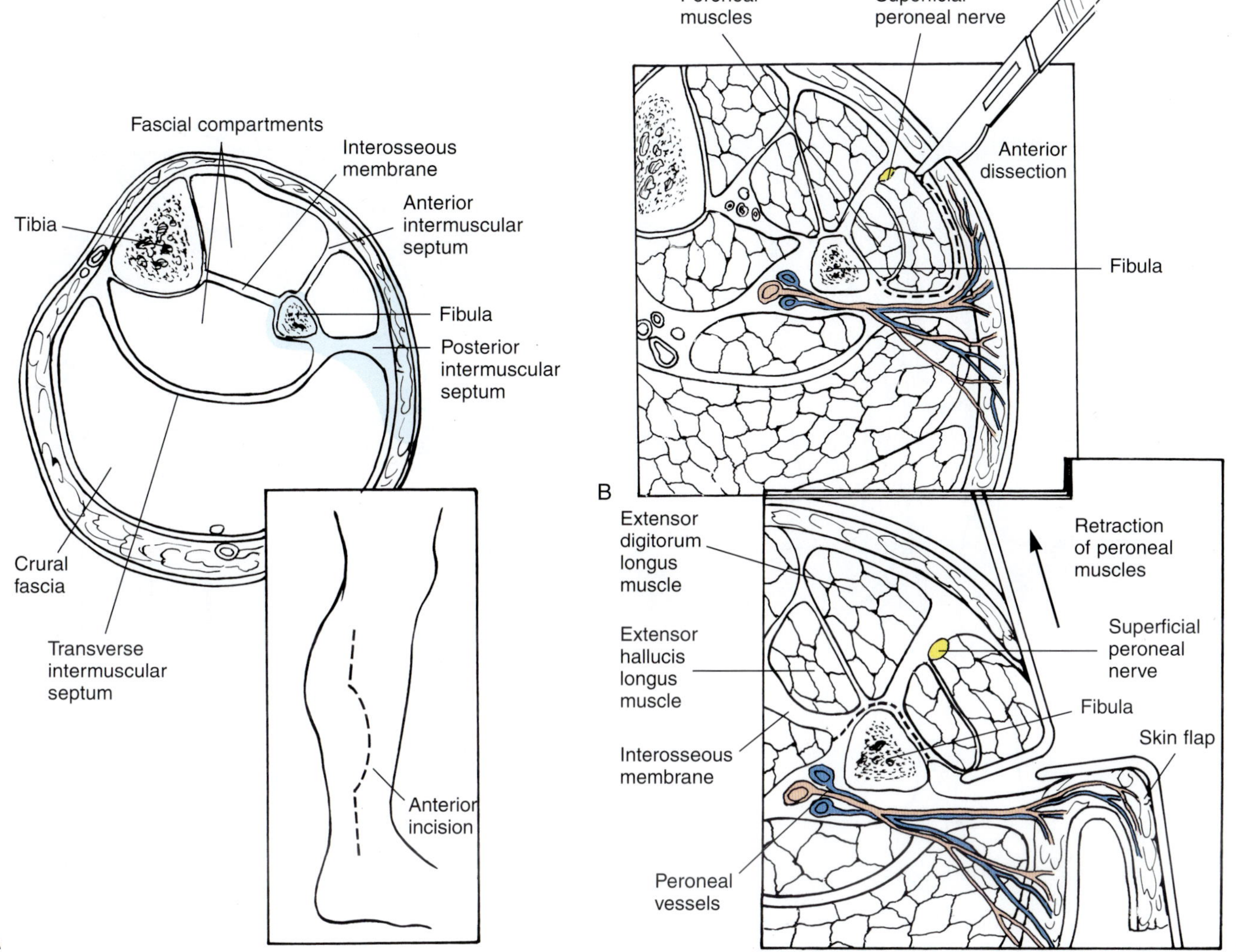

FIG. 12A. The flap harvest is approached from the lateral aspect of the leg.

FIG. 12B,C. B: The anterior incision is made over the peroneal musculature, with care taken to avoid injury to the superficial branch of the peroneal nerve. **C:** The incision is made down through the deep muscle fascia and the flap is then elevated toward the posterolateral intermuscular septum, which is preserved, since the skin perforators travel in this fascia.

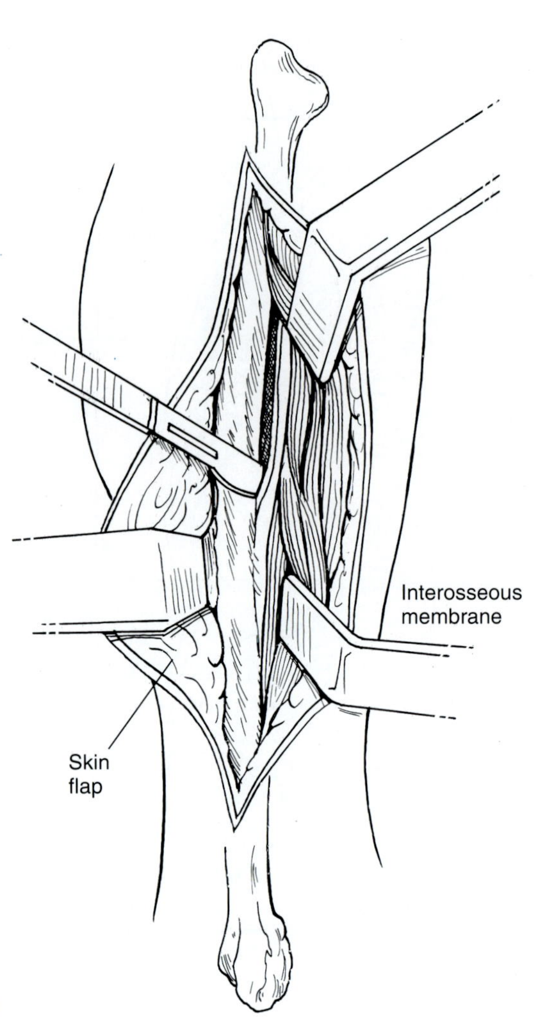

FIG. 12D. The muscles are elevated from the septum up over the top of the fibula, dividing the anterolateral intermuscular septum and the interosseous membrane.

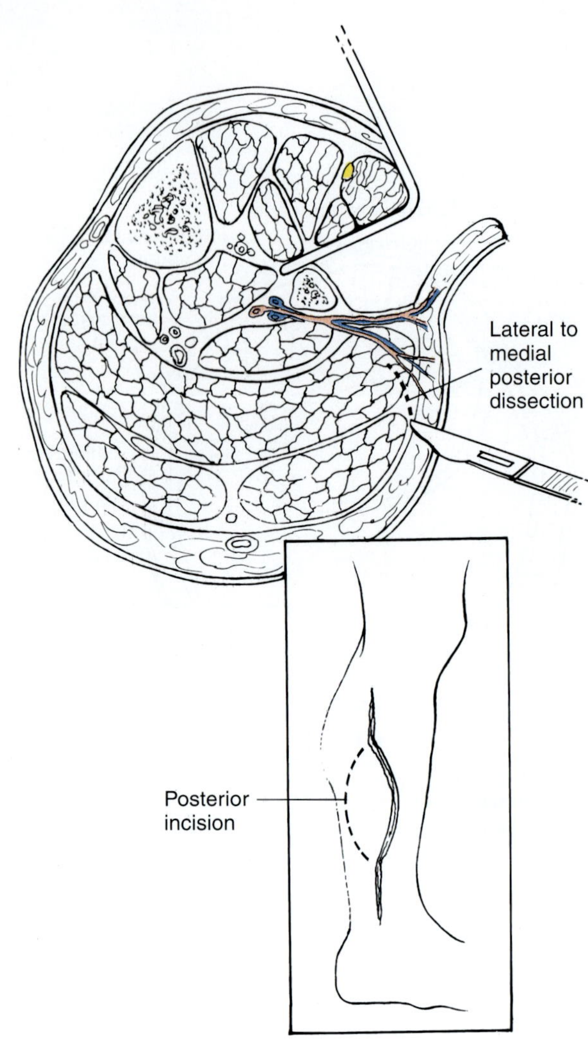

FIG. 12E. After the interosseous membrane has been divided, the posterior skin incision is made again including the deep muscle fascia, but the elevation is stopped 1 cm from the edge of the soleus. At that point the soleus muscle is incised for a depth of about 1m, then the bone cuts are made.

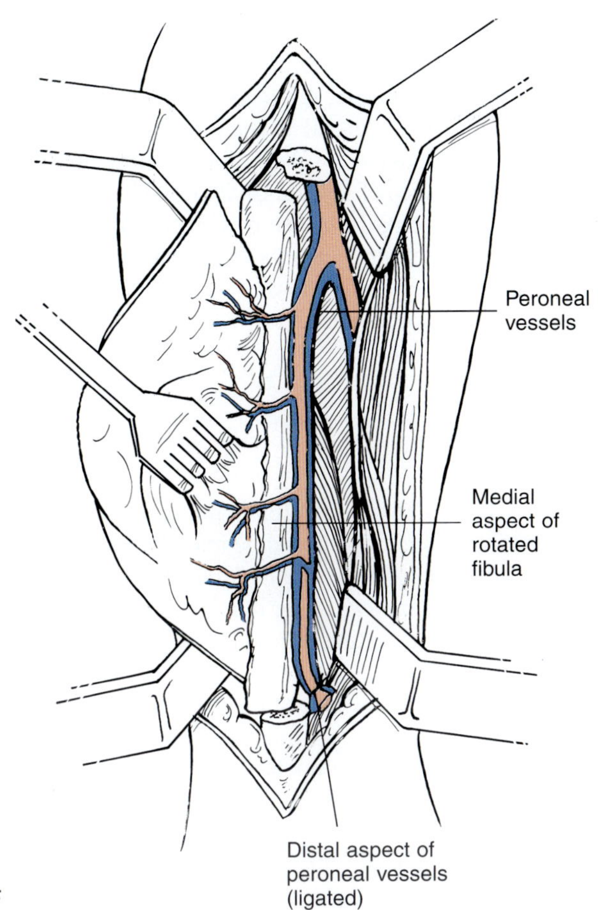

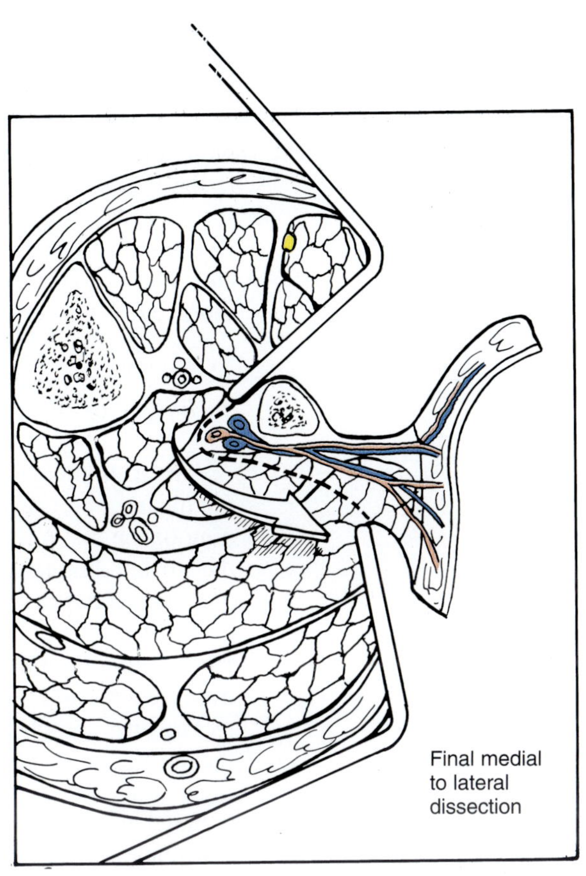

FIG. 12F. The osteotomies are done, allowing for traction on the flap that exposes the deep musculature and helps with the medial dissection. The peroneal vessels are ligated distally, and the musculature is then divided from distal to proximal, taking care to avoid injury to the flap vessels.

FIG. 12G. The remainder of the posterior dissection can then be done from medial to lateral, which helps prevent injury to the skin perforators.

broad, and triangular in shape, with a length of 38 cm, a width of 20 cm, and a thickness of 0.8 cm.

The dominant blood supply to the muscle is the thoracodorsal artery, which arises as a continuation of the subscapular artery. The entrance of the thoracodorsal artery to the muscle is located 8.7 cm distal to the origin of the subscapular artery and 2.6 cm medial to the lateral border of the muscle. Before its entrance, the thoracodorsal artery gives off one or two branches to the serratus muscle. After its entrance in the muscle, the thoracodorsal artery divides in medial and lateral branches. The medial branch courses parallel to the upper margin of the muscle, while the lateral branch continues along the lateral edge of it. Both branches give off several divisions. The blood supply to the latissimus dorsi is also provided segmentally by the posterior paraspinatus perforators, which are seen as two rows of segmental vessels. There are usually four to five vessels in each segmental row, and their individual size is about 1.5 mm in diameter. The venous drainage is supplied by a single vena comitantes accompanying the thoracodorsal artery.

Technique of Dissection

A measurement of the size of the defect to be reconstructed and the decision regarding the use of muscle versus musculocutaneous flap should be made prior to the beginning of the dissection. Recipient vessels should be evaluated and dissected free from the surrounding tissue. If two surgical teams are available, it is possible to perform the preparation of the recipient vessel and flap harvesting simultaneously. Once an appropriate plan is established, the patient is placed on his side with the donor side upward, the shoulder joint abducted, and the hip and knee joints semiflexed. The arm is passed over the head and secured to a support, a roll is placed under the opposite axilla to protect against compression of the brachial plexus. The posterior and anterior margin of the muscle as well as the angle of the scapula are marked. If the flap is elevated including a skin paddle, this should be marked within the edges of the muscle. An incision is then carried posterior and parallel to the lateral margin of the muscle, and the fascial plane of the muscle is found. If the flap includes a skin paddle, the incision is placed along its marked edge. The dissection continues in the fascial plane superiorly and laterally to identify the superior and lateral edges of the latissimus. Then the entire muscle is exposed in its lateral border, close to the serratus anterior muscle. Care is taken to coagulate all perforators directed to the skin flaps. The dissection is continued inferiorly to include the all muscle, and medially to the midline insertion. Carefully, the lateral border of the muscle is separated from the chest wall, and care is taken not to include part of the serratus muscle and to coagulate all perforators between the chest wall and the latissimus. The lateral branch of the thoracodorsal artery can be identified at this stage. The medial edge of the latissimus is also dissected free of the chest wall and all branches from the lumbar and intercostal arteries are coagulated. The distal edge of the muscle is then separated from its insertion on the thoracolumbar fascia and the muscle is elevated, exposing the vascular pedicle. If the main pedicle is not visible, its presence may be confirmed by using an ultrasonic Doppler. In the axillary dissection, the thoracodorsal vascular pedicle is identified approximately 2 to 3 cm medial to the lateral border of the muscle. One or two branches to the serratus are ligated, and the thoracodorsal pedicle is isolated and marked with a loop. After the identification of the circumflex scapular artery, the thoracodorsal pedicle is dissected up to the origin of the subscapular vessels. The thoracodorsal artery is gently dissected from the vein with care not to provoke the vessel spasm, and the artery and vein are marked with vessel loops. The proximal portion of the muscle is then divided near its insertion. After inspection of the recipient vessel, the thoracodorsal pedicle is ligated and divided, and the flap is transferred to the recipient area. The donor site is closed in layers. Two closed-suction drains are left in the subcutaneous space.

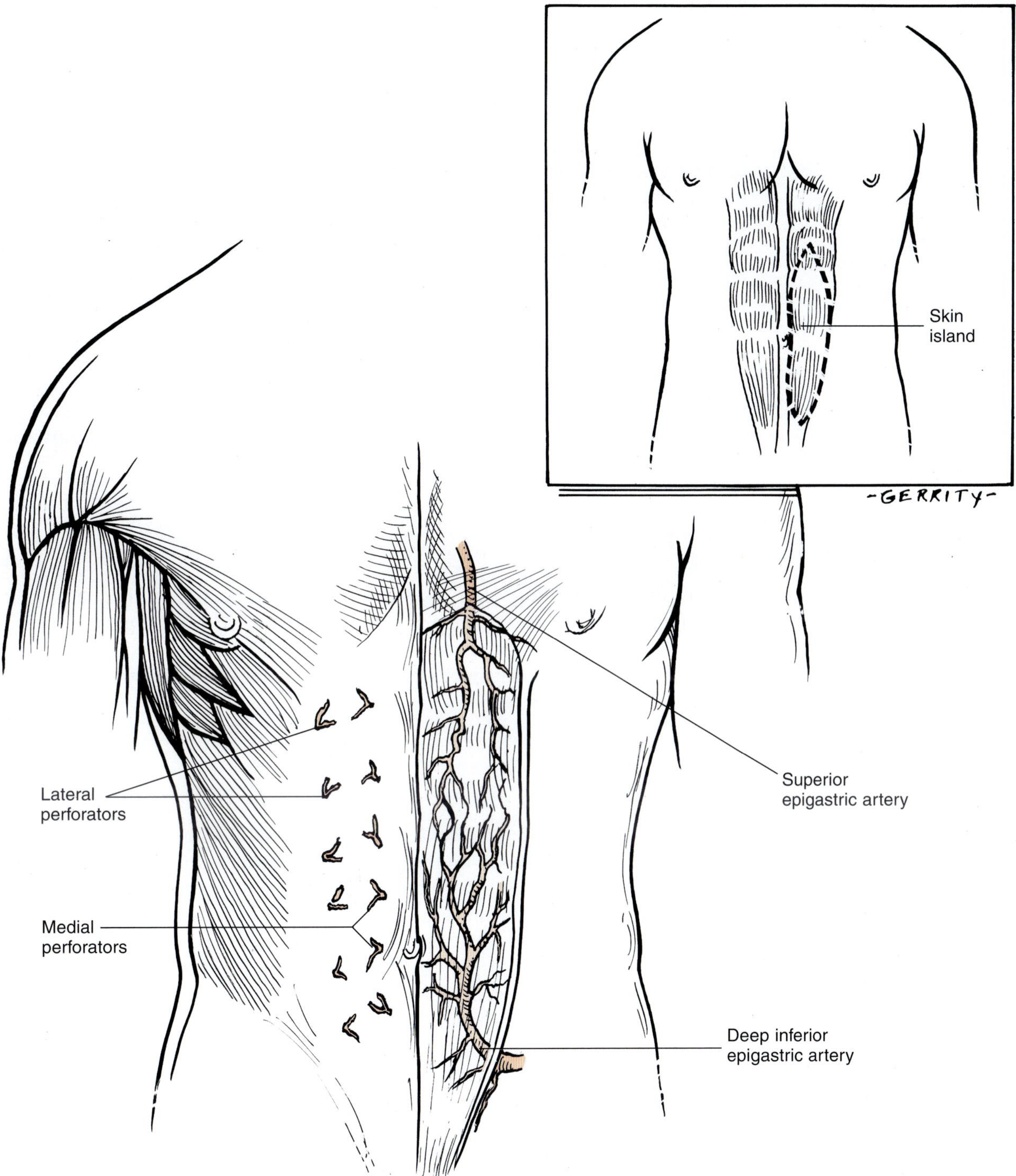

FIG. 13. The anatomy of the rectus abdominis muscle flap, vertical skin paddle orientation.

Flap Inset

The flap is draped across the defect and oriented to allow the vascular pedicle to reach the recipient vessels without tension. It is partially inset by suturing around the periphery with absorbable sutures. After this, the flap may be revascularized by anastomosis of the vein followed by the artery. The inset may be completed by securing the periphery of the flap to the tissues surrounding the defect. If a skin paddle is used with the flap, then care must be used to avoid too tight closure that might compress the flap against the unyielding cranium, causing ischemia. Allowance must be made for the flap swelling postoperatively. The muscle may be folded to fill contour depressions, but care must be taken to avoid compression at the fold to prevent ischemia in the folded tissue. Again, closed suction drainage catheters may be placed beneath the flap. Most often, the muscle is used alone and requires a split-thickness skin graft, which is then dressed lightly (e.g., Xeroform or Adaptic and antibiotic ointment) to prevent desiccation, but no compressive dressing is used because it may cause compromise to the blood supply of the flap. The blood flow of the flap is then again assessed using an ultrasonic Doppler and a reliable point for Doppler reading on the skin graft is marked using a nonabsorbable suture.

Radial Forearm Flap

Skull defects requiring skin resurfacing can be successfully treated by using the radial forearm flap. This thin flap is particularly suitable when a pliable soft tissue is required to resurface a contour deformity that will later be restored using a maxillofacial prosthesis. An osteocutaneous flap is also available for reconstruction of soft/hard tissue defects in the midface.

Pertinent Anatomy

The territory of this flap may extend from the wrist flexion crease to the lower third of the arm. The flap is based on the radial vessel, which courses through the anterior lateral intermuscular septum, with drainage from the venae comitantes or a superficial vein such as the cephalic vein (Fig. 19A–C). The skin is supported by small multiple perforators through the fascial septum. The radial artery is a terminal branch of the brachial artery. It courses deeply between the pronator teres muscle and the brachioradialis muscle in the upper forearm and between the brachioradialis muscle and the flexor carpis radialis in the lower forearm. Distally it contributes to the deep palmar arch, passing through the anatomic "snuff box" between the tendons of the abductor pollicis longus and extensor pollicis brevis muscles. A rich vascular network is derived from the radial artery in the forearm. The venous drainage is based on superficial and deep veins. The deep system is composed of the comitantes veins accompanying the radial artery. These veins have an average diameter of 1.3 mm and are considered too small for the microvascular anastomosis. When possible, the superficial system should be included in the flap. The superficial system includes the cephalic and the basilic veins. The cephalic vein arises from the radial border of the forearm and receives tributaries from both sides of the forearm. It is usually the preferred vein in transferring this flap. The basilic vein ascends along the ulnar border of the forearm and then travels forward along the medial bicipital groove where it joins the cephalic vein. An anterolateral segment of the radial bone (10 cm) can be harvested in the flap. This bone is particularly suitable for reconstructions of the midface involving the orbital and maxillary bones and for bony contour defects. The blood supply to the bone is derived from the fascioperiosteal branches, through the intermuscular septum and musculoperiosteal branches, and through the flexor pollicis longus and pronator quadratus muscles from the radial artery.

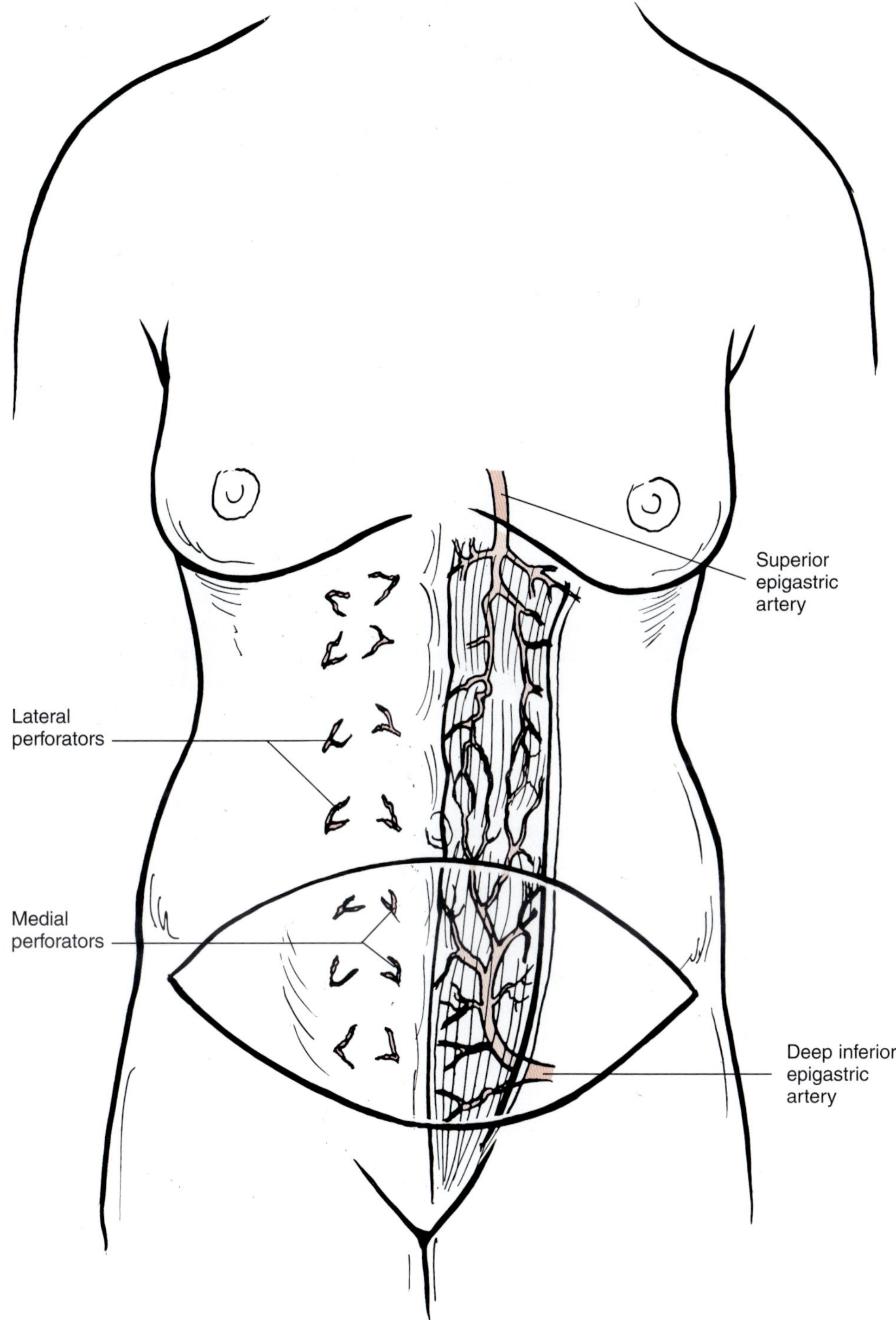

FIG. 14. The anatomy of the rectus abdominis flap depicting the horizontal skin orientation.

Flap Dissection

The flap should be designed as far proximally on the forearm as possible to prevent excessive exposure of the distal tendons of the forearm. The dimensions of the defect are determined, and the necessary pedicle length is assessed by measuring the distance from the planned recipient vessels to the closest point on the defect. This distance is plotted on the forearm beginning 4 cm distal to the elbow flexion over the approximate origin of the radial artery. The proximal margin of the flap is thus determined, and the remainder of the flap is designed on the skin overlying the radial artery and cephalic vein.

The flap is elevated by first incising distally to identify the radial artery and venae comitantes lying between the flexor carpi radialis and brachioradialis tendons (Fig. 20A–D). These vessels are ligated and divided. The lateral margins of the flap are then elevated in the subfascial plane. The superficial veins of the cephalic system are included. The superficial branch of the radial nerve is located and protected. Special care must be taken when approaching the interval between the brachioradialis and the flexor muscle group to preserve the septum between the radial artery and the skin paddle. It is thin and easy to injure, particularly when the flap is elevated under tourniquet control. Numerous perforating vessels on the deep surface of the radial artery enter the forearm musculature and interosseous membrane. These are carefully controlled with hemoclips or bipolar cautery and divided. Once the skin paddle is elevated, the dissection continues proximally to obtain adequate pedicle length. The dissection is complete when the bifurcation of the brachial artery is reached. The tourniquet is deflated and the flap allowed to perfuse for 20 minutes prior to dividing the pedicle for transfer.

Meticulous care must then be given to the donor site. The paratenon must be preserved during flap elevation and protected from desiccation when attention is focused on transfer and revascularization of the flap. During closure, the wound edge is advanced to protect the superficial branch of the radial nerve, and muscle bellies are mobilized to cover as much of the exposed tendons as possible. A full-thickness graft harvested from the inguinal crease provides the best coverage of the remaining open wound. A bulky dressing and a forearm splint is applied, which prevents wrist and finger movement.

When bone is required, soft tissue attachments are maintained between the radial artery pedicle and the periosteum of the bone. The periostium of the radius is reached by dividing the muscle bellies of the flexor pollicis longus and pronator quadratus muscles. The bone is then cut in a beveled fashion approximately 0.5 cm on either side of the radial vessels. The excision should not be greater than one-third of the diameter of the radius.

Flap Inset

Usually this flap is selected for midface reconstructions. The flap is oriented to fill the defect and allow approximation of the vascular pedicle and the recipient vessels. If bone is included in the flap, it is fit into the defect first. Bone from the radial forearm flap is especially well suited for nasal or infraorbital rim reconstruction (see Fig. 2). The surfaces are shaped with a powered saw or bur, and the bone is fixed using microplates and screws. Next, the soft tissue of the flap is partially inset using absorbable sutures. If external coverage and internal lining are needed, the skin paddle may be folded to restore both surfaces. Insetting of the internal lining is performed first, followed by partial insetting of the outer skin. Revascularization of the flap is then performed using standard microsurgical techniques as described above. The vascular pedicle may be passed through the subcutaneous tissues of the cheek to reach the margin of the mandible or the cervical vessels. After revascularization, the inset may be completed. Postoperative swelling is not as great as in flaps containing muscle, so a more precise inset is allowed. Care should be taken not to create a reconstruction that

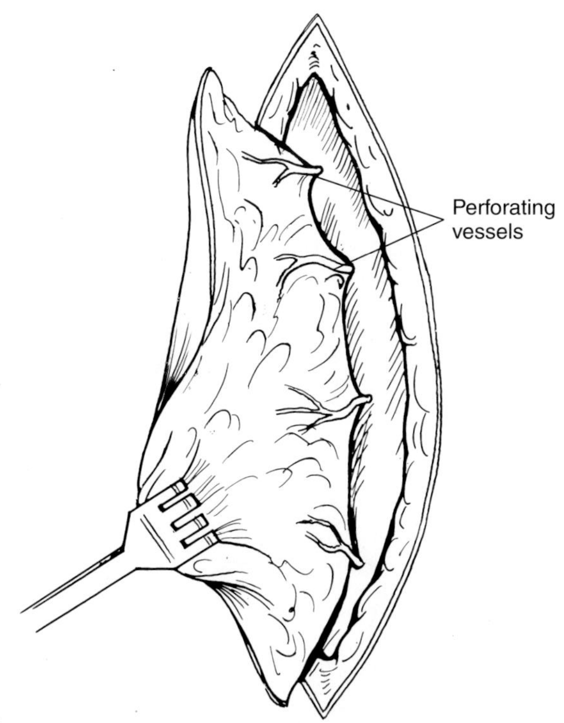

FIG. 15A. Elevation of the rectus abdominis flap using the vertical skin paddle (vertical rectus abdominis muscle [VRAM]) design. The perforators are exposed laterally and medially.

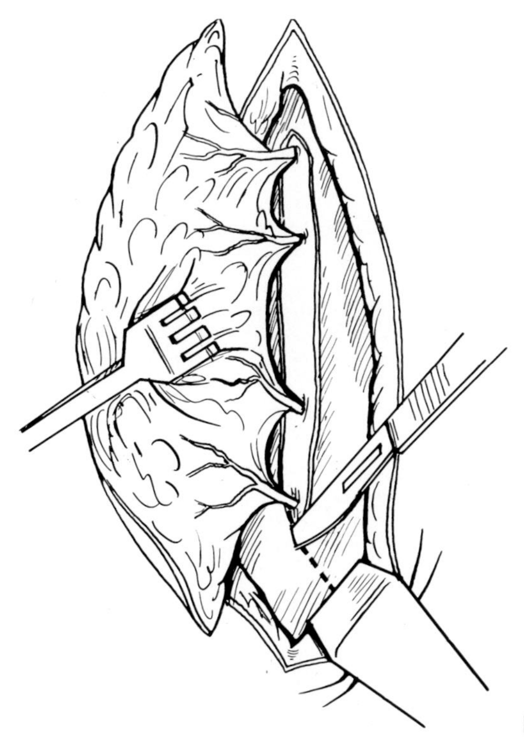

FIG. 15B. The fascia is incised circumferentially.

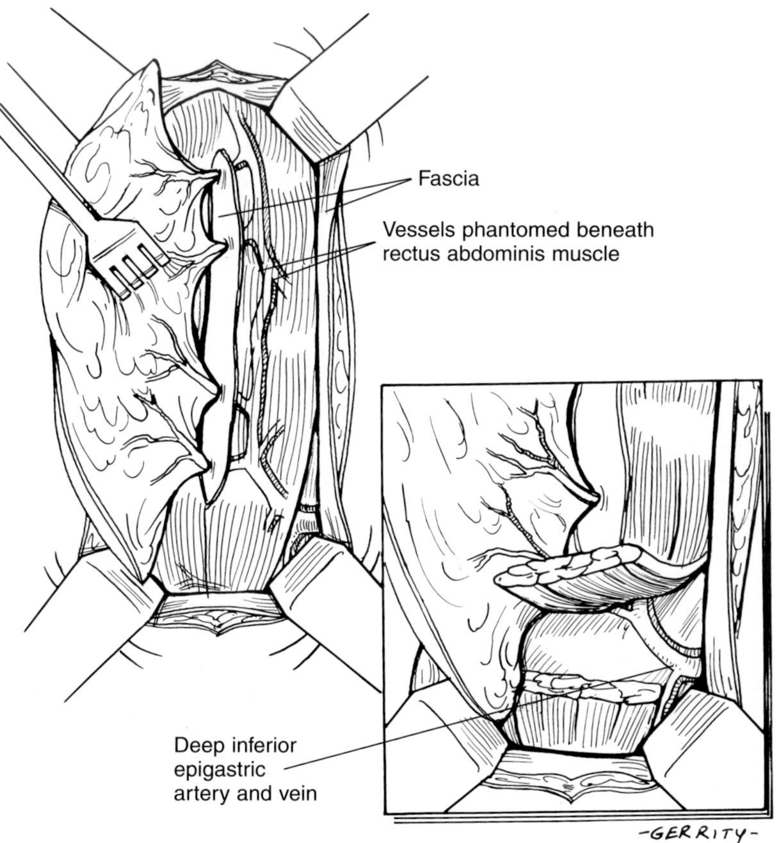

FIG. 15C. The deep inferior epigastric vessels are identified in the lower lateral aspect of the muscle. **Inset:** Once the lower aspect of the muscle is divided, the vessels are traced to their origin.

C

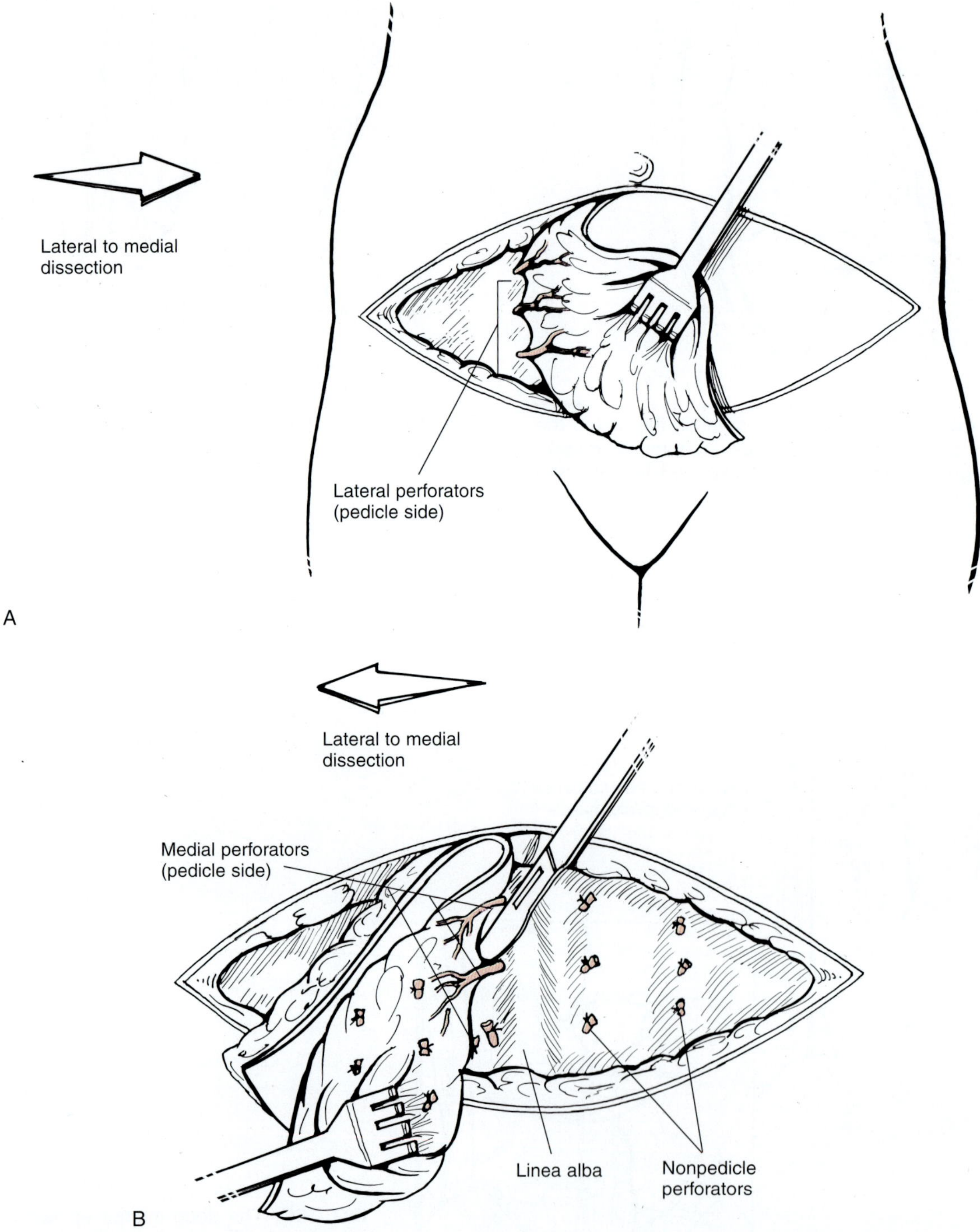

FIG. 16A,B. A: Elevation of the transverse rectus abdominis myocutaneous (TRAM) flap is begun from lateral to medial. When the lateral perforators are encountered, they are spared and the dissection is then started on the opposite side. **B:** The perforators on the contralateral side are sacrificed and, in order to spare more fascia, one may also sacrifice the medial perforators on the ipsilateral side.

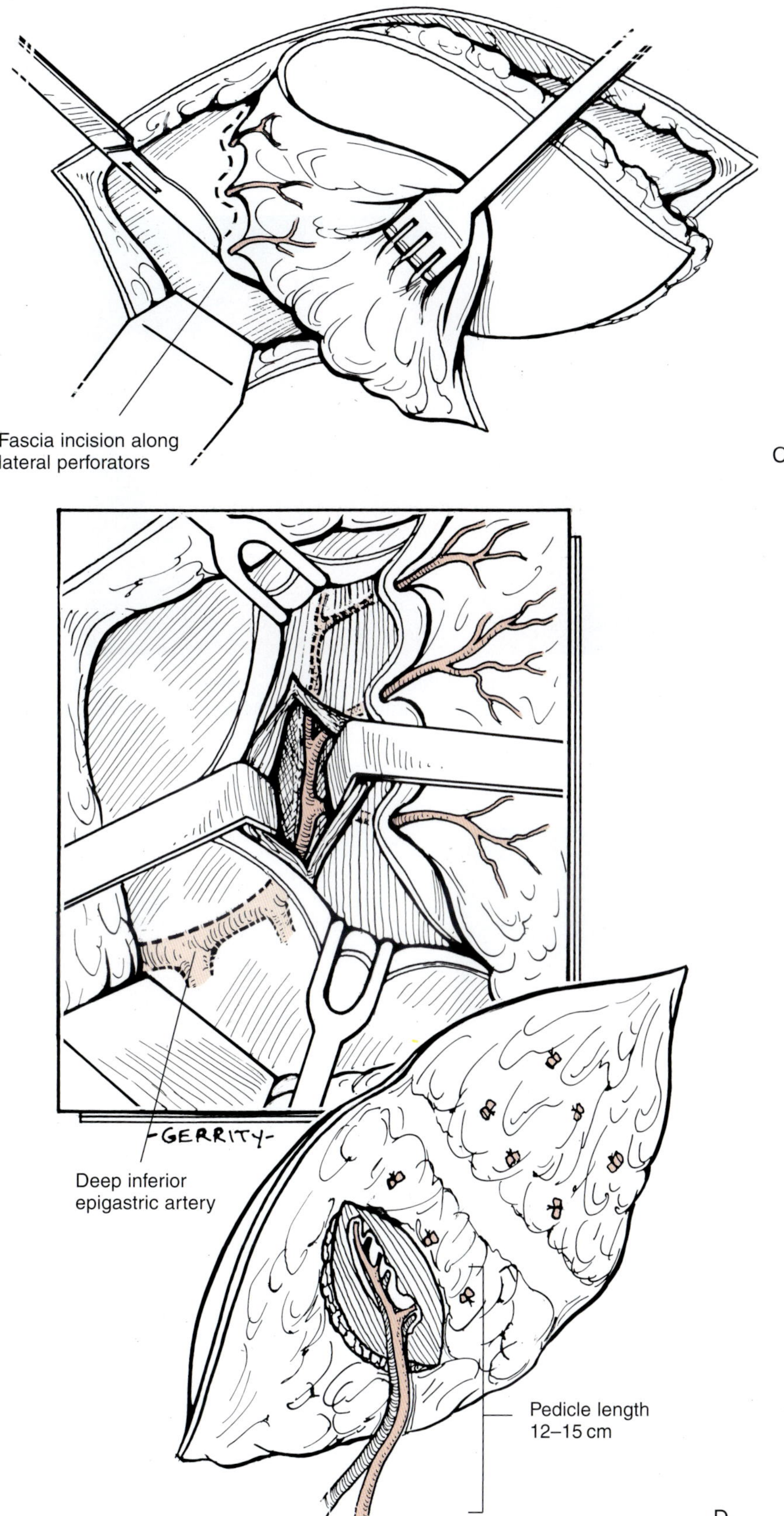

FIG. 16C,D. C: Next the fascia is incised circumferentially around the perforators and the muscle is dissected. **D:** The lateral portion of the muscle is split and the deep inferior epigastric vessel is identified. This is then traced to its origin. By splitting the muscle, one can achieve a pedicle length of 12 to 15 cm with minimal abdominal wall sacrifice.

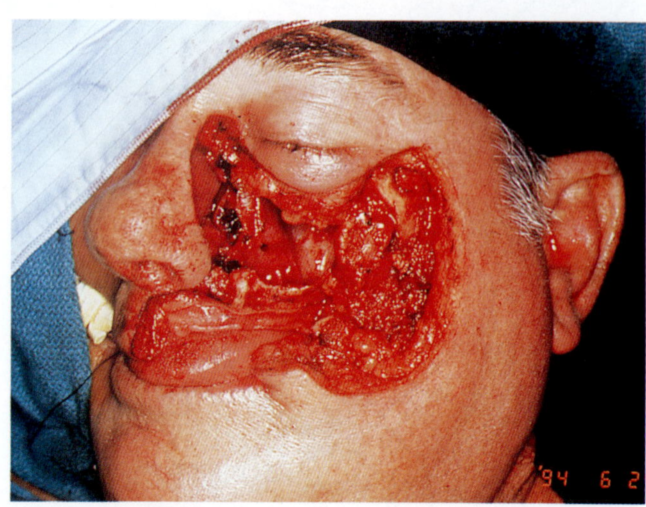

FIG. 17A. Maxillary defect closed with rectus abdominis muscle flap and skin graft. Intraoperative view of defect after tumor resection.

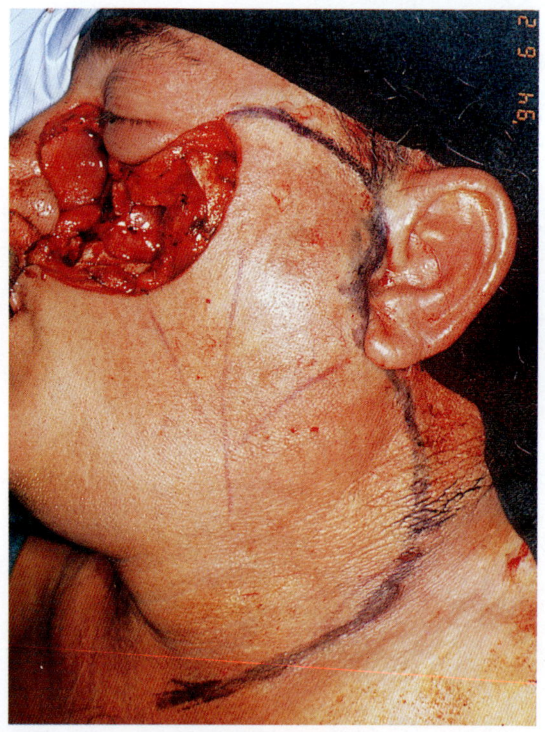

FIG. 17B. Surgical plan for cervicofacial flap elevation. Use of this flap will help to expose the recipient vessels and facilitate closure of the inferior part of the defect.

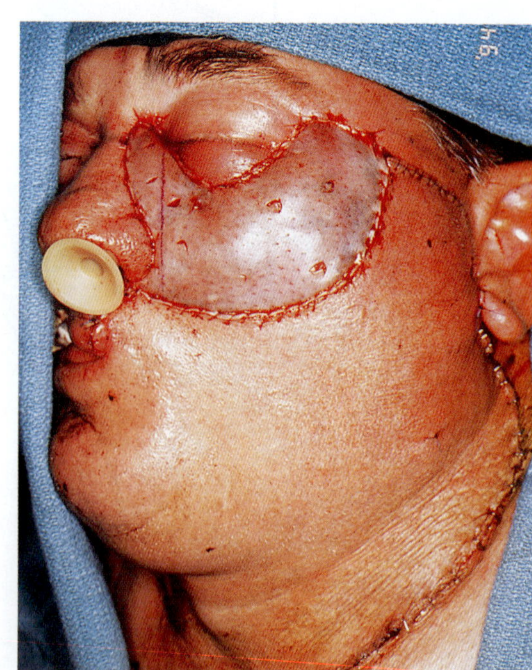

FIG. 17C. After flap transfer, placement of skin graft and skin flap closure.

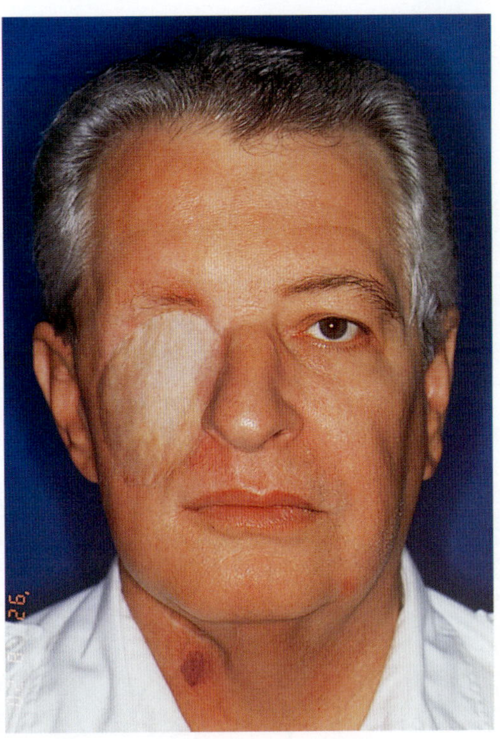

D

FIG. 17D. Similar case with long-term follow-up. Note well-healed skin graft.

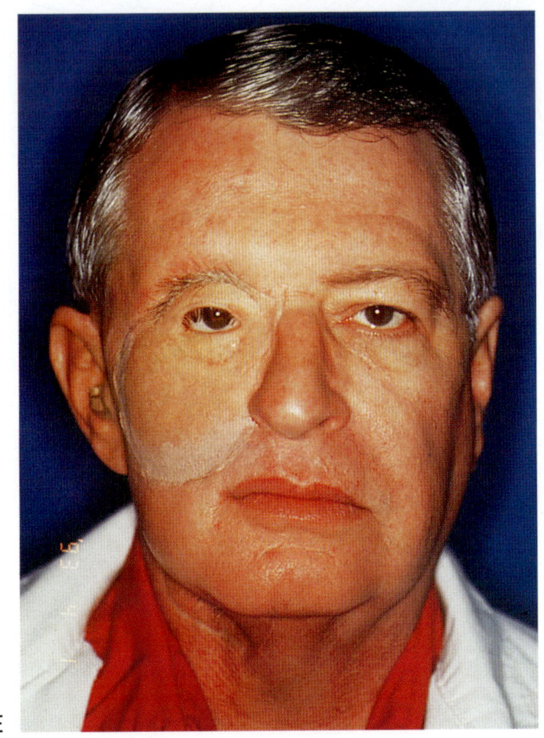

E

FIG. 17E. Prosthesis in place.

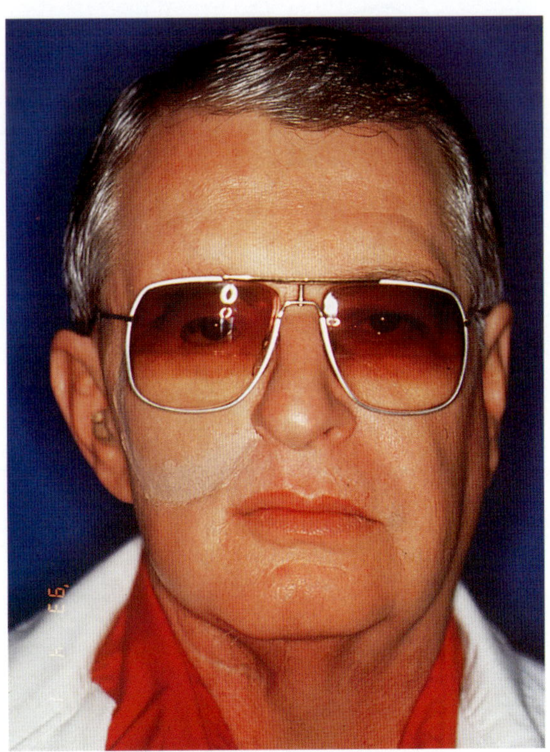

F

FIG. 17F. Use of sunglasses gives increased camouflage of defect.

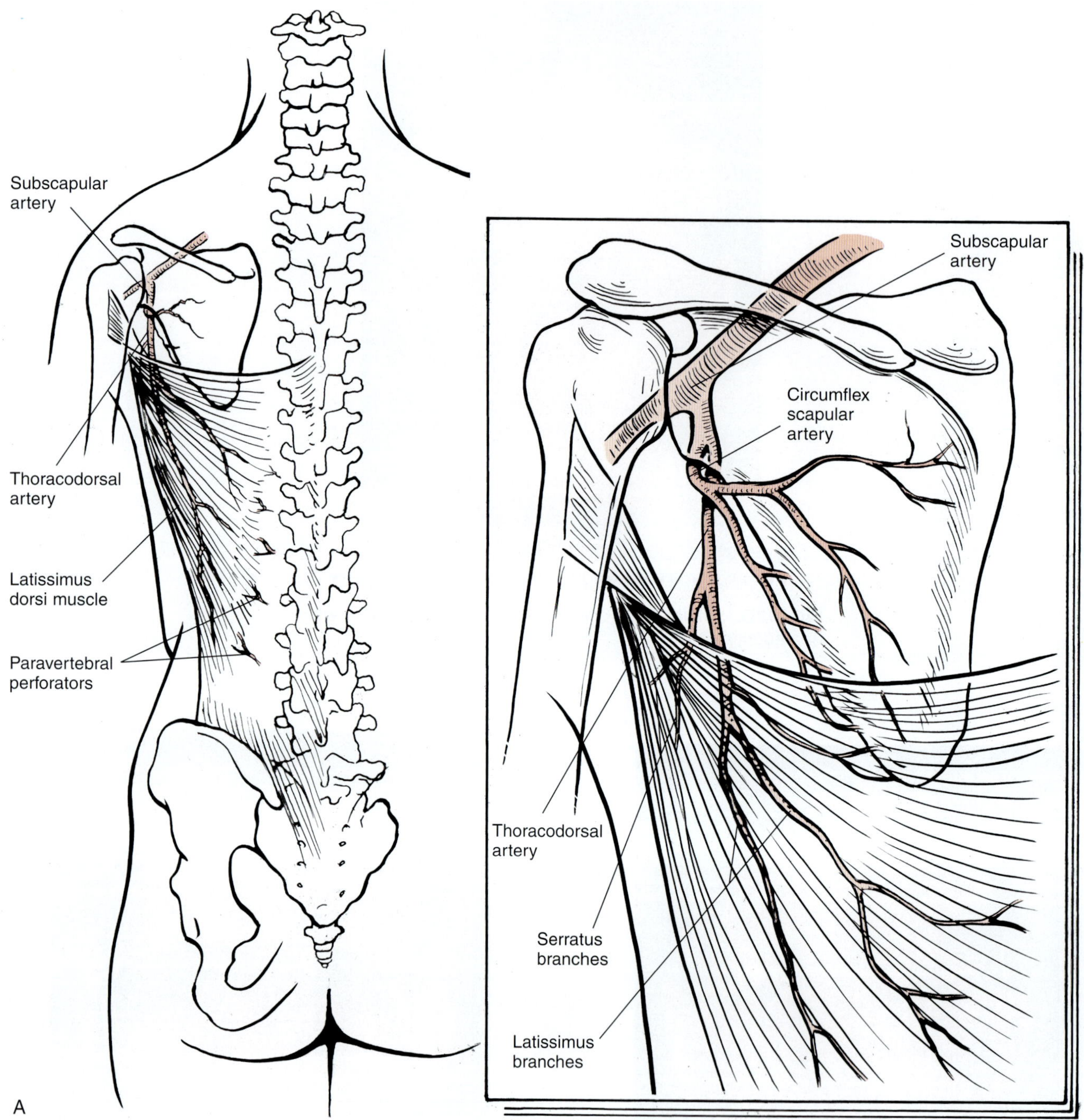

FIG. 18A–C. The latissimus dorsi muscle flap is based on the thoracodorsal vessels. It can be transferred as a myocutaneous flap, or a muscle flap that requires skin graft coverage.

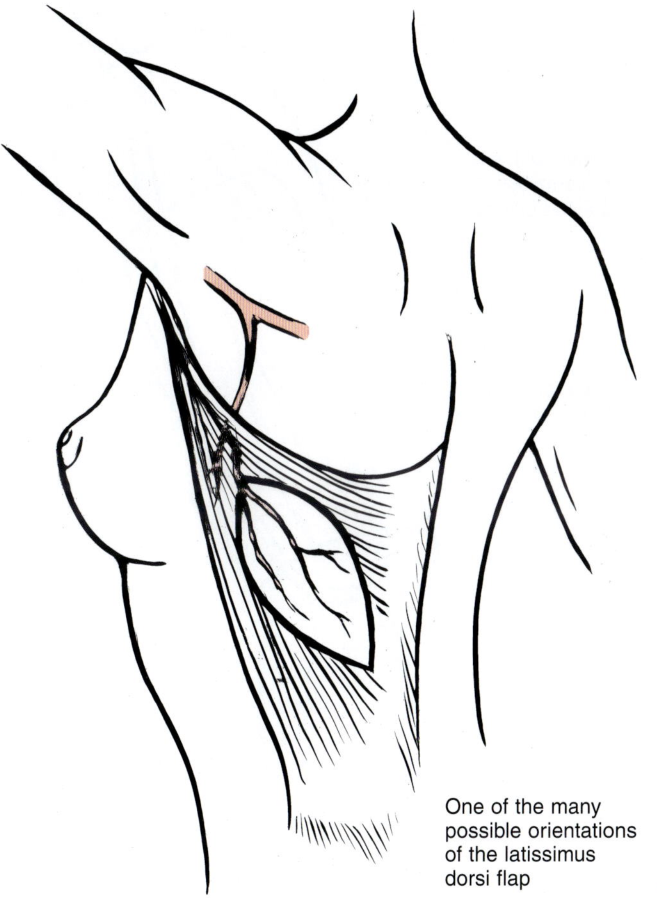

FIG. 18A–C. *Continued.*

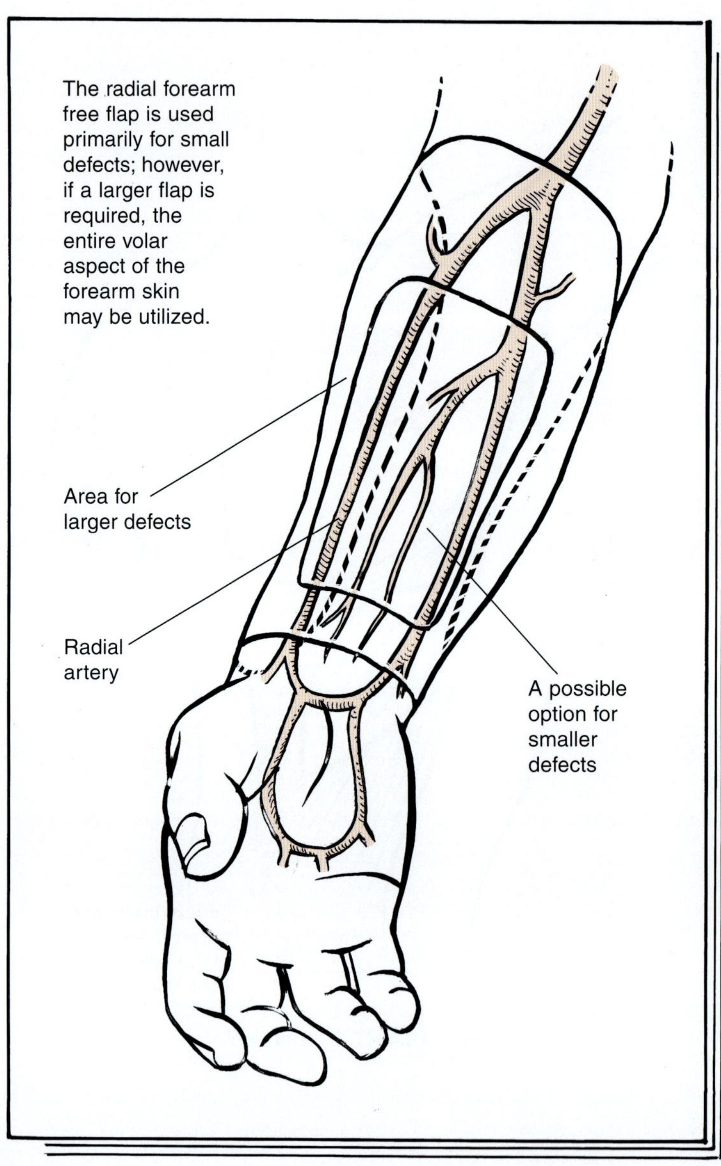

FIG. 19A. Anatomy of the radial forearm flap. Flap design is located over radial vessels.

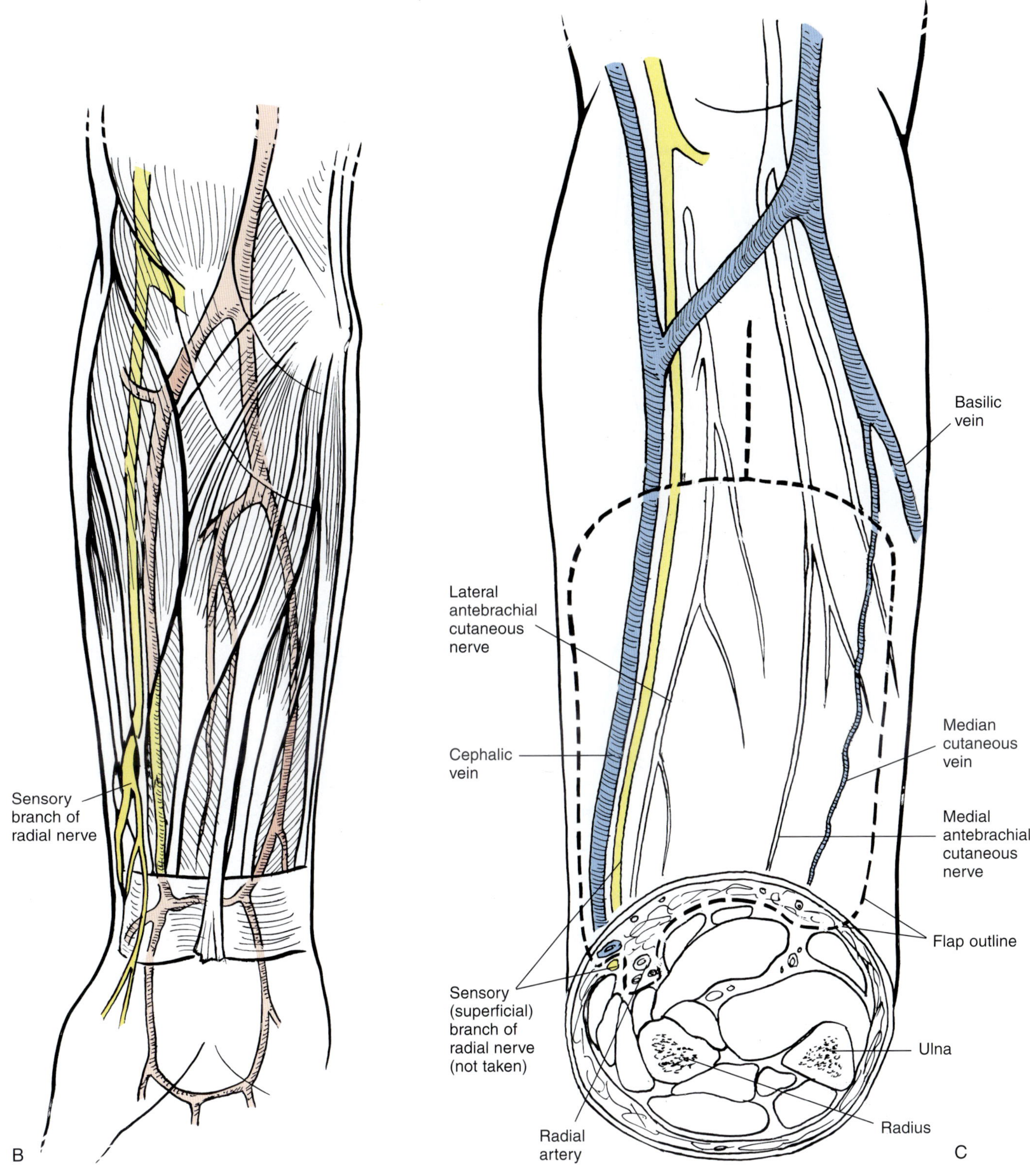

FIG. 19B. Vascular anatomy of the radial forearm flap. Note location of superficial radial nerve.

FIG. 19C. Cross-sectional anatomy of proposed flap elevation.

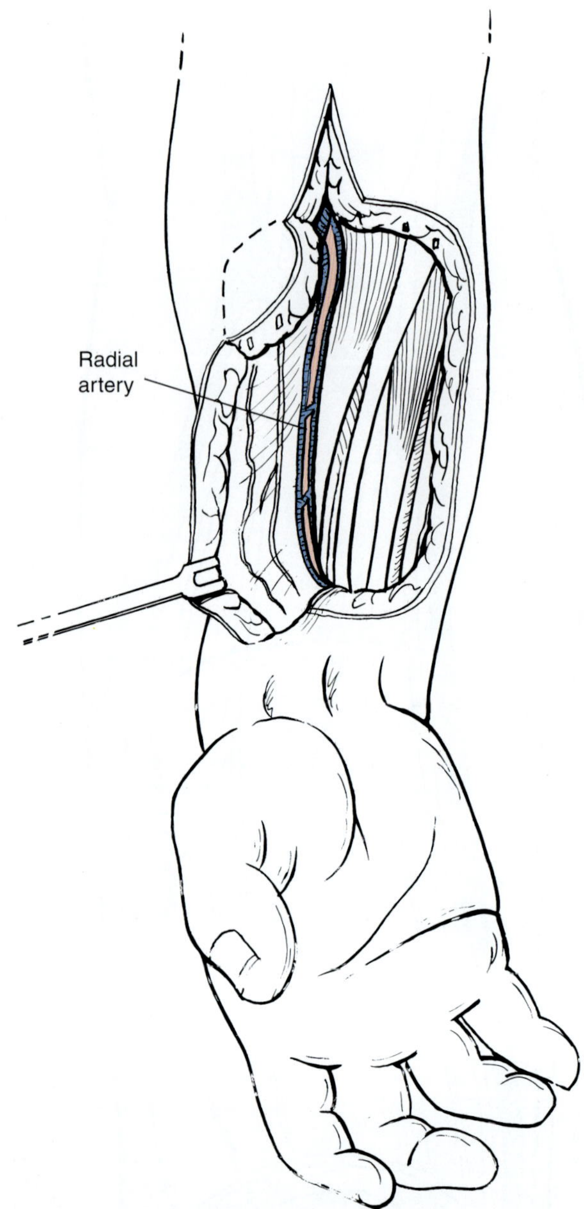

FIG. 20A. Radial forearm flap elevation. Medial incision and flap elevation with exposure of radial vessels.

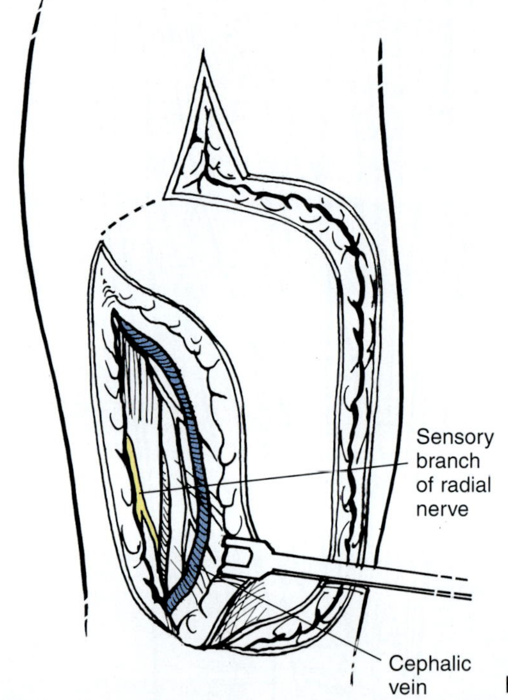

FIG. 20B. Lateral incision with exposure of cephalic vein and identification and preservation of radial nerve.

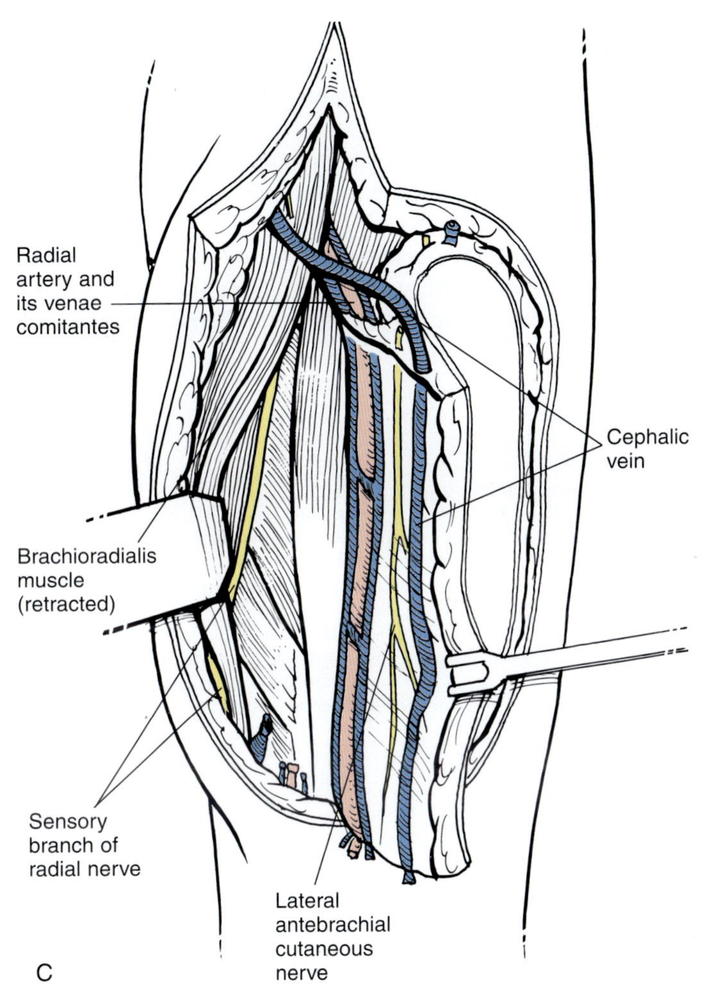

FIG. 20C. Ligation of vessels distally, with elevation of remainder of flap.

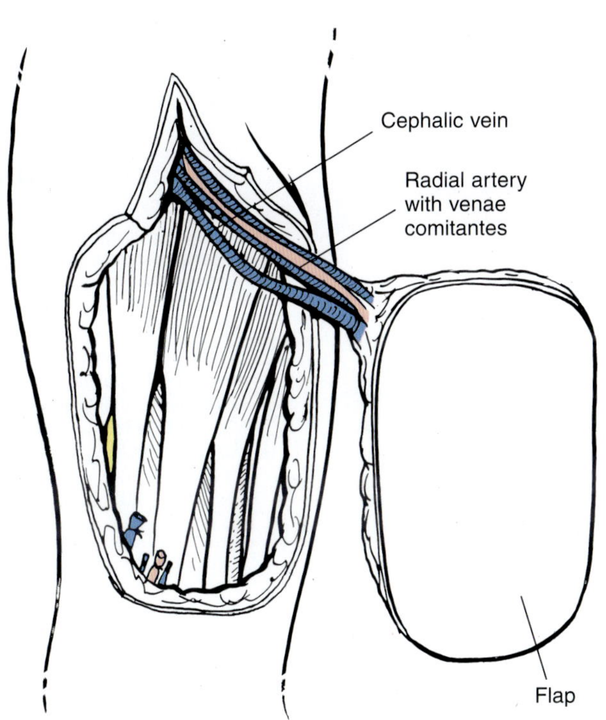

FIG. 20D. Donor vessels are then traced to their origin.

has a higher contour than normal, so as to allow fabrication of maxillofacial prosthetics. No dressing is applied at the end of the procedure. A suitable location is identified for postoperative monitoring of the flap perfusion.

SUMMARY

This chapter demonstrates the use of free flaps for reconstruction of the midface and scalp. For reconstruction of scalp and cranial defects, generally large flaps such as the latissimus dorsi muscle or rectus abdominis muscle flap are utilized. Large defects of the midface can be reconstructed with the scapula or fibula osteocutaneous flaps, with the goal being to provide a foundation for maxillofacial prosthetics. Smaller defects of the orbit can be reconstructed with the radial forearm osteocutaneous flap. For defects involving the cranial base, which require separating the intracranial contents from the upper aerodigestive tract, most commonly the rectus abdominis muscle flap is utilized.

Although the superficial temporal and facial vessels may be suitable as recipient vessels, preferential use of the external carotid artery and internal jugular vein, utilizing a vein graft if necessary, actually increases the reliability of the flaps by augmenting the flow (Fig. 5).

SELECTED READINGS

Jones NF, Hardesty RA, Swartz WM, et al. Extensive complex defects of the scalp, middle third of the face, and palate: the role of microsurgical reconstruction. *Plast Reconstr Surg* 1988;82:937.

McLean DH, Bunke HJ. Autotransplant of the omentum to a large scalp defect with microsurgical revascularization. *Plast Reconstr Surg* 1972;49:268.

Miller MJ, Schusterman MA, Reece GP, Kroll SS. Microvascular craniofacial reconstruction in cancer patients. *Ann Surg Oncol* 1995;2:145.

Robson MC, Zachary LS, Schmidt DR, et al. Reconstruction of large cranial defects in the presence of heavy radiation damage and infection utilizing tissue transferred by microvascular anastomosis. *Plast Reconstr Surg* 1989;83:438.

Schusterman MA, Reece GP, Miller MJ. Osseous free flaps for orbit and midface reconstruction. *Am J Surg* 1993; 166:341.

Swartz WC, Banis JC. *Head and neck microsurgery.* Baltimore: Williams and Wilkins, 1992;121.

Microsurgical Reconstruction of the Cancer Patient, edited by M.A. Schusterman.
Lippincott-Raven Publishers, Philadelphia © 1997.

6

Microneurovascular Reconstruction for Facial Reanimation

Geoffrey L. Robb

One of the most difficult challenges in the head and neck cancer patient is reconstruction of facial reanimation after paralysis of the facial nerve. Patients undergoing resections for extensive cancers involving the parotid gland or adjacent structures may require excision of the facial nerve when it is involved with the malignancy. In many cases, although the main trunk of the seventh nerve and the majority of the nerve divisions are sacrificed, a reasonable length of the proximal and distal nerves will be available for immediate interpositional nerve grafting, which should be the procedure of choice, if possible. In some cases, however, a more extensive resection is needed and the proximal or distal (or both) stumps of the facial nerve are unavailable for grafting. If the proximal facial nerve is missing, nerve grafting from an intact cranial motor nerve donor site can be an excellent reconstructive option. Two options are currently available. One site that has been used is the hypoglossal nerve. The successful functional outcomes of end-to-side hypoglossal-facial nerve neurorrhaphies with minimal to absent speech or swallowing morbidity demonstrate the excellent potential of achieving very good resting facial tone and nonspontaneous facial motion, with the disadvantage that the patient's facial movements based on the tongue can frequently be distracting (talking), unpredictable (chewing), and asymmetric to the normal side of the face. The second option, and the one that is preferable, is to use the contralateral facial nerve. This technique involves use of some of the distal branches of the facial nerve grafting across the face to power the affected side. The donor branches

G. L. Robb: Department of Plastic Surgery, The University of Texas, M.D. Anderson Cancer Center, Houston, Texas 77030.

used are those that are redundant, such as the buccal branches. The use of this technique allows for more spontaneous facial activity, and, by slightly weakening the contralateral facial nerve, better symmetry is obtained. Because of these benefits, this is the technique that is described in this chapter.

If the distal facial nerve segments or facial musculature are missing or the facial paralysis is beyond 18 months to 2 years in duration, facial motor unit replacement is necessary for rehabilitation of facial motion. This can be achieved directly through the use of pedicled regional muscle redirection to the paralyzed eye, upper lip, and commissure. These muscle transfers (temporalis or masseter) depend on trigeminal nerve activation for successful resting tone and nonspontaneous facial movement. These transfers are more prone to becoming only modestly active static commissure slings.

The facial motor replacement can often be more effectively accomplished in a one- or two-stage microneurovascular procedure using a free muscle transfer in conjunction with a cross-facial nerve graft (spontaneous facial motion) or a hypoglossal nerve transfer (nonspontaneous facial motion). It is a matter of surgical preference whether to use a first-stage cross-facial nerve graft and only inset the muscle transfer at a second stage when the axon crossing is complete versus insetting a muscle (rectus femoris) in one stage with a long enough nerve supply to act as a simultaneous cross-facial nerve graft, anticipating reinnervation of the muscle prior to muscle end-plate atrophy.

FACIAL PARALYSIS MORBIDITY

Following sacrifice of the facial nerve, patients typically endure an indefinite period of facial paralysis characterized by ipsilateral brow ptosis, eye irritation secondary to corneal dryness from incomplete eyelid closure, and chronic epiphora from loss of lower eyelid tone and support. An early priority for corneal protection and eye rehabilitation is most important to minimize potentially severe ocular complications that can occur in this paralytic state. Simple procedures such as taping the lid at night, in conjunction with adequate moisture from lubricating drops or ointment as needed, can help protect the cornea for an indefinite period. Some patients can develop more significant ocular problems from chronic corneal exposure that may require some form of lid surgery to improve corneal coverage, such as upper lid gold weight placement for lagophthalmos or lower lid tightening or cartilage strut placement for ectropion.

RECONSTRUCTIVE OPTIONS AND PATIENT SELECTION

A number of important considerations affect the selection of the reconstructive option for facial expression rehabilitation in the individual patient. In delayed cases, each patient with facial paralysis presents a unique example of an established seventh nerve functional and cosmetic deficiency. An accurate cranial nerve examination will document the current functional status of the facial nerve bilaterally, identifying any weakness or absence of function in relation to the patient's normal facial expression. Patients should be asked to describe the deficiency of facial motion that most bothers them and what their rehabilitative expectations are. This will help guide the surgeon as to the best course of reconstruction to offer the patient.

In both immediate and delayed cases, the patient's age and anticipated medical prognosis directly influence the decision regarding the extent of the reconstructive effort. Physical factors, such as the presence or absence of the main facial nerve trunk and the division branches, and the condition of the facial musculature and overlying facial soft tissues especially impact the possibilities for facial rehabilitation. If the paralysis is over 2 years old, the native facial musculature has atrophied such that simple nerve grafting will not be sufficient, and replacement of the motor units is necessary. Prior radiation will often mandate soft tissue replacement to provide a well-vascularized bed for nerve graft placement.

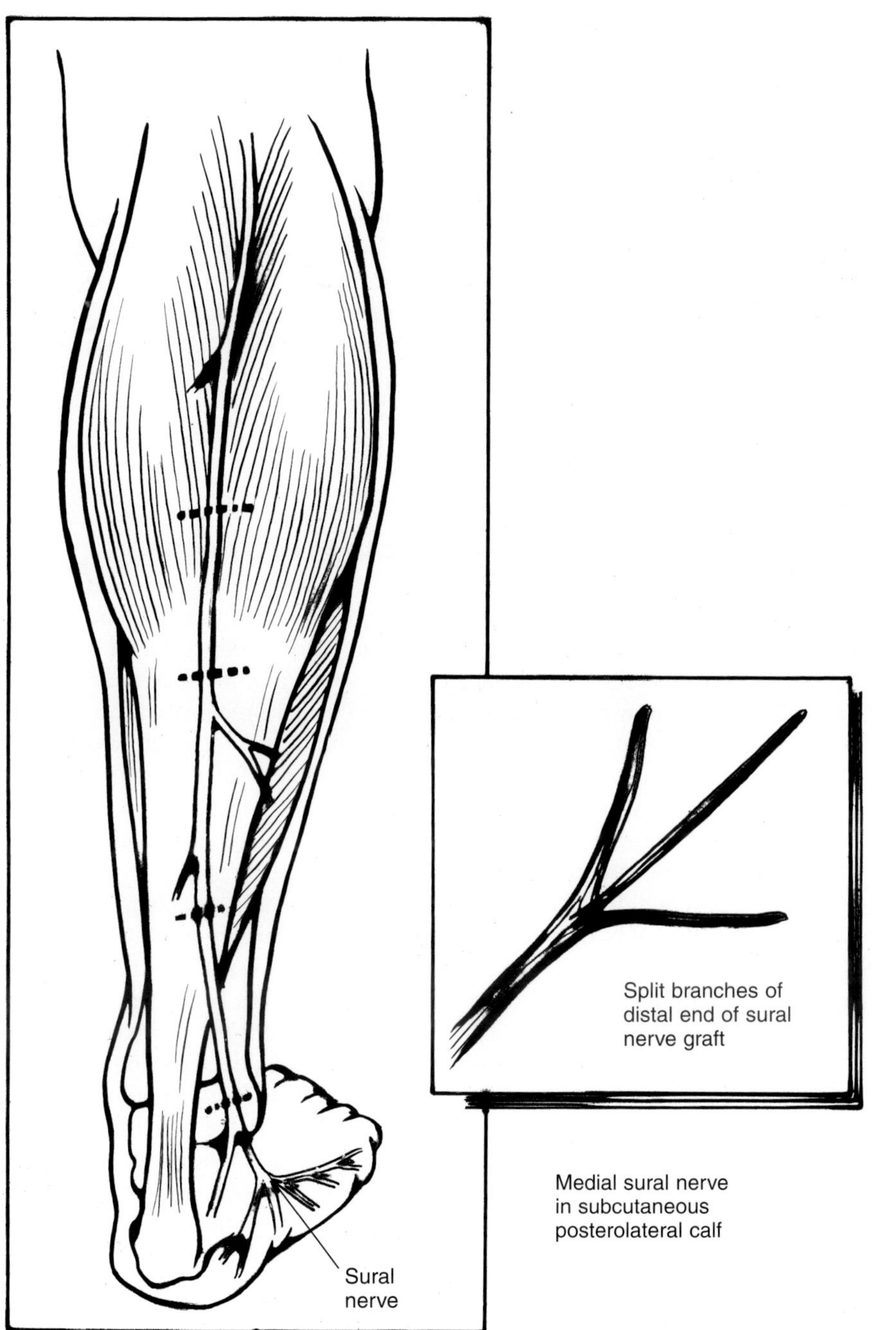

FIG. 1. Medial sural nerve in subcutaneous posterolateral calf. **Inset:** Split branches of distal end of sural nerve graft.

Reconstruction of the facial nerve paralysis involves either a dynamic or static solution (i.e., fascial sling), depending primarily on the desires of the patient and what can realistically be accomplished in the rehabilitation. In most cases of facial nerve deficiency, where possible, the reconstructive objective is dynamic functional recovery with spontaneous animation of the face, which can only be achieved using the facial nerve. However, clinical conditions can also occur in which no dynamic facial recovery may be possible. For example, if an advanced tumor requires a massive resection of the cheek, there may not be any facial muscles or even features left to reanimate. In such a case, static fascial or Gortex slings (WL Gore and Associates, Flagstaff, Arizona) placed within the cheek reconstruction can help maintain indefinite elevation of the oral commissure and minimize drooling from the loss of oral tone. The static sling can also be used as a temporizing functional and cosmetic aid in conjunction with a dynamic muscle procedure in which facial motion is anticipated in the future. Of course, aesthetic procedures can also be used to enhance the patient's overall recovery and facial rehabilitation.

MICRONEUROVASCULAR RECONSTRUCTION

Delayed lower facial spontaneous movement can also be the reanimation goal in other circumstances. In some situations, an immediate facial nerve reconstruction may not have been done for oncologic reasons, and the patient, as a head and neck cancer survivor, now presents for delayed facial nerve reconstruction. In other cases, primary nerve grafting may not have been successful in providing any spontaneous muscle activity, and the patient requests additional spontaneous facial rehabilitation. Many patients can also present with facial paralysis that has been chronic beyond several years in duration so that natural facial muscle reinnervation is beyond probable recovery. Of course, for any of these circumstances, a regional muscle transposition can be used for static facial support and dynamic movement, but no spontaneous facial activity can result.

Probably the most popular method currently used to restore spontaneous movement to the upper lip, alar base, and oral commissure complex (separate from the eye) and attain a reasonably symmetric smile in these situations is the staged free muscle transfer following cross-facial nerve grafts from the normal side of the face. To optimally attain spontaneous motion for the affected side, the opposite, healthy facial nerve is used as a donor for the nerve grafts. The reconstructive goal therefore becomes the development of static, resting mouth symmetry with the dynamic aspects of spontaneous, involuntary facial motion, such as smiling and laughing, made as symmetric as possible.

This one- or two-stage microneurovascular muscle transfer procedure, when successful, can accomplish several important aspects of the facial reconstruction simultaneously. Besides providing the oblique smile movement for the commissure complex in the lower face, the muscle is also perfectly located to add desirable subcutaneous bulk in the anterolateral cheek, which is otherwise atrophic following the facial nerve denervation. The surgical challenge is to avoid an excessive volume in the cheek while providing enough muscle power for adequate facial motion.

Many individual muscles have been described for this facial reanimation technique, including the latissimus dorsi, extensor digitorum brevis, pectoralis minor, serratus anterior, rectus abdominis, gracilis, and the rectus femoris (used for the one-stage procedure because of a long neural leash to act as a cross-facial graft). The gracilis is probably the preferred muscle for the two-stage transfer due to the ease of harvest, minimal donor site morbidity, and appropriate amount of muscle contraction attained with reinnervation, while using only a small section of the muscle to avoid cheek bulk.

FACIAL RECONSTRUCTION PLANNING

One of the most important aspects of the free tissue transfer reconstruction of the smile mechanism is the preoperative planning specific to the individual patient. After

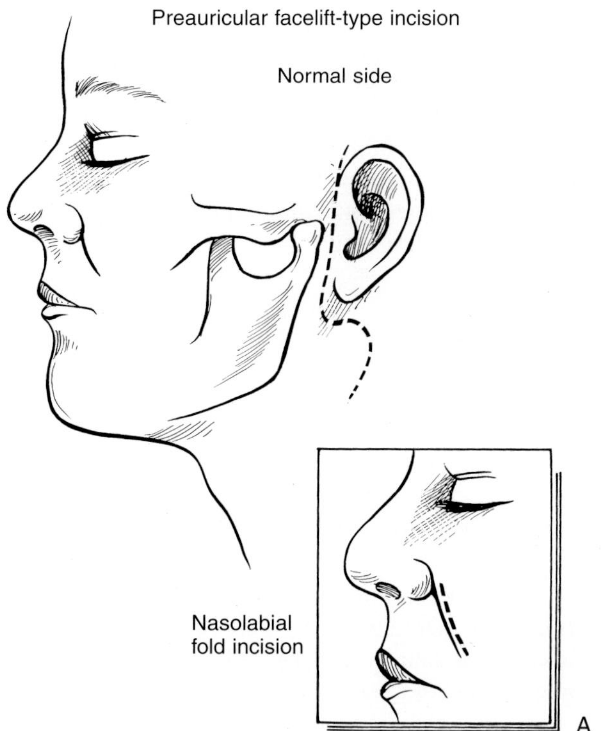

FIG. 2A. Preauricular facelift-type incision. **Inset:** Nasolabial fold incision.

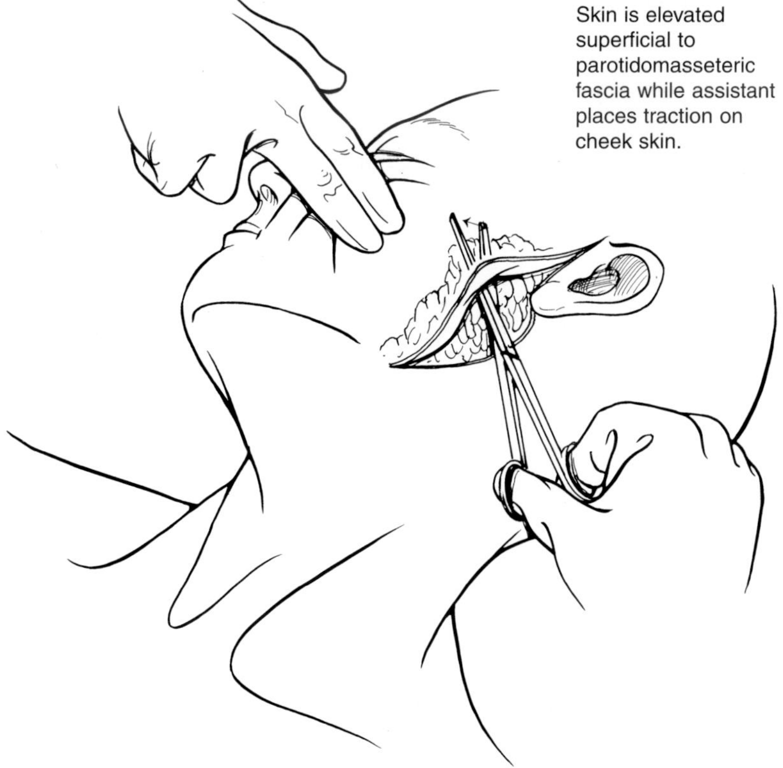

FIG. 2B. Preauricular skin is elevated superficial to parotidomasseteric fascia while assistant places traction on cheek skin.

the first priority of eye protection has been completed, most patients' next concern is lip and commissure symmetry, both at rest and when smiling. Planning is begun by selecting the method of innervation of the free muscle transfer. Appropriate innervation of the muscle may not result if a proximal facial nerve stump on the affected side is used, because multiple conflicting motor functions could be routed to the transferred muscle. If no more distal facial nerve stump such as the buccal branch is available on the affected side (not common in delayed reconstructions), the best motor nerve source is usually a commissure facial nerve branch on the normal side.

First Stage of Reconstruction

The first stage of the reconstruction is the placement of one or two cross-facial nerve grafts, either over or under the nose, in the upper lip, or below the lower lip. The nerve grafts are usually harvested from the posterior calf from the medial sural nerve, because a long nerve graft can be obtained with relatively little donor site morbidity (Fig. 1). The graft should be harvested through a stocking seam incision with direct exposure of the entire medial sural nerve. Each side branch is directly ligated with 4-0 silk, with a continuous effort to minimize stretching, overmanipulation, and desiccation of the nerve graft. This harvest can also be accomplished endoscopically through one or two small incisions with appropriate instruments to maintain an optical space and harvest the graft atraumatically. The donor site should be closed with a subcuticular suture technique to minimize incisional scarring.

The buccal facial nerve branches are identified distal to the parotid gland on the normal side, where several branches specific to the commissure or lateral upper lip can be sacrificed with no detectable functional loss. The approach can be either through a preauricular incision or more medially via a small incision in the nasolabial fold area, through which adequate exposure is much more difficult (Fig. 2A,B). Once the nerve branch exposure is accomplished, low-amperage stimulation allows the surgeon to explore and test the nerves multiple times, finally selecting the most appropriate nerve branches, considering size of the nerve and motor action accomplished, preferring the largest nerves with actual commissure or very lateral upper lip movement (Fig. 3A,B). Usually half of the branches peripheral to the parotid border for any particular function can be used as donor nerves without clinical functional loss. With this in mind, the microsurgeon should perform several cross-facial nerve grafts, in case one graft is not successful.

Generally two nerve grafts are used, each one to an isolated nerve donor on the normal side and then routed subcutaneously to the preauricular area of the normal side of the face, with a permanent large black suture tied at the end of the nerve to facilitate identification of the graft at the second-stage procedure. The subcutaneous nerve tunnel pathways should be initially infiltrated with epinephrine and small incisions made at the alar bases for the upper lip route or in the labiomental crease for the lower lip tunnel to facilitate the subcutaneous dissection and make it easier to pass the nerve gently across to the other cheek (Fig. 4A). A long, straight hemostat can be used to bluntly spread subcutaneously from the donor nerve area directly across, high on the upper lip or low on the lower lip to the opposite cheek area directly in front of the ear (Fig. 4B). With the nerve grafts reversed and in place through the subcutaneous tunnels, the neurorrhaphies can then be performed.

The neurorrhaphies between the nerve grafts and the donor facial nerve branches must be performed meticulously, under microscopic magnification, utilizing very small sutures (11-0). The most important technical consideration should be the absence of tension at the neurorrhaphy. The incisions are all closed in layers and the skin approximated with fine simple sutures. No drains are used for the face or leg. A compressive dressing is placed on the leg, secured with a 6-inch Ace bandage. A face-lift soft compression dressing is used overnight on the face and then discontinued.

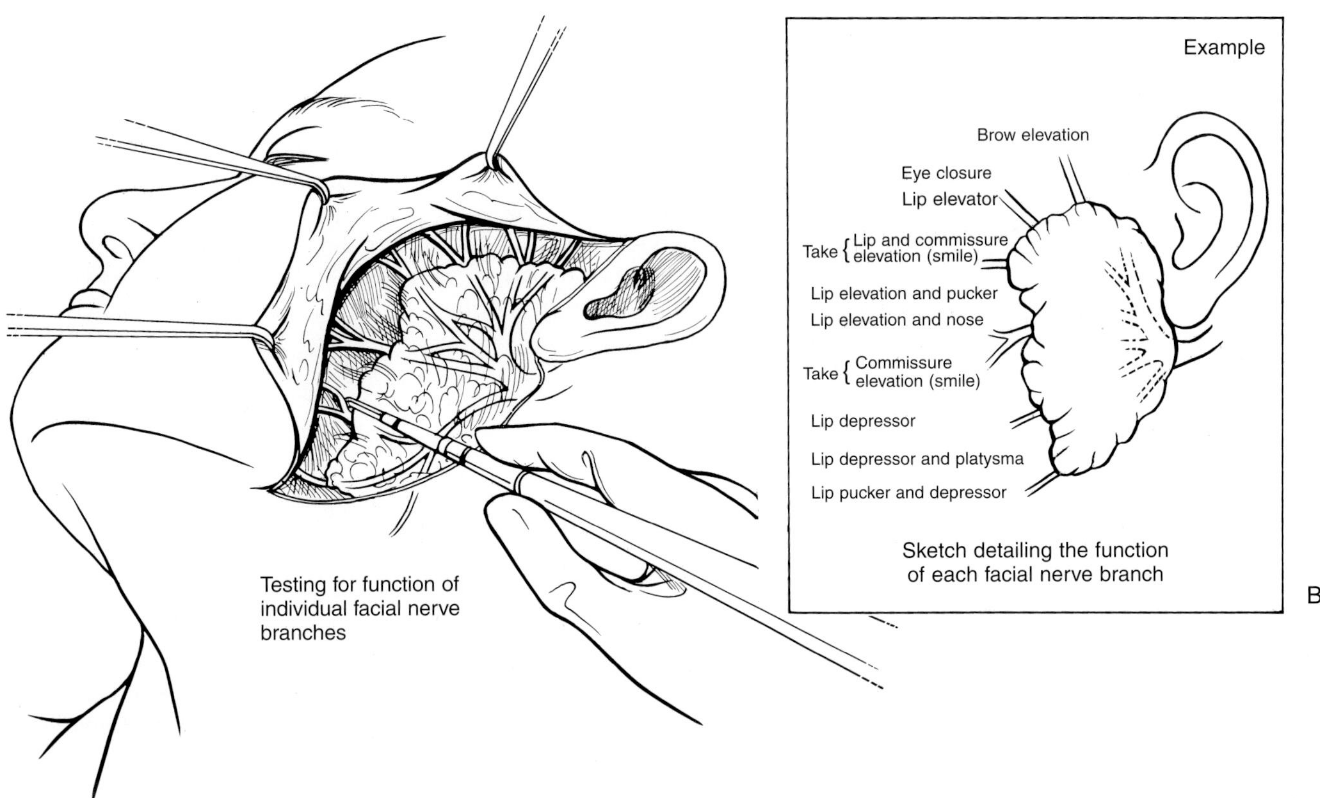

FIG. 3A,B. A: Testing function of individual facial nerve branches. **B:** Intraoperative sketch detailing the function of each facial nerve branch.

A delay of 9 to 12 months should be anticipated before sufficient nerve growth occurs to allow the second stage to be completed. As the nerve grows, the patient can usually feel a tingling sensation (Tinel's sign) when a finger is tapped along the course of the nerve graft as it courses to the affected side of the face. Most patients will feel the tingling directly where tapped along the course of the graft as well as some referred tingling simultaneously to the area of the neurorrhaphy. When the Tinel's sign is positive at the distal end of the nerve graft placed just anterior to the tragus, the patient is ready for the second stage, which is the free muscle transfer. The subsequent ability of the patient to achieve dynamic, spontaneous facial movement will then depend on the successful outcome of the microneurovascular muscle transfer to the cross-facial nerve grafts.

Second Stage of Reconstruction

The most important part of the preoperative evaluation for the second stage is the smile analysis. The smile shape and the direction vector of the commissure movement on the normal side should be closely analyzed to determine the best size and orientation of the muscle transfer on the paralyzed side. Indelible markings should be made on the face denoting the appropriate smile direction vectors, location of the nasolabial fold, and the intended position and extent of the muscle on the affected side. The end of the nerve graft as determined by the Tinel's sign should be marked. The location of the facial recipient vessels on the paralyzed side can also be marked from palpation or transcutaneous Doppler sonography.

The actual muscle should be short (4–7 cm) and it should have the ability to contract at least 1 to 2 cm. A reliable vascular pedicle of satisfactory diameter and length is necessary to improve the probability of a successful outcome. Currently, this single muscle transfer is restricted to the reconstruction of the lower face (smile complex), with the eye rehabilitation accomplished as previously described with local techniques to avoid the disturbing problem of facial synkinesis.

The muscle used for the facial reconstruction should ideally leave no significant donor site deficiency. In part because of minimal donor site morbidity, we prefer the gracilis muscle. It is easily accessible in the medial thigh, with adequate vascular pedicle length and diameter for microvascular anastomoses. The obturator nerve branches innervating the muscle are easily harvested and tested to determine which nerve branch controls the muscle around the pedicle entry and which is the portion of muscle to be isolated for transfer, along with the neurovascular bundle (Fig. 5).

At the surgical procedure, a cheek flap on the paralyzed side is elevated in the standard fashion from a preauricular incision to locate the end of the nerve graft with the black suture in the preauricular area (Fig. 6) and to prepare the medial cheek recipient area for the muscle flap. Once the nerve graft is identified, a portion of the distal graft is sent for a frozen section to identify viable peripheral nerve. The facial vessels in the submandibular space are isolated and prepared as recipient vessels in the usual fashion. In most cases, the vessel size match and location for the gracilis pedicle to the facial vessels is ideal.

A small portion of the gracilis muscle with its neurovascular pedicle is harvested simultaneously by a second surgical team. The medial circumflex femoral vascular pedicle of the gracilis is isolated between the adductor magnus and the adductor longus after the gracilis muscle has been dissected free from all of the surrounding soft tissues (Fig. 7A). There is more friable, fibrofatty tissue around the neurovascular pedicle, which obstructs easy visualization of the vessels and makes isolation of the nerve and vessels more difficult. Careful dissection with tenotomy scissors and the bipolar cautery allows safe separation of the obturator nerve and the vascular pedicle close to the muscle. The vascular pedicle seems particularly prone to spasm with manipulation, so early and generous application of papaverine is a recommended preventative measure. The vascular pedicle runs between the adductor group of muscles

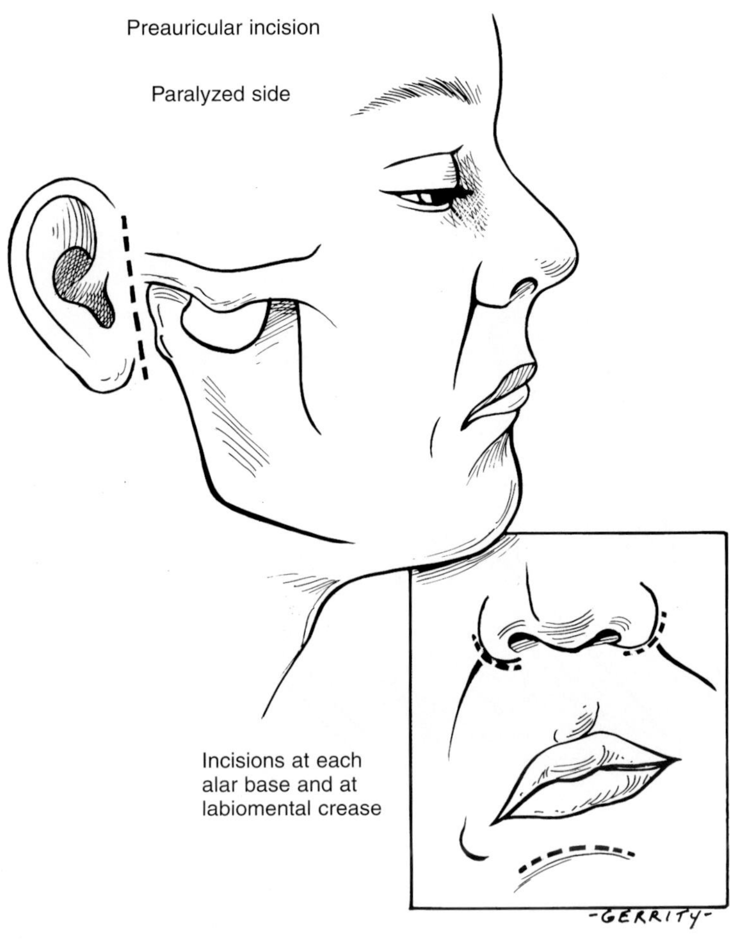

FIG. 4A. Paralyzed side: preauricular incision. **Inset:** Incisions at each alar base and labiomental crease.

A

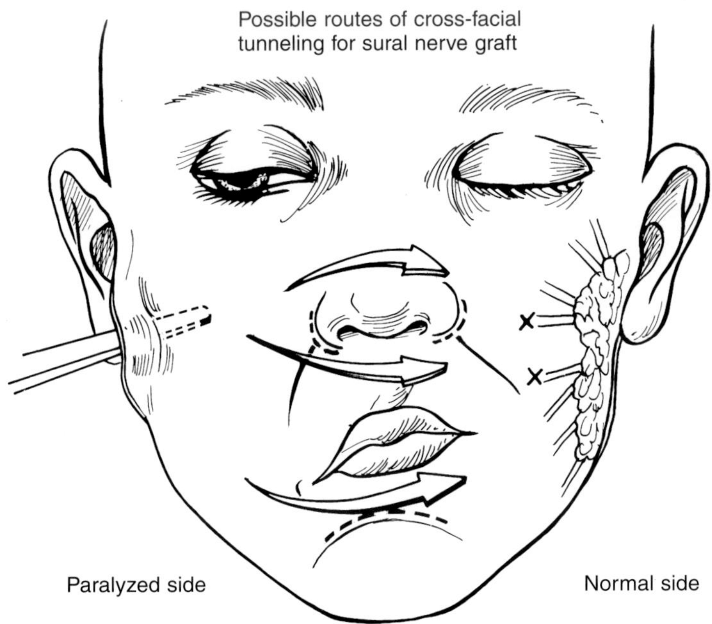

FIG. 4B. Possible routes of cross-facial nerve tunneling for sural nerve graft.

B

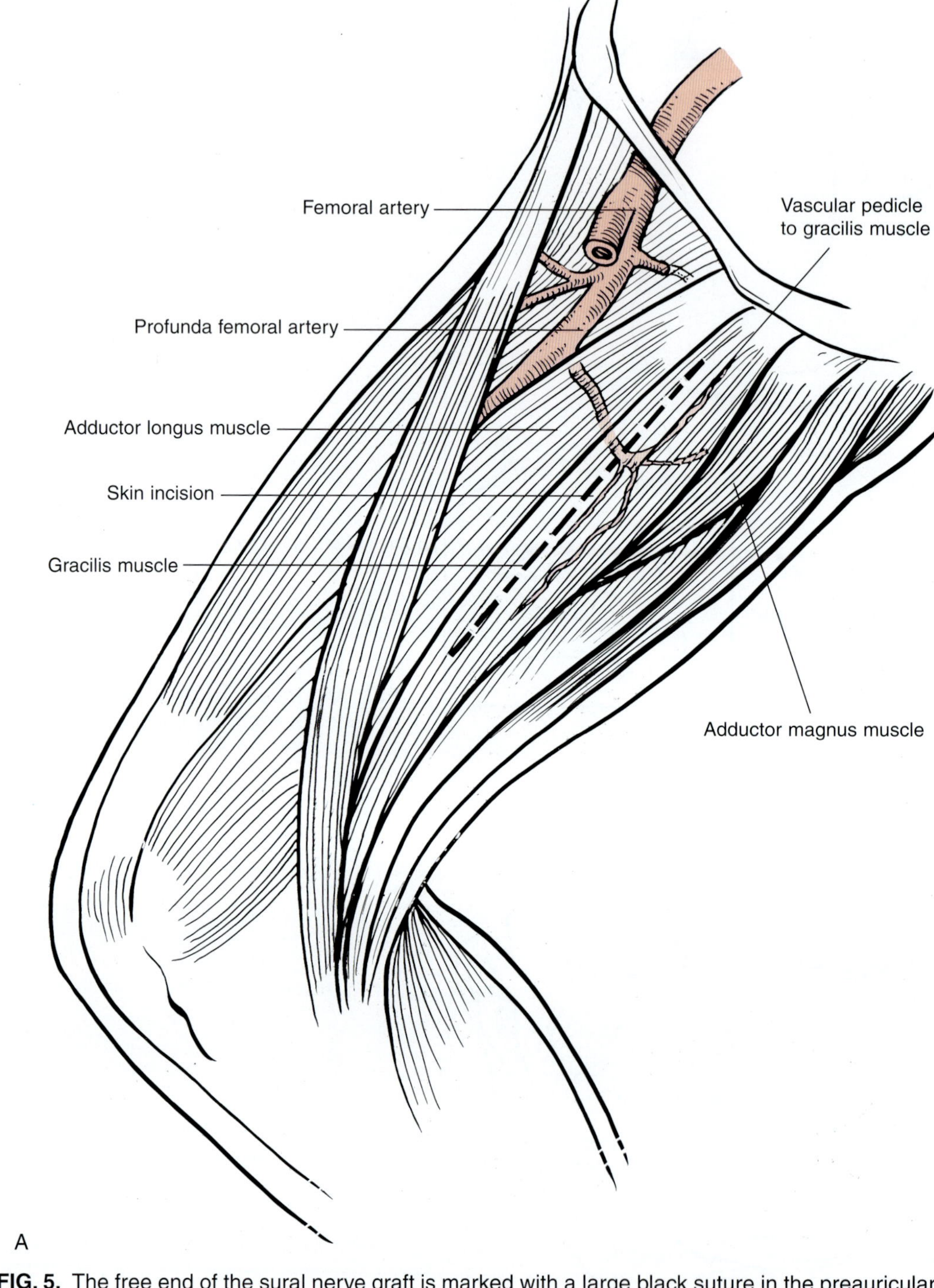

FIG. 5. The free end of the sural nerve graft is marked with a large black suture in the preauricular area of the normal side of the face for easy identification at the time of the muscle transplantation.

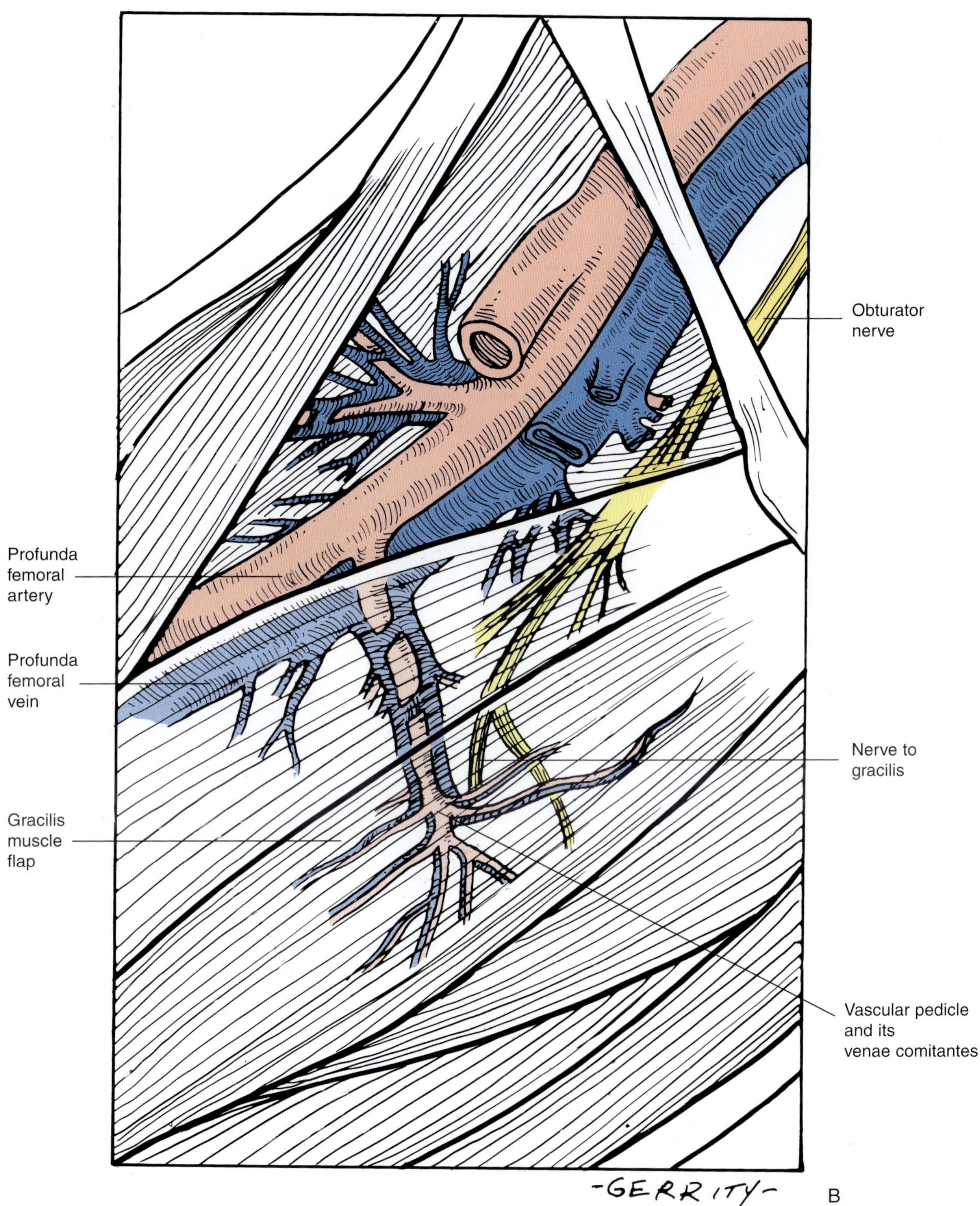

FIG. 5. *Continued.*

and immediately gives off a very short pedicle to the adductor longus muscle. If the interval between the adductor muscles is aggressively opened above and below the circumflex pedicle as it goes under the adductor longus, the exposure of the more proximal portion of the circumflex pedicle as it branches from the profunda femoris vessel is vastly improved. The ligation of the short muscle pedicle into the adductor longus should be very gingerly performed so that the main circumflex vessels are not injured (Fig. 7B). The remainder of the pedicle is then further isolated down to the profunda vessels and then left to perfuse the muscle.

Next, the obturator nerve is isolated and separated into branches, the fascicles of which are individually stimulated to identify the fascicles supplying the anteriormost portion of the muscle where the neurovascular pedicle enters (Fig. 7B). It is important to plan to harvest several centimeters of extra muscle and then trim any excess during the actual inset of the muscle, so that there is adequate pedicle length with some flexibility in the orientation of the muscle in the cheek. Prior to the final harvest of the gracilis muscle segment, sutures should be placed in the muscle edge at 1-cm intervals from the proximal to the distal end of the segment, so that this same resting length of the muscle can be restored in the transfer (Fig. 7C,D).

The donor muscle is then inset into the fibers of the orbicularis oris muscle above and below the oral commissure and into the lateral upper lip (Fig. 8A–C). A medial tongue of the donor muscle can be tailored into the alar base to facilitate resting alar symmetry and improve the patency of the ipsilateral nostril (Fig. 8C). Taking into account the shape of the smile on the normal side, the optimal locations of the muscle fixation points on the lip and alar base are determined by the shape of the mouth when traction is placed on the long ends of the fixation sutures (Fig. 8A). The malar end of the muscle flap is tested for the necessary length to reach the zygoma, with the excess trimmed. The bulk of the muscle is also assessed at this point and thinned appropriately from the side opposite the pedicle (Fig. 8C).

With the majority of the muscle flap manipulation completed, the vascular anastomoses of the flap pedicle to the facial recipient vessels are accomplished in an end-to-end fashion (Fig. 8D). The neurorrhaphy is completed with 11-0 nylon with the obturator nerve end as close to the muscle as possible to reduce reinnervation time (Fig. 8D). Monitoring of the transferred flap can then be set up with an internal 20-MHz Doppler probe. The probe is attached to the vein distal to the vascular anastomosis, providing continuous computerized monitoring of the flow through that vessel. If either the artery or vein of the pedicle is occluded, flow through the vein will cease, and the change in flow will be noted by the monitoring equipment.

The preoperative markings direct the final orientation of the muscle along the preplanned vector. The appropriate amount of pull is placed on the commissure and upper lip complex to achieve the correct mouth shape. Additional sutures may have to be placed to improve the contour of the upper lip in relation to the commissure. Deep orbicularis sutures seem to hold the upper lip at the correct angle when the commissure complex is pulled upward, without too much eversion of the lip, which predominates with more superficial orbicularis sutures. The malar attachments are then completed, restoring the original resting length of the muscle simply by measuring out the 1-cm intervals previously marked with silk sutures with slight tension on the muscle before the final inset suturing (Fig. 8D). There will intentionally result a notable overcorrection of the commissure height on the paralyzed side at the completion of the procedure. Some surgeons feel a temporary splint supporting the commissure aids in the early healing of the muscle flap, reducing the possibility of the sutures tearing through the muscle.

The perioral tone is immediately improved following surgery from the static sling effect. After approximately 6 months, some motion may be apparent at the commissure that progressively increases with time. If no motion is seen by 6 to 9 months postoperatively, an electromyogram (EMG) can be obtained to determine the electrophysiologic status of the muscle transfer. As the transplanted muscle begins to function, the patient can aid in the recovery of facial movement by performing facial exercises

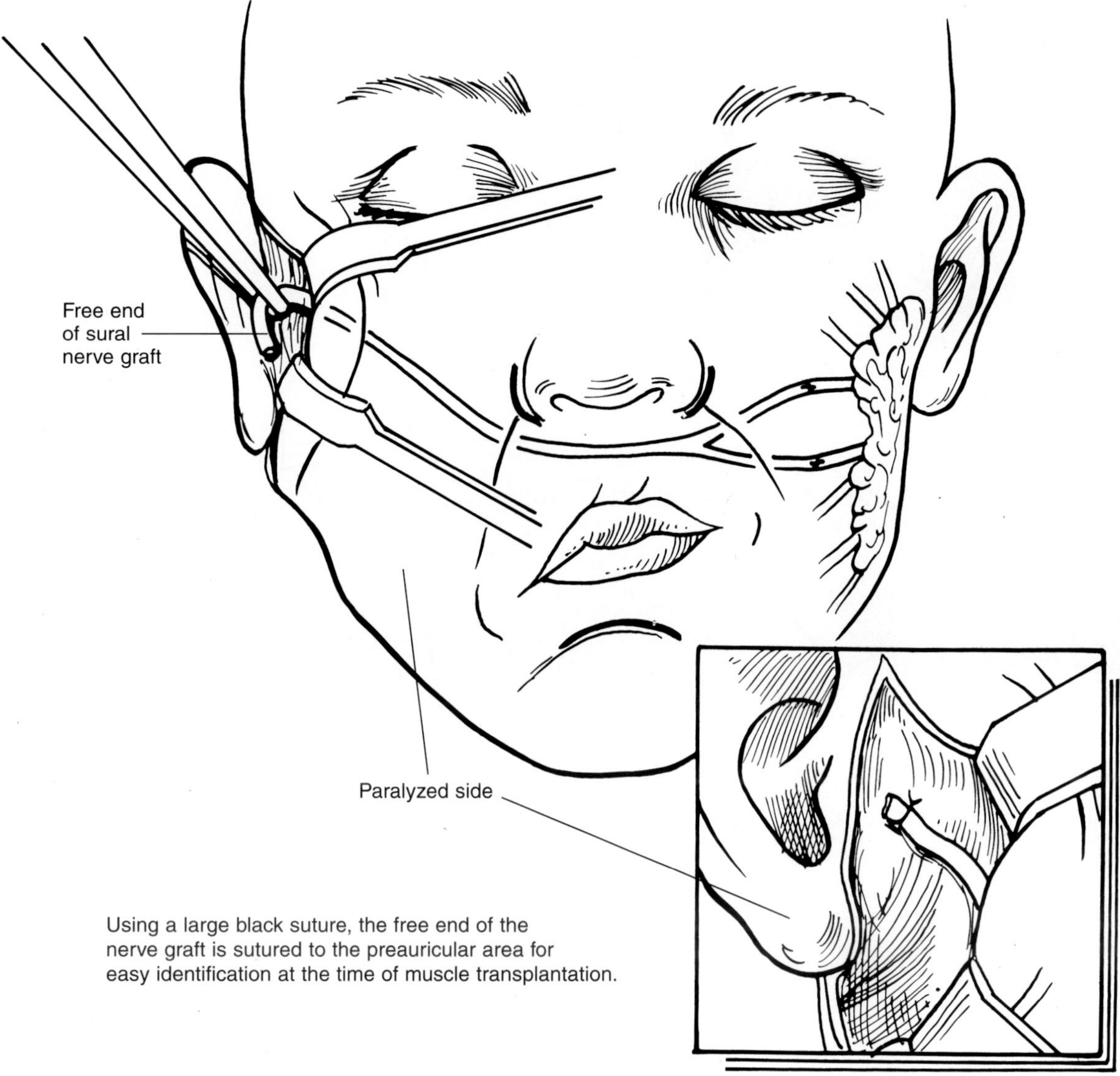

FIG. 6. Medial thigh incision over the gracilis muscle. **Inset:** Medial circumflex femoral vascular pedicle to the gracilis muscle, just inferior to the obturator nerve.

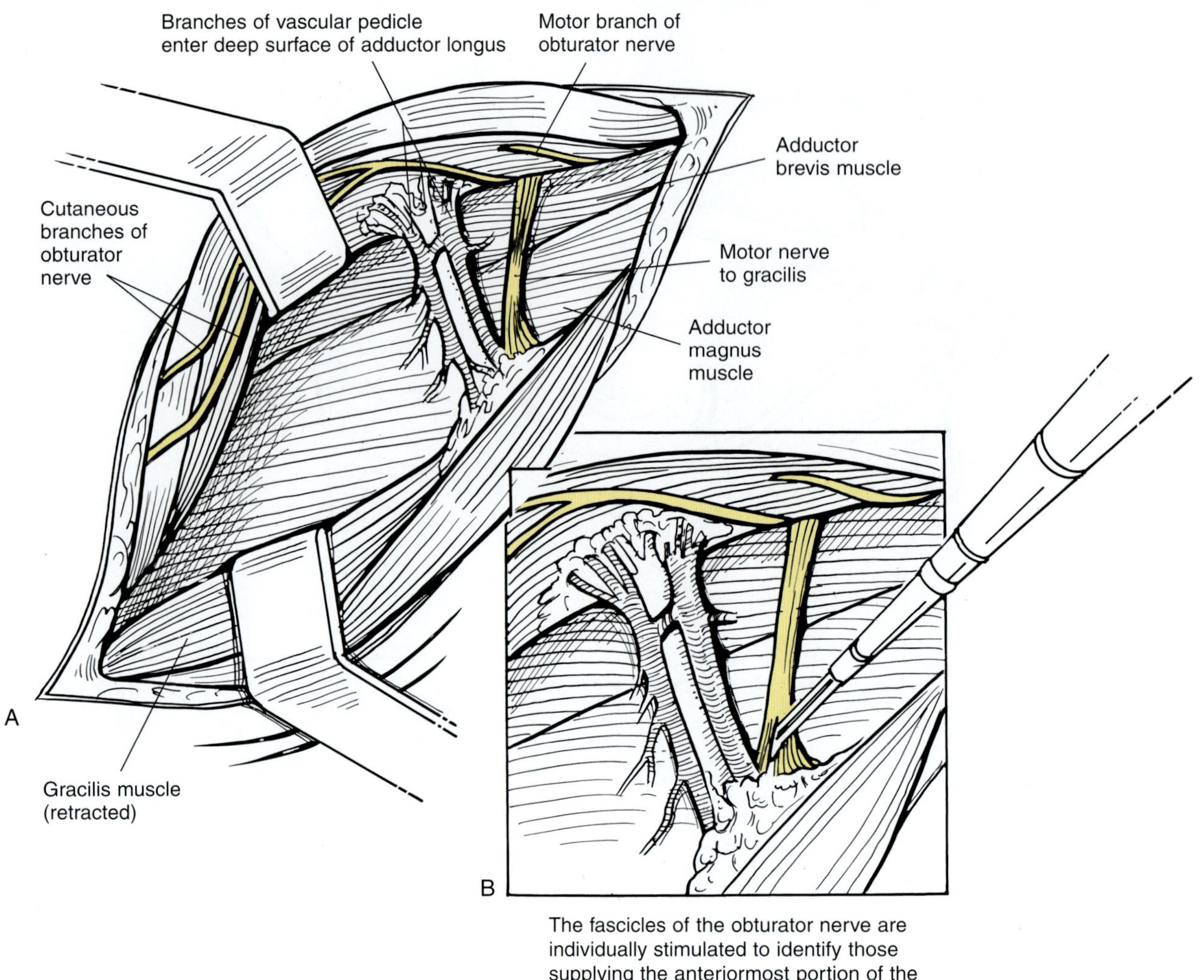

The fascicles of the obturator nerve are
individually stimulated to identify those
supplying the anteriormost portion of the
muscle, where the pedicle enters.

FIG. 7A,B. A: Relationship of the adductor longus and magnus muscles to the gracilis muscle neurovascular pedicle. **B:** The branches of the obturator nerve are individually stimulated to identify those innervating the anteriormost portion of the muscle where the neurovascular pedicle enters.

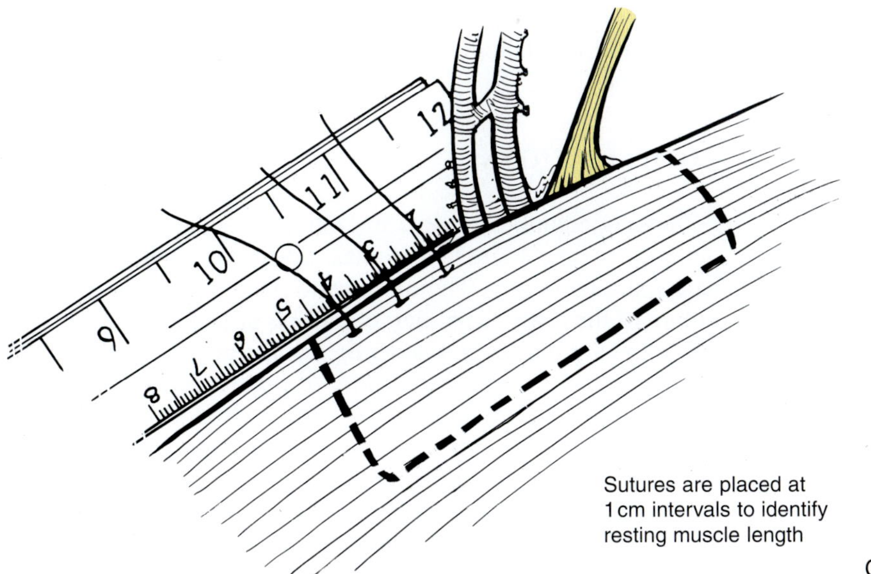

FIG. 7C. Sutures placed at 1 cm intervals to identify the resting muscle length.

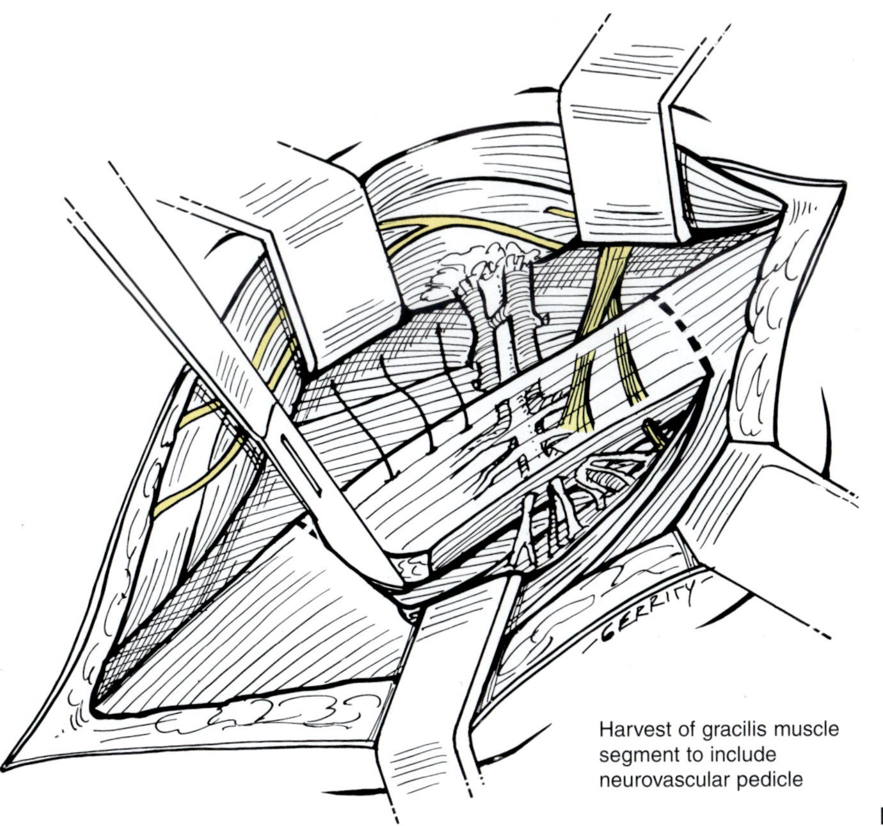

FIG. 7D. Harvest of the gracilis muscle segment to include the neurovascular pedicle.

in front of a mirror. These exercises are quite valuable in strengthening the muscle contraction and helping to achieve the final symmetric appearance of spontaneous expressions.

COMPLICATIONS

Surgical complications of microneurovascular facial reanimation, such as typical donor or recipient site hematomas, infections, or healing problems in general, fortunately, are quite rare. The more serious problems occasionally encountered relate to failure of the cross-facial nerve grafting or lack of movement of the transferred muscle following the second stage of reconstruction. These results would require facial exploration to determine the cause of failure, such as nerve graft neuroma formation or thrombosis of the muscle flap, which would usually be recognized early after its occurrence. Nerve graft revisions or redo flaps could be done in hopes of salvaging the facial reanimation effort in these situations.

Some patients might complain of excessive muscle bulk in the cheek following successful facial reanimation. The muscle lymphedema slowly resolves over a period of 3 to 6 months, and, in most cases, the muscle should probably be observed for a year prior to any consideration to thin or revise the flap, which may affect the functional animation outcome achieved up to that time.

SUMMARY

Facial nerve paralysis is a serious physical and emotional problem for the cancer patient. It holds a significant challenge for the surgeon and an uncertain future for the patient. The first priority, early in the course of the paralysis, is protection of the eye. Without eye protection measures, the risk of permanent damage to the vision and even complete loss of the eye is quite high. The next priority is to stabilize the lower face and eliminate facial sagging and, if reasonable, restore active volitional, spontaneous movement to the mouth. Numerous reconstructive options are available for the individual patient, ranging from simple to complex. The particular choice for the individual patient strongly depends on functional need, overall health and prognosis, and what the most reasonable approach is in relation to the patient's goals. Function and cosmesis must complement one another well to achieve a satisfactory outcome for what otherwise is a devastating condition.

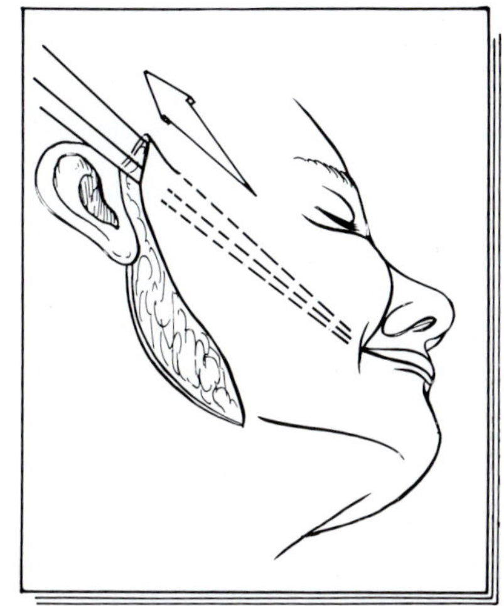

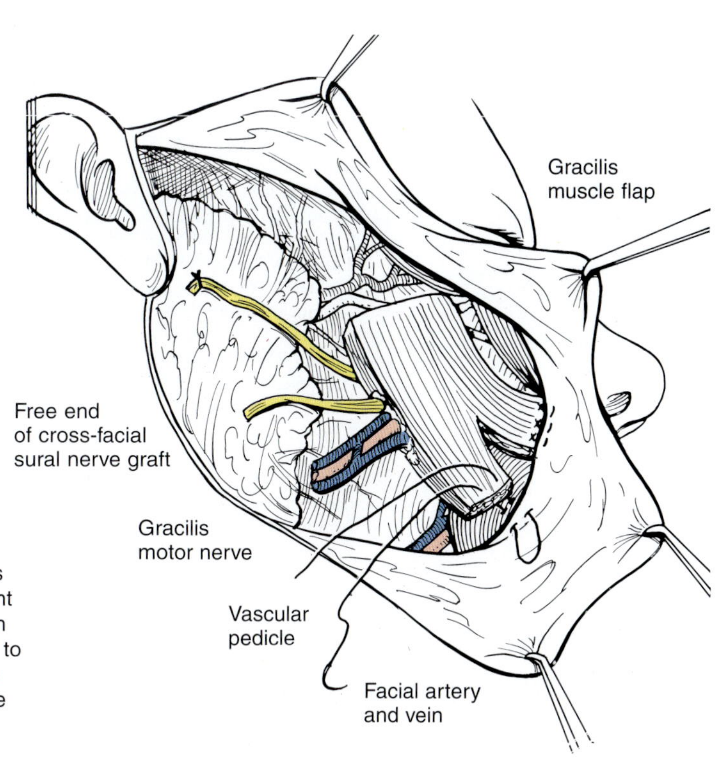

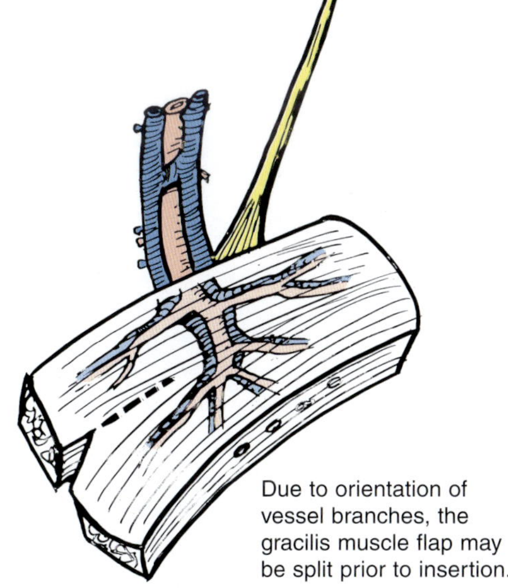

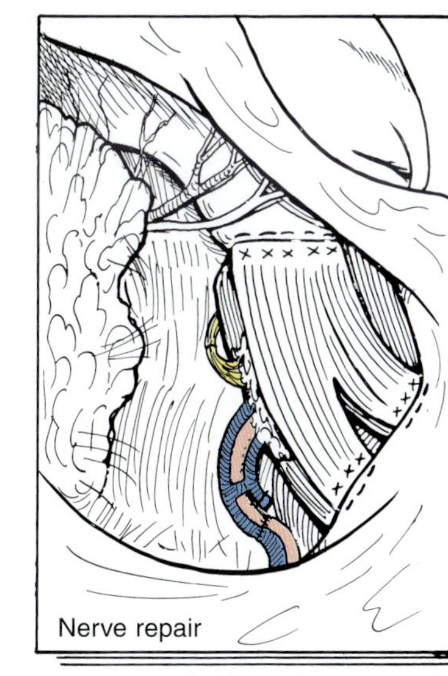

FIG. 8A–D. A: The ends of the insertion sutures for muscle placement are initially left long. Traction can then be applied to assess the resulting smile prior to the muscle transplantation. **B:** Due to the longitudinal orientation of the vessel branches, the gracilis muscle flap may be split as necessary prior to insertion. **C:** Inset of the muscle into the lip/alar base complex using mattress sutures. **D:** Upper muscle inset at the zygoma followed by end-to-end vessel anastomosis and nerve graft neurorrhaphy.

SELECTED READINGS

Fisch U. Facial nerve grafting. *Otolaryngol Clin North Am* 1974;7:517.

Freilinger G. A new technique to correct facial paralysis. *Plast Reconstr Surg* 1975;56:44.

Hamilton SGL, Terzis JK. Surgical anatomy of donor sites for free muscle transplantation to the paralyzed face. *Clin Plast Surg* 1984;11:197.

Harii K, Ohmori K, Torri S. Free gracilis muscle transplantation with microneurovascular anastomoses for the treatment of facial paralysis. *Plast Reconstr Surg* 1976;57:133.

Harrison D. The pectoralis minor vascularized muscle graft for the treatment of unilateral facial palsy. *Plast Reconstr Surg* 1985;75:206.

Manktelow R. Free muscle transplantation for facial paralysis. *Clin Plast Surg* 1984;11:215.

Manktelow RT. Facial paralysis reconstruction. In: Manktelow RT, ed. *Microvascular reconstruction.* New York: Springer-Verlag, 1986:128–144.

Millesi H. Nerve suture and grafting to restore the extra-temporal facial nerve. *Clin Plast Surg* 1979;6:333.

O'Brien BM, Franklin JD, Morrison WA. Cross-facial nerve grafts and microneurovascular free muscle transfer for long established facial palsy. *Br J Plast Surg* 1980;33:202.

Rubin LR. The anatomy of a smile: its importance in the treatment of facial paralysis. *Plast Reconstr Surg* 1974;53:384.

Rubin LR, ed. *Reanimation of the paralyzed face.* St. Louis: Mosby–Year Book, 1979.

Spector JG, Lee P, Peterin J, Roufa D. Facial nerve regeneration through autologous nerve grafts: a clinical and experimental study. *Laryngoscope* 1991;101:537.

Van Laeken N, Manktelow RT. Facial paralysis: principles of treatment. In: Georgiade GS, ed. *Textbook of plastic, maxillofacial and reconstructive surgery.* Philadelphia: Williams and Wilkins, 1992:581–595.

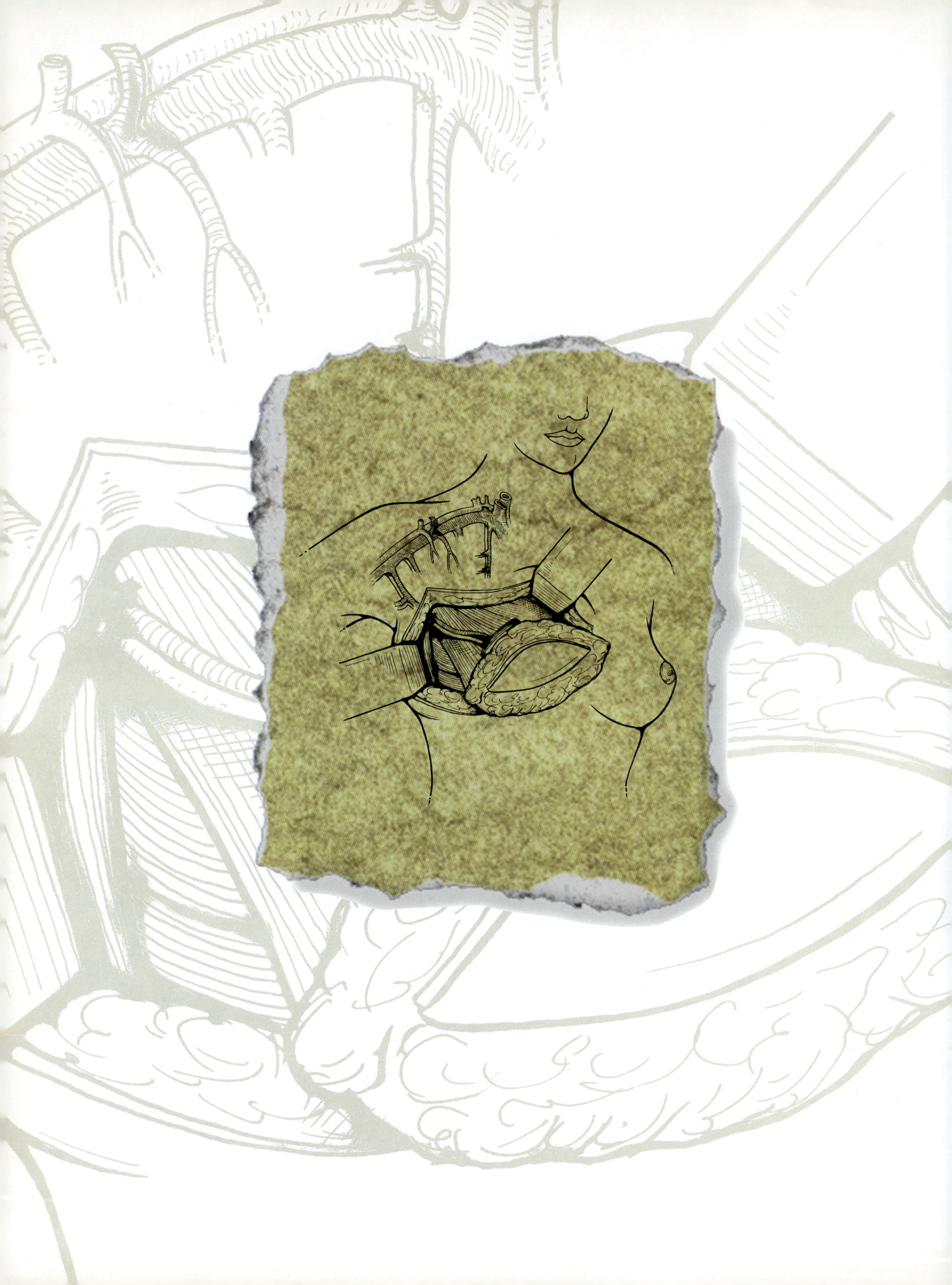

The Breast

Microsurgical Reconstruction of the Cancer Patient, edited by M.A. Schusterman.
Lippincott-Raven Publishers, Philadelphia © 1997.

7

General Principles of Free Flap Breast Reconstruction

Stephen S. Kroll

RATIONALE

Reconstruction of postmastectomy defects with free tissue transfer is a concept that often meets resistance from surgeons who are not used to working with free flaps on a regular basis. The need for microvascular surgery adds complexity to autologous tissue breast reconstruction, a process that already is far from simple. Why would a surgeon choose a free flap to transfer tissue to the breast when other options are available? The answer is in two parts: blood supply and donor site morbidity.

The most important reason to prefer free flaps for breast reconstruction is the improved blood supply to the flap. Using a pedicled transverse rectus abdominis myocutaneous (TRAM) flap, blood flow from the superior epigastric artery is attenuated by its need to pass through "choke vessels" in the muscular pedicle. Perfusion of the flap itself is indirect, and not always sufficient to ensure flap survival. In patients who smoke, partial flap loss after conventional TRAM flaps is sufficiently common that the double-pedicle technique is usually recommended, an alternative that significantly increases donor site morbidity. The use of a free flap eliminates the "choke vessel" problem because blood vessels that supply the flap directly are used as the pedicle. Provided that the anastomosis remains patent, blood supply is usually excellent and significant partial flap loss is rare, even in patients who smoke. The key to success is obviously a successful anastomosis, a goal that is manifestly achievable and one that is further addressed in subsequent chapters.

Another reason to use free flaps is the reduced donor site morbidity. When harvesting a pedicled TRAM flap, the function of at least one entire rectus abdominis muscle

S. S. Kroll: Department of Surgery, The University of Texas, M.D. Anderson Cancer Center, Houston, Texas 77030.

must be sacrificed. In contrast, when harvesting a free TRAM flap only a minimal amount of muscle tissue is removed, and the superior half of the rectus abdominis muscle is undisturbed. This minimizes postoperative pain and loss of muscle strength, so that most patients who undergo free TRAM flap surgery, even when it is bilateral, can perform situps once they have finished their convalescence. As a general principle, free flaps of all types, including those used for breast reconstruction, require sacrifice of only that muscle that surrounds the vascular pedicle of the flap, and loss of function in the donor site is correspondingly reduced.

FLAP CHOICE IN AUTOLOGOUS BREAST RECONSTRUCTION

The Free TRAM

There are a number of different flaps that can be used successfully to reconstruct a breast, but the most popular flap by far is the free TRAM flap. The free TRAM flap is technically easy to elevate, can be harvested with the patient in the supine position at the same time that the patient is undergoing her mastectomy, and has minimal donor site morbidity. Moreover, it is very pliable and compared with other alternatives is relatively easy to shape into a facsimile of a breast. The donor scars are symmetrical and well tolerated. Provided that both breasts are reconstructed simultaneously, the TRAM flap can be split in half and used to accomplish bilateral reconstruction. For these reasons, the free TRAM flap is the overwhelming favorite of patients and surgeons alike at the University of Texas M.D. Anderson Cancer Center, and the vast majority of our breast reconstructions are performed with that technique.

For patients who have already had a unilateral TRAM flap reconstruction, patients who have had a prior abdominoplasty, or for patients with a "pot-belly" habitus for whom sacrifice of rectus abdominis muscle and fascia would be unwise and who are not candidates for a TRAM flap, other alternatives must be considered. These alternatives include the superior and inferior gluteal free flaps, the lateral thigh free flap, and the Rubens fat pad free flap. The extended latissimus flap may be a good choice for selected patients even though it leaves a rather conspicuous donor site scar, but it is not a free flap and will not be discussed here. The remaining alternatives, however, are reviewed along with their respective advantages and disadvantages.

The Superior Gluteal Free Flap

The superior gluteal free flap has a donor scar that is covered by clothing and usually provides abundant tissue for breast reconstruction. It has the disadvantage of a very short vascular pedicle so that the use of a vein graft is almost always required, especially if the surgeon wishes to use the thoracodorsal vessels as recipients. Flap elevation cannot be performed with the patient in the true supine position, so that simultaneous bilateral reconstruction is difficult. The fatty tissue transferred with this flap is less malleable than that of a TRAM flap, so that shaping of the breast is more difficult. Elevation of the flap is technically more complex than elevation of a TRAM flap, with blood vessels being more fragile and having many branches. For these reasons, the superior gluteal free flap is not often used in our institution. Nevertheless, it must be said that some outstanding results have been obtained with it, and for some patients it remains an excellent choice.

The Inferior Gluteal Free Flap

The inferior gluteal free flap has some of the advantages of the superior gluteal free flap—adequate fatty tissue and a covered donor site—but without the disadvantage of a short vascular pedicle. In most cases, the pedicle is sufficiently long that a vein graft

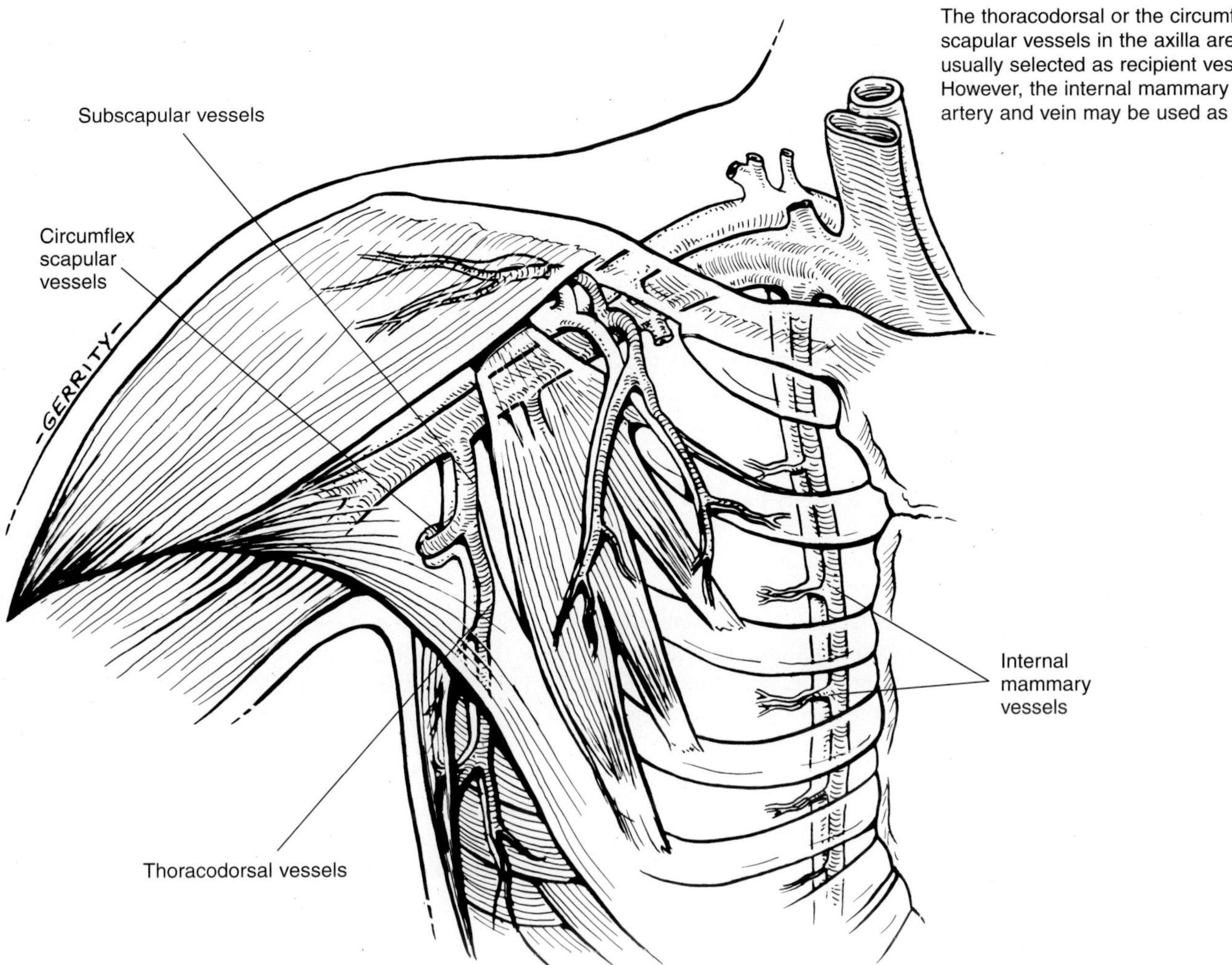

FIG. 1. Possible choices for recipient vessels for free flap breast reconstruction. The thoracodorsal vessels are usually the first choice, especially for free flap reconstruction.

is not required. For this reason, it is technically easier than the superior gluteal, and is therefore a preferable choice. As in the superior gluteal flap, the vein is fragile, and has many branches. The fatty tissue is less pliable than that of the TRAM flap, and positioning requirements are such that simultaneous bilateral reconstruction is difficult. Nevertheless, the technique is capable of yielding very satisfactory results and for some patients is an excellent choice.

The Transverse Lateral Thigh Flap

This is a modified tensor fascia lata free flap that can be used for patients who have excess tissue in the "saddlebag" area of the lateral thigh. It can be successful in creating a good breast mound, but the donor site scars are significant and not easily hidden. Because of this, the flap is rarely selected unless the patient has an unusual excess of lateral thigh tissue and is also willing to accept the visible donor scar.

The Rubens Fat Pad Free Flap

This method of autogenous breast reconstruction, described by Hartrampf and colleagues, uses redundant fatty tissue in the flank vascularized by the deep circumflex iliac vessels. It is essentially an iliac crest composite free flap, as used for mandibular reconstruction, but without the bone. The donor scar is relatively inconspicuous, and the fatty tissue is pliable, as in the TRAM flap. Bilateral reconstruction is much easier than with the gluteal flaps, and the pedicle is of adequate length. The main benefit to the Rubens flap is the donor site aesthetics, which, like the TRAM flap but unlike the gluteal or thigh flaps, are often enhanced due to the flap harvest. In addition, previous abdominoplasty or TRAM flap does not preclude use of the Rubens flap. For these reasons, the Rubens flap has become our alternative of choice to the TRAM flap for autogenous tissue reconstruction of the breast.

PATIENT EVALUATION

Most patients who consult a plastic surgeon about breast reconstruction do not have to be convinced of its value. They wish to avoid deformity, avoid the need for an external prosthesis, and be able to wear regular clothing. Nevertheless, it should be clearly understood by the patient from the beginning that the goal of the surgeon is to make the patient look normal in her clothing, not in the nude. Although the surgeon's real goal may well be to make the patient look as normal as possible in the nude, the promised goal should be more limited and unrealistic expectations discouraged. Patients are never unhappy when they are given a result better than promised, while the reverse can lead to disappointment and unhappiness.

Most women with breast cancer are candidates for reconstruction, but not every patient is a candidate for a free flap. Patients who are very obese will have a high complication rate, and for them it is often preferable to use a simpler technique like the extended latissimus dorsi flap, accepting the scar on the back as the price of a reconstructed breast. For patients who are older or in poor health, the long-term advantages of autogenous tissue reconstruction may not be pertinent, and an implant-based reconstruction may be preferable.

Cigarette smoking is not a contraindication to breast reconstruction with a free flap. In fact, smokers have far less trouble with flap survival after a free TRAM flap than when a conventional TRAM flap has been performed, so a positive smoking history can be an indication for use of a free TRAM. Smoking does increase the risk of necrosis in the umbilicus, abdominoplasty flap, and mastectomy flaps, however; patients should be warned about this prior to surgery. The presence of moderate obesity, although it does increase the risk of minor complications, is also not a contraindica-

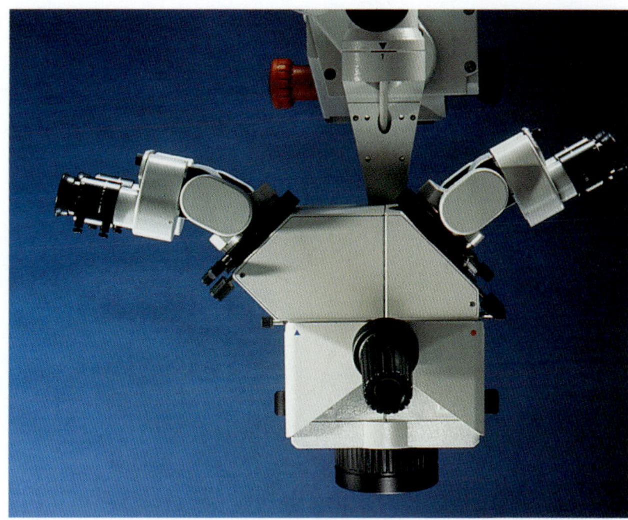

FIG. 2. The Wild Leitz 680 microscope.

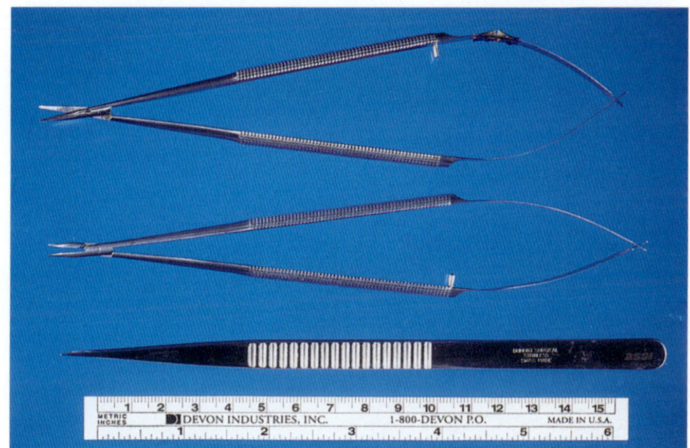

FIG. 3. Long microsurgical instruments 15 cm in length are necessary to perform the anastomosis deep in the axilla.

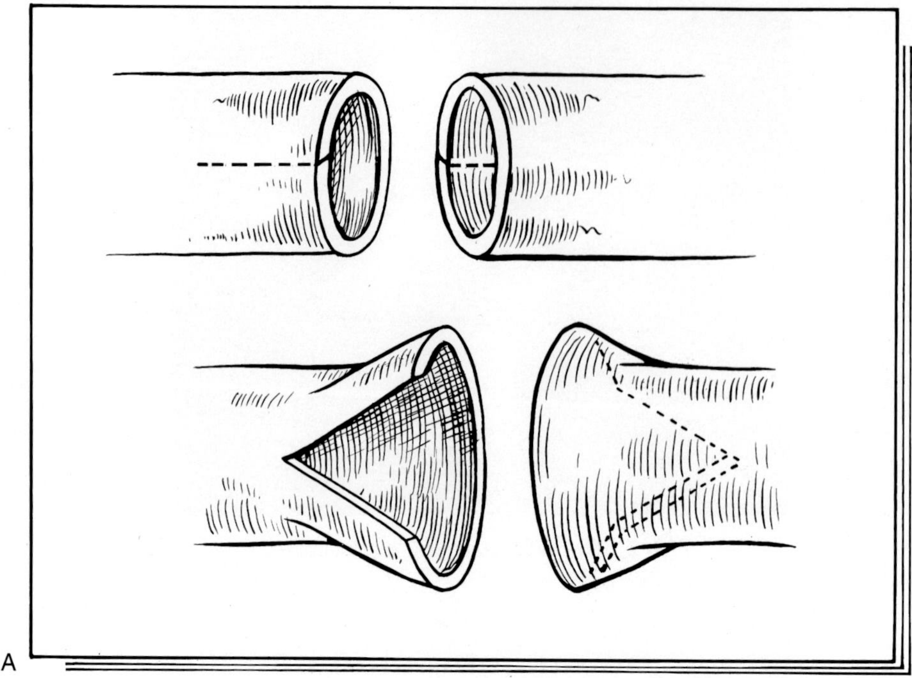

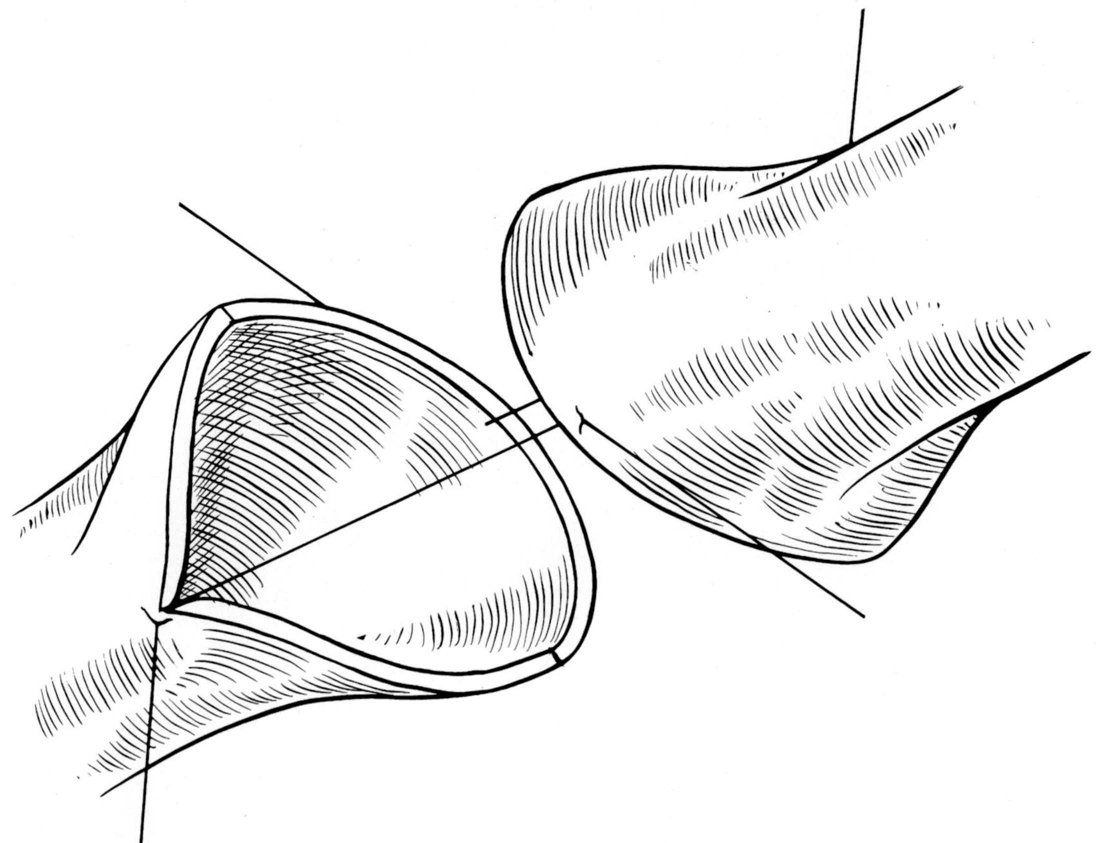

FIG. 4A–D. An end-to-end spatulated anastomosis is performed using two running sutures as the preferred technique.

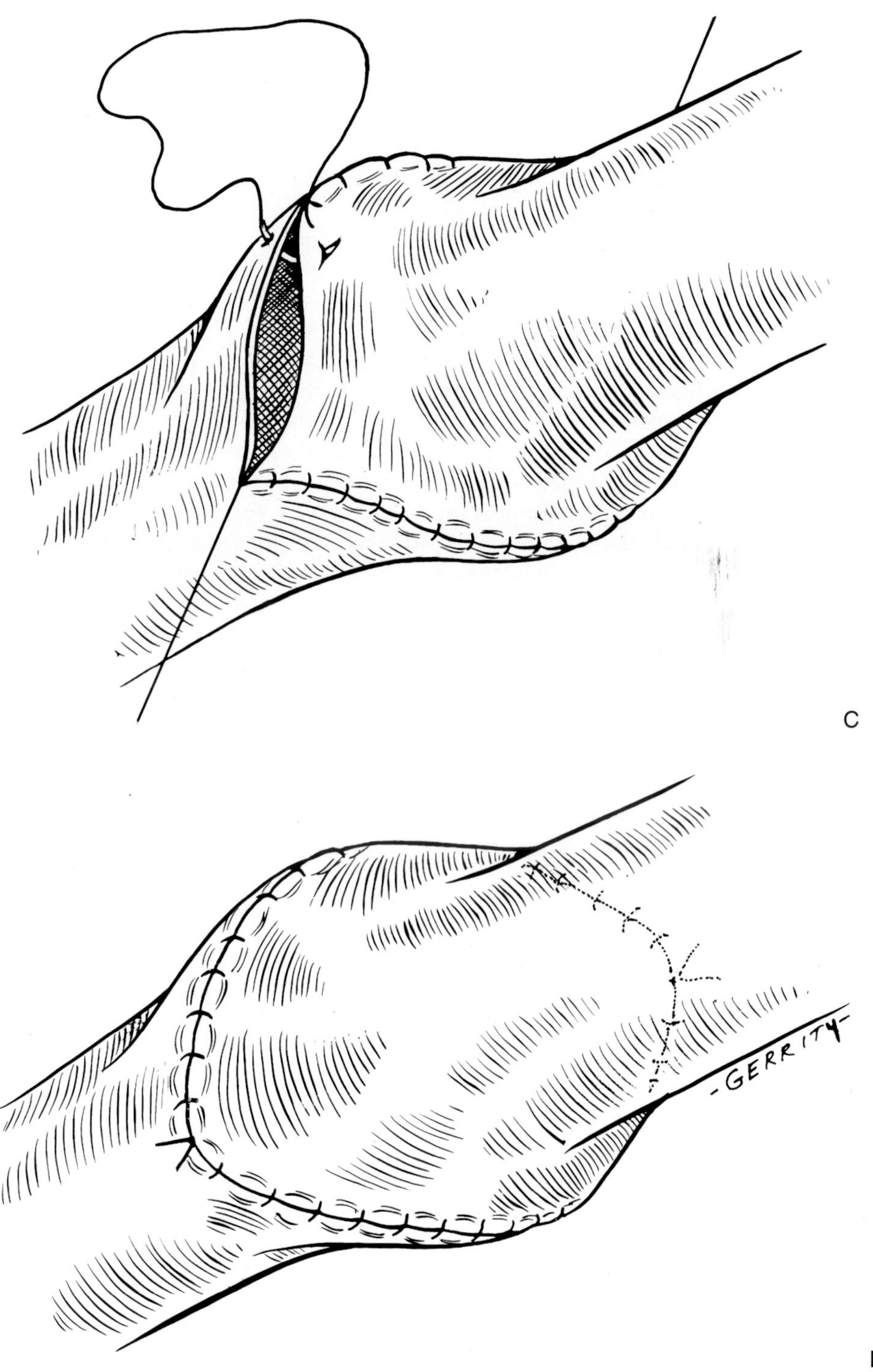

FIG. 4A–D. *Continued.*

tion to free flap reconstruction. Most such patients will get satisfactory results, albeit with more effort than would be required to reconstruct a thin patient. Extremely thin patients may also be candidates for free flap reconstruction. Although there is less donor tissue available in such patients, they usually have small breasts so less tissue is required. Especially if a free TRAM flap is used, the excellent circulation allows the flap to be extended laterally as far as necessary to provide sufficient tissue to reconstruct one or even two breasts.

CHOICE OF RECIPIENT VESSELS

The choices available for recipient vessels are the thoracodorsal vessels, the internal mammary vessels, and the axillary vessels (Fig. 1). Our recipient vessels of choice are the thoracodorsal vessels, because they are almost always present and of adequate caliber. In the case of immediate reconstruction, the vessels are often exposed by an axillary dissection, facilitating execution of a free flap. In candidates for delayed reconstruction, if the patient has had a previous axillary dissection the surgeon should palpate the latissimus muscle while the patient contracts it, to see if it is innervated. If the nerve is functioning, the thoracodorsal vessels will usually be intact and a free flap can be planned. Even so, the decision to commit the patient to a free flap (by dividing the rectus abdominis muscle superiorly, for example) should not be made irrevocably until the surgeon has confirmed the presence of recipient vessels in the operating room. If the thoracodorsal vessels are inadequate, use of the internal mammary vessels can be attempted. The internal mammary artery is usually present and satisfactory, but the vein may be very small and for this reason the internal mammary vessels are not usually our first choice as recipient vessels. If both the thoracodorsal and internal mammary vessels are not available, then one may choose to use the axillary vessels. These vessels are usually accessible since the axillary dissection stops at the inferior aspect of the axillary vein. One needs to use caution when dissecting the artery to avoid injury to the branches of the brachial plexus. Although the pedicle of the free TRAM is sometimes long enough to reach the axillary vessels, if any of the other flaps are used a vein graft will be required.

Required Equipment

The availability of good equipment contributes significantly to achieving success with free flaps. A high-quality microscope with good optics and light source, such as the Wild Leitz 680 microscope, is essential (Fig. 2). The longer objective lens (250 mm) is necessary due to the deepness of the axilla in which the anastomosis is often performed. Although there are reports of good results using only loupe magnification, our experience has been that visualization with the microscope is far superior and that when performing an anastomosis on very small vessels, in particular, use of an operating microscope is vastly preferable. Loupes are necessary, however, for dissection of the recipient vessels in the axilla. We use 3.5× or 4.5× loupes for this purpose, and have found either magnification satisfactory.

The availability of microsurgical instruments is obviously a prerequisite for microvascular surgery. Long (15 cm) instruments are essential to reach sufficiently far into the axilla (Fig. 3). It is helpful to have several extra pairs of fine jeweler's forceps because their tips become damaged very easily, rendering them useless. Fortunately, jeweler's forceps are inexpensive, so maintaining a supply of extra pairs is not burdensome.

For the overwhelming majority of our microvascular anastomoses, we use 9-0 nylon suture. If the vessel walls are thickened with plaque or calcifications, we substitute 8-0 nylon. If the vessels are very small (in the range of 1 mm) we use 10-0 suture instead. An end-to-end spatulated anastomosis is performed using a running technique

(Fig. 4A–D). We have used coupling devices, for venous anastomoses particularly, but most surgeons in our group continue to prefer suture anastomoses.

Operating Room Setup

If reconstruction is to be immediate, the patient must be supine on the operating room table with the anesthesiologist at the head. The arms are extended laterally on arm boards, which must be positioned high enough that the surgeon has access to the axilla, but not so high that the brachial plexus is stretched. If there is foam padding under the axilla, it should be cut away sufficiently that it does not impede the surgeon's access. The patient should be placed symmetrically on the table, straight enough so that symmetry will be maintained when the back is elevated to the sitting position. The table must be capable of sitting the patient nearly upright, so that ptosis can be checked while the breast is being shaped. The table should also be capable of being "banked" to the right or the left like an airplane, to improve visualization of the axilla during the anastomosis.

If a gluteal flap is being performed, the surgeon must be able to access both the breast and the buttock. This is accomplished by having the patient supine, but with the legs crossed and one hip elevated. The torso will not remain straight, but the table can be "banked" toward the mastectomy side to improve access to the breast, then away from it to gain access to the buttock later in the procedure.

Regardless of what technique is used, we recommend the use of antiembolic ankle boots during and after the surgery to reduce the risk of deep venous thrombosis.

Postoperative Monitoring

Postoperative monitoring is an important part of free tissue transfer. The majority of thrombotic events occur during the first three days, so we monitor our flaps hourly during that period. Clinical monitoring by an experienced nurse is crucial, so that the flap can be rapidly explored if color or temperature changes suggest obstruction of the pedicle. In addition, Doppler signals are measured at least hourly. We prefer the simplicity of the hand-held pencil Doppler if there is a good signal available on the exposed skin paddle; otherwise, a laser Doppler is used. If there is no exposed skin paddle, a continuous buried 20-MHz Doppler probe can be used, but this is required only rarely for reconstruction of the breast.

Regardless of what technique is used to monitor the flap, it is essential that the flap be explored rapidly if flap changes suggest possible vascular occlusion. If there is doubt about flap perfusion, explore the anastomosis. Flap salvage is possible only through early intervention, and it is better to perform many unnecessary explorations than to not perform one that was truly necessary, and thereby lose a flap. Free flap breast reconstruction can be highly rewarding for patients and their surgeons alike, but only if a high success rate is maintained, and failures remain rare.

SELECTED READINGS

Codner MA, Nahai F. The gluteal free flap breast reconstruction: making it work. *Clin Plast Surg* 1994;21: 289–296.

Elliott LF, Beegle PH, Hartrampf CR Jr. The lateral transverse thigh free flap: an alternative for autogenous-tissue breast reconstruction. *Plast Reconstr Surg* 1990;85:169–181.

Grotting JC, Urist MM, Maddox WA, Vasconez LO. Conventional TRAM flap versus free microsurgical TRAM flap for immediate breast reconstruction. *Plast Reconstr Surg* 1989;83:842–844.

Hartrampf CR Jr, Noel RT, Drazan L, Elliott LF, Bennett GK, Beegle PH. Rubens fat pad for breast reconstruction: a peri-iliac soft-tissue free flap. *Plast Reconstr Surg* 1994;93:402–407.

Hidalgo DA, Jones CS. The role of emergent exploration in free-tissue transfer: a review of 150 consecutive cases. *Plast Reconstr Surg* 1990;86:492–498.

Holmstrom H. The free abdominoplasty flap and its use in breast reconstruction. *Scand J Plast Reconstr Surg* 1979;13:423.

Ishii CH, Bostwick J, Raine TJ, Coleman JJ, Hester TR. Double-pedicle transverse rectus abdominis myocutaneous flap for unilateral breast and chest-wall reconstruction. *Plast Reconstr Surg* 1985;76:901–907.

Kroll SS, Schusterman MA, Reece GP, Miller MJ, Robb GL, Evans GRD. Abdominal wall strength, bulging, and hernia after TRAM flap breast reconstruction. *Plast Reconstr Surg* 1995;96:616–619.

McCraw JB, Papp C, Edwards A, McMellin A. The autogenous latissimus breast reconstruction. *Clin Plast Surg* 1994;21:279–288.

Moon HK, Taylor GI. The vascular anatomy of rectus abdominis musculocutaneous flaps based on the deep superior epigastric system. *Plast Reconstr Surg* 1988;82:815–829.

Nahai F. Inferior gluteus maximus musculocutaneous flap for breast reconstruction. *Perspect Plast Surg* 1992; 6:65.

Schusterman MA, Kroll SS, Miller MJ, et al. The free TRAM flap for breast reconstruction: a single center's experience with 211 consecutive cases. *Ann Plast Surg* 1994;32:234–242.

Schusterman MA, Kroll SS, Weldon ME. Immediate breast reconstruction: why the free TRAM over the conventional TRAM flap? *Plast Reconstr Surg* 1992;90:255–262.

Shaw WW. Breast reconstruction by superior gluteal microvascular free flaps without silicone implants. *Plast Reconstr Surg* 1983;72:490.

Shaw WW. Microvascular free flap breast reconstruction. *Clin Plast Surg* 1984;11:333–341.

Swartz WM, Izquierdo R, Miller MJ. Implantable venous Doppler microvascular monitoring: laboratory investigation and clinical results. *Plast Reconstr Surg* 1994;93:152–163.

Wagner DS, Michelow BJ, Hartrampf CR Jr. Double-pedicle TRAM flap for unilateral breast reconstruction. *Plast Reconstr Surg* 1991;88:987–997.

Microsurgical Reconstruction of the Cancer Patient, edited by M.A. Schusterman.
Lippincott-Raven Publishers, Philadelphia © 1997.

8

Free Transverse Rectus Abdominis Myocutaneous Flap for Breast Reconstruction

Mark A. Schusterman

The development of the transverse rectus abdominis myocutaneous (TRAM) flap allowed for routine postmastectomy breast reconstruction using autogenous tissue. As originally described, the TRAM flap consisted of the rectus abdominis muscle and lower abdominal skin perfused by the deep superior epigastric vessel via the periumbilical musculocutaneous perforators. Despite widespread acceptance of this flap, partial flap necrosis due to flap ischemia and lower abdominal weakness were consistent problems. Anatomical studies have demonstrated that the dominant blood supply of the lower abdominal skin comes actually from the inferior system rather than the superior system, so in theory an improvement in blood supply could be realized if the flap were based on the deep inferior epigastric vessels (Fig. 1). Use of the inferior system required transfer of the tissue as a free flap, which caused concern among some surgeons about the possible increase in risk of total flap loss due to vessel thrombosis, a risk that was low to negligible with the pedicled TRAM flap. If the free TRAM flap could be transferred with a vessel patency rate approaching 100%, this would then be the desired method of breast reconstruction. This chapter discusses and illustrates our method for transfer of the free TRAM flap, which has a success rate in our hands of more than 99%.

M. A. Schusterman: Department of Plastic Surgery, The University of Texas, M.D. Anderson Cancer Center, Houston, Texas 77030.

PATIENT SELECTION AND EVALUATION

The accepted contraindications for the standard pedicled TRAM flap include obesity, cigarette smoking, and previous upper abdominal surgery. Use of the free TRAM flap does not eliminate these contraindications but it does make them less absolute. The improved vascular supply to the free flap allows patients with an obese body habitus or history of tobacco use to be considered candidates for an autogenous tissue reconstruction. In addition, patients who have had upper abdominal surgery with division of the superior aspect of the rectus abdominis muscle can still be candidates for autogenous tissue reconstruction using the free TRAM flap.

This operation is well tolerated and ideal for the immediate setting (i.e., for perfomance at the time of mastectomy). A skin-sparing mastectomy facilitates the reconstruction by retaining the skin "brassiere," thus only tissue volume needs to be replaced in order to achieve a natural and normal appearance of the breast. The axillary dissection commonly done during mastectomy prepares the thoracodorsal vessels for use as recipient vessels, thus further facilitating the free tissue transfer.

Skin marking for the free TRAM flap is the same as for the conventional pedicled TRAM flap (Fig. 2). The desired final breast contour determines whether the right or left rectus abdominis muscle will be used. If the ipsilateral muscle is used, the surgeon can orient the flap vertically, fold the lower part of the flap underneath the upper part to increase the projection, and thus create a more youthful-appearing breast mound (Fig. 3A). Use of the contralateral rectus abdominis muscle requires horizontal positioning of the flap, resulting in a more mature, relaxed, or pendulous breast (Fig. 3B).

ROOM SETUP

In the operating room, the table is reversed so the patient's head is at the foot. This allows adequate room for the surgeons' legs if they wish to sit during the microanastomoses. The patient's arms are slightly abducted and placed on arm boards, with ample foam padding at the elbows and wrists. Extra padding is placed under the wrists so that the arms are slightly flexed at the elbows. Both arms are then secured to the arm boards with gauze rolls. The patient is placed on a foam mattress, and a portion of the mattress is removed at the axilla to facilitate the axillary dissection.

One must be sure that the patient is lying symmetrically and straight on the table and that the waist is at the proper bend on the table so that the patient can be placed in the sitting position during flap shaping and insetting. The flap harvest and the breast resection are accomplished simultaneously to reduce operating time. After the patient is draped, the surgical oncology team stands on either side of the ipsilateral arm board, while the plastic surgeon stands on the contralateral side at the level of the abdomen (Fig. 4). The plastic surgical assistant stands below the surgical oncologist, on the ipsilateral side at the level of the patient's hips. The anesthesiologist is at the patient's head; the ether screen is draped to allow enough room so that surgeons may stand on either side of the arm boards. This is imperative for assisting during the microanastomoses.

OPERATIVE TECHNIQUE

The skin flap is elevated off of the deep muscle fascia, from lateral to medial starting on the pedicle side (Fig. 5A). When the lateral perforating vessels are reached, the dissection is switched to the nonpedicle side, and the flap is elevated to the linea alba and umbilicus. The position of the perforating vessels is carefully noted because the anatomy on the pedicle side is often a mirror image. The umbilicus is detached from the skin flap and retained on its vascular stem.

As the dissection passes the midline, care should be taken to preserve the medial perforators. Once the medial and lateral perforators have been exposed, one may fur-

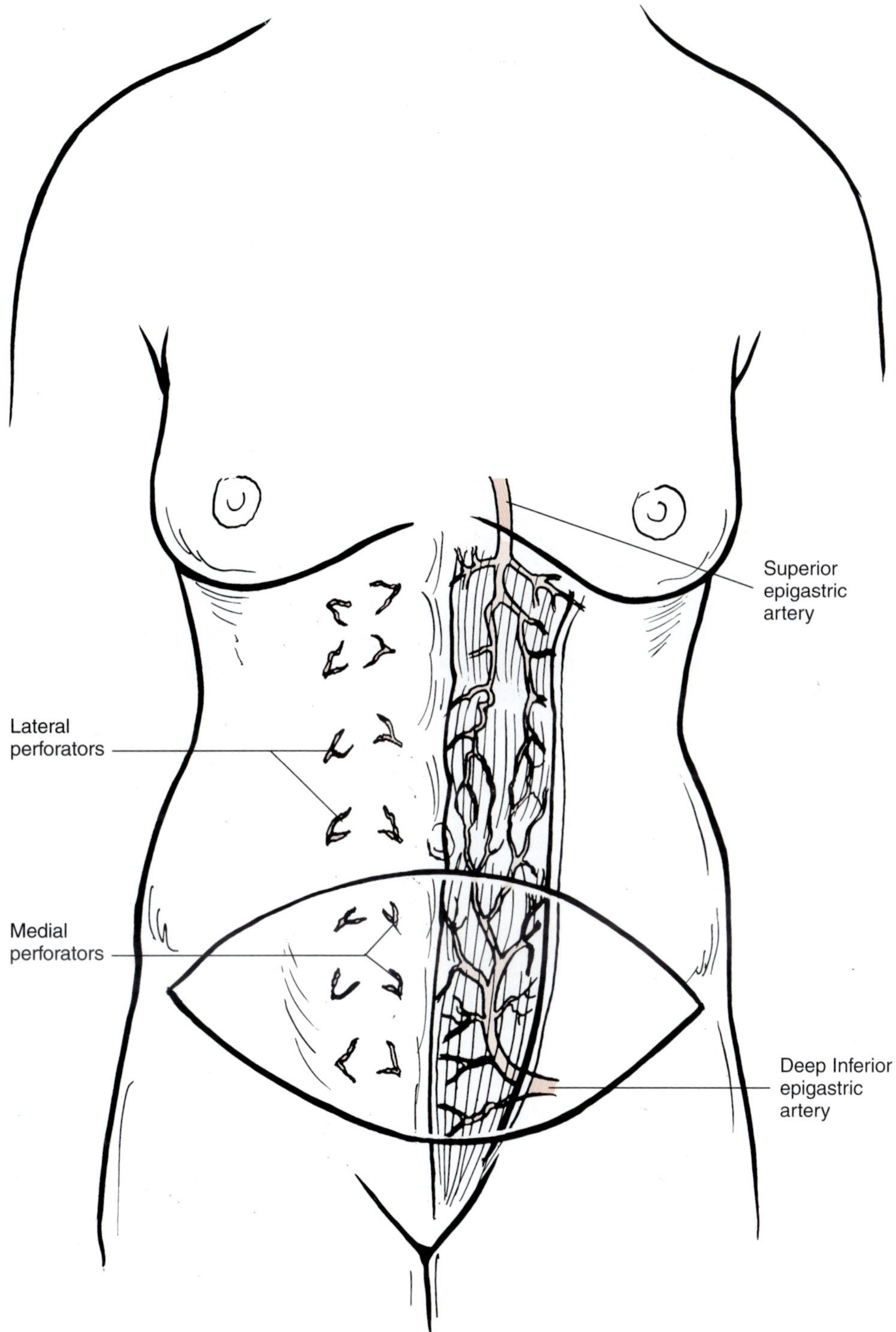

FIG. 1. Diagram of vascular supply to the free TRAM flap. Note the proximity of the deep inferior upper gastric vessels to the flap and the presence of choke vessels in the course of the superior epigastric vessels to the flap. It has been shown that the dominant blood supply to the skin island is from the deep inferior epigastric vessels.

ther reduce the amount of fascia sacrificed by harvesting only one row of perforators (Fig. 5B). This is facilitated by the anatomy of the deep inferior epigastric pedicle, which divides into a medial and lateral branch at the inferior point of its inframuscular course (Fig. 2). These medial and lateral branches correspond to medial and lateral perforators; thus, the flap can be subdivided into a medial or lateral perforator flap. Since the deep inferior epigastric vessels enter the muscle laterally, it is usually easier to use the lateral row of perforators. Once the selection of perforators has been made, the fascia is incised circumferentially around the perforators (Fig. 5C), and the lower lateral part of the rectus abdominis muscle is split longitudinally to find the vascular pedicle, which is then dissected toward its origin (Fig. 5D). Once the pedicle is deemed acceptable, the remaining muscle is divided. One should not divide the superior muscle and thus mandate transfer of the TRAM as a free flap until both the recipient and the donor vessels have been dissected and deemed optimal for free tissue transfer.

If the reconstruction is immediate, the thoracodorsal vessels will have already been prepared by the axillary dissection. If the reconstruction is delayed, these vessels must be located, their suitability confirmed, and their preparation for microanastomosis completed. If the thoracodorsal vessels are unsatisfactory, several options exist. The axillary vessels can be used, although, sometimes inadequate pedicle length may preclude their use. Using the muscle sparing TRAM flap harvest technique, an average pedicle length of 12 to 15 cm is obtainable, and this is generally adequate to reach the axillary vessels without a vein graft (Fig. 6). The axillary vessels lie in a tissue plane that will not have been disturbed by the axillary dissection, so their dissection is generally straightforward.

The internal mammary vessels have also been advocated for use as recipient vessels, especially in delayed reconstructions. One removes the 4th or 5th costal cartilage, and the vessels are just underneath the perichondrium. The main problem with these vessels is inadequate diameter, especially on the left side, but exploration for these vessels in worthwhile if the thoracodorsal vessels are unsuitable.

The flap vessels are not divided and ligated until the recipient vessels are prepared; then the flap is transferred to the chest wall (Fig. 7). The end-to-end microvascular anastomoses are accomplished using 9-0 nylon sutures. A running, spatulated technique is utilized (Fig. 8A–D). Our average ischemia time is approximately 1 hour. The flap is checked for adequate revascularization, shaped appropriately, and inset.

The abdominal donor site is closed either during the microanastomosis or after, depending on the availability of team members and the comfort of the surgeon. The closure is facilitated by the limited fascial sacrifice and may be done with a running #1 nonabsorbable suture (Figs. 9 and 10). Plastic mesh is rarely used except when bilateral flaps have been harvested; in that situation, some reinforcement may be required. The abdominal wall integrity is ensured by suturing the internal oblique fascia firmly and compactly to the midline fascia deep to the linea alba. Two closed suction drains are used and brought out through the pubic area so that the scars are hidden.

Once the abdomen has been closed completely, the integrity of the microanastomoses are checked. The artery should be pulsating vigorously along its entire length and up into the muscle. The vein should be pale blue and soft. The flap itself should be pink with good capillary refill, and any bleeding points should show bright red blood. Only after the surgeon is convinced that these clinical signs of healthy reperfusion are present should the flap shaping and insetting be undertaken.

Flap shaping is facilitated in the immediate setting by the skin-sparing mastectomy. Appropriate flap size may be estimated by weighing the mastectomy specimen, but more often flap size and shape is determined by trial and error: placing the flap in the skin envelope, closing the wound with a skin stapler, and raising the back of the table to the sitting position to observe the result.

As stated previously, use of the ipsilateral pedicle facilitates a more vertical orientation and use of the contralateral pedicle a lateral orientation. I tend to use the ipsilateral/vertical orientation most often, since this allows the flap to be folded under

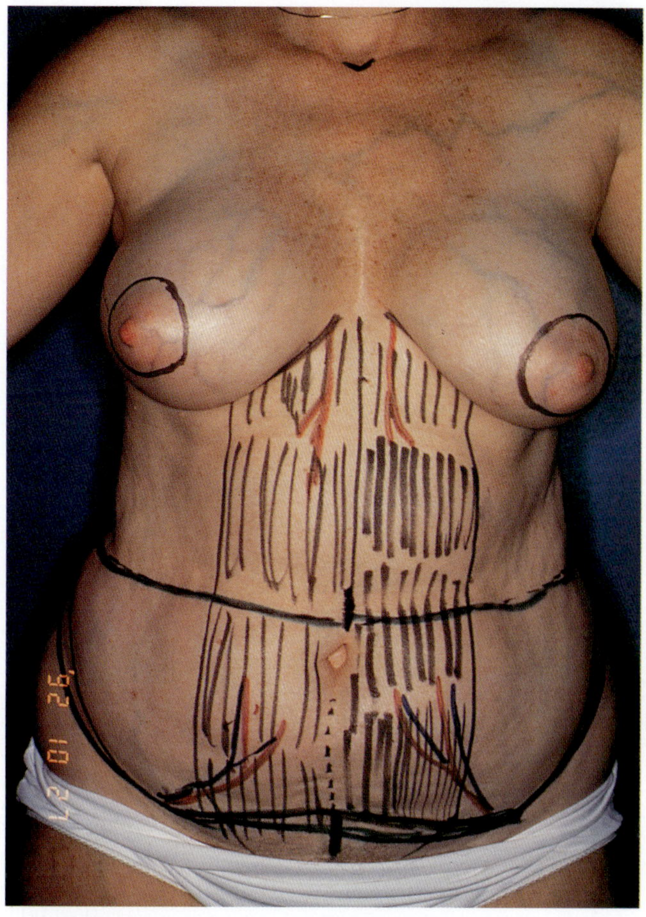

FIG. 2. Skin marking for the free TRAM flap.

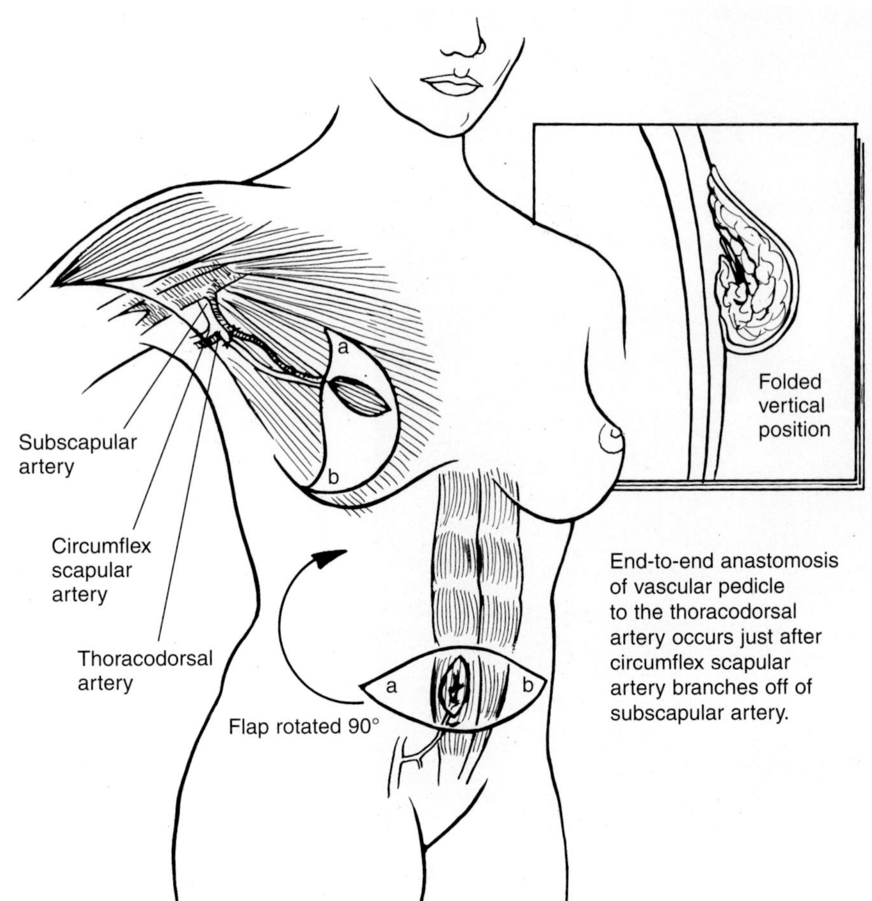

FIG. 3A. Use of the ipsilateral pedicle allows for a verticle orientation of the flap after turning the flap 90° to orient the vessels in the axilla. Note this allows for the flap to be folded under itself in order to give better projection.

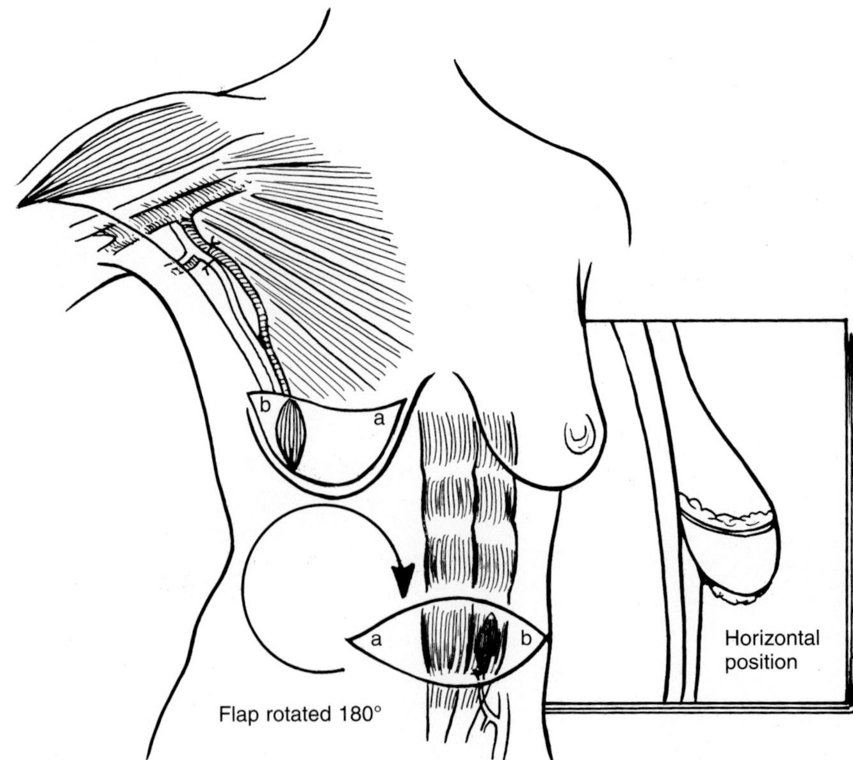

FIG. 3B. Use of the contralateral pedicle requires the flap be turned 180° to orient the vessels so that they are in the axilla and that this position of the flap creates a more mature, relaxed, and pendulous breast.

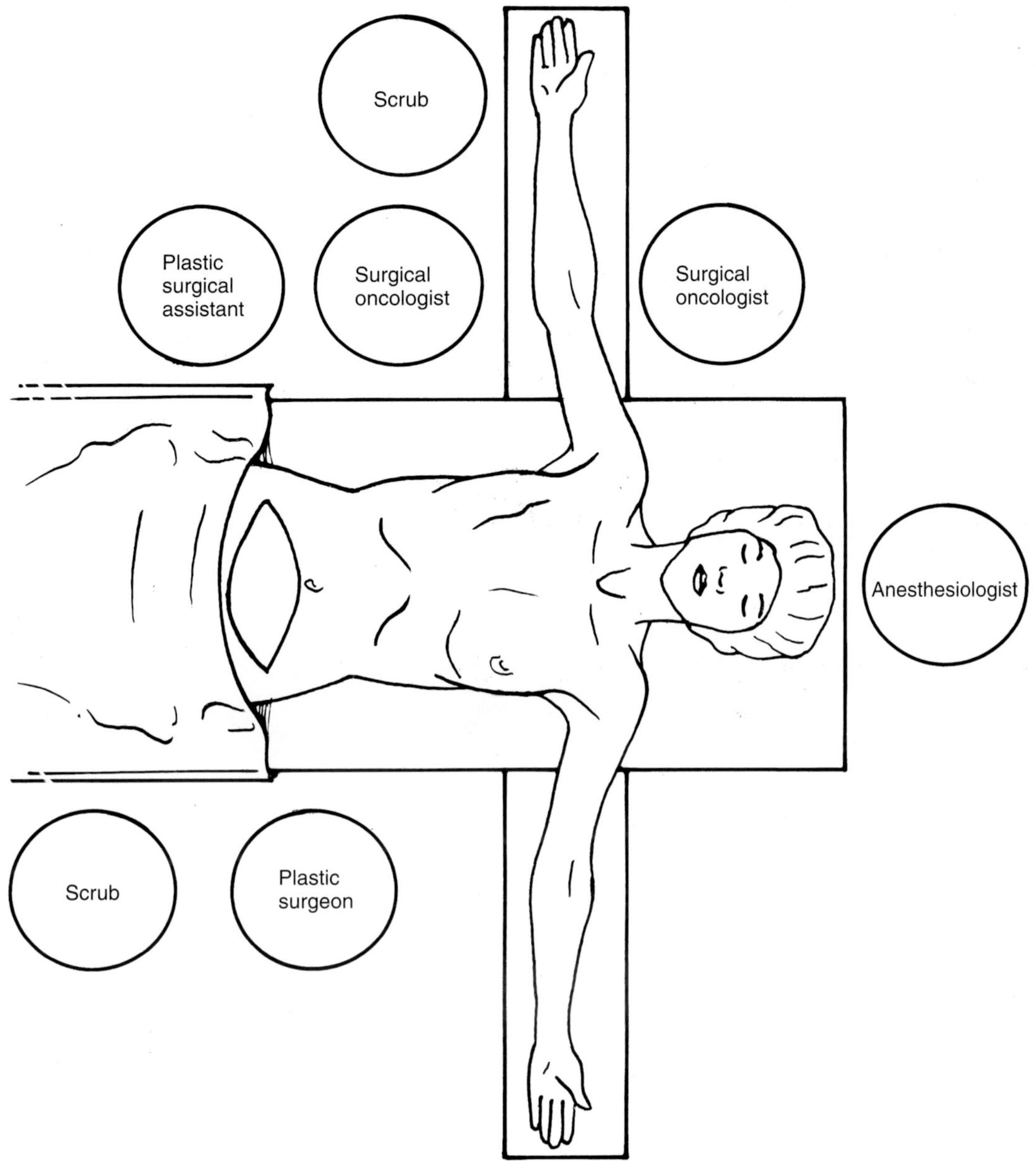

FIG. 4. Diagram of the positioning of the surgical teams for performance of a simultaneous mastectomy and free TRAM flap.

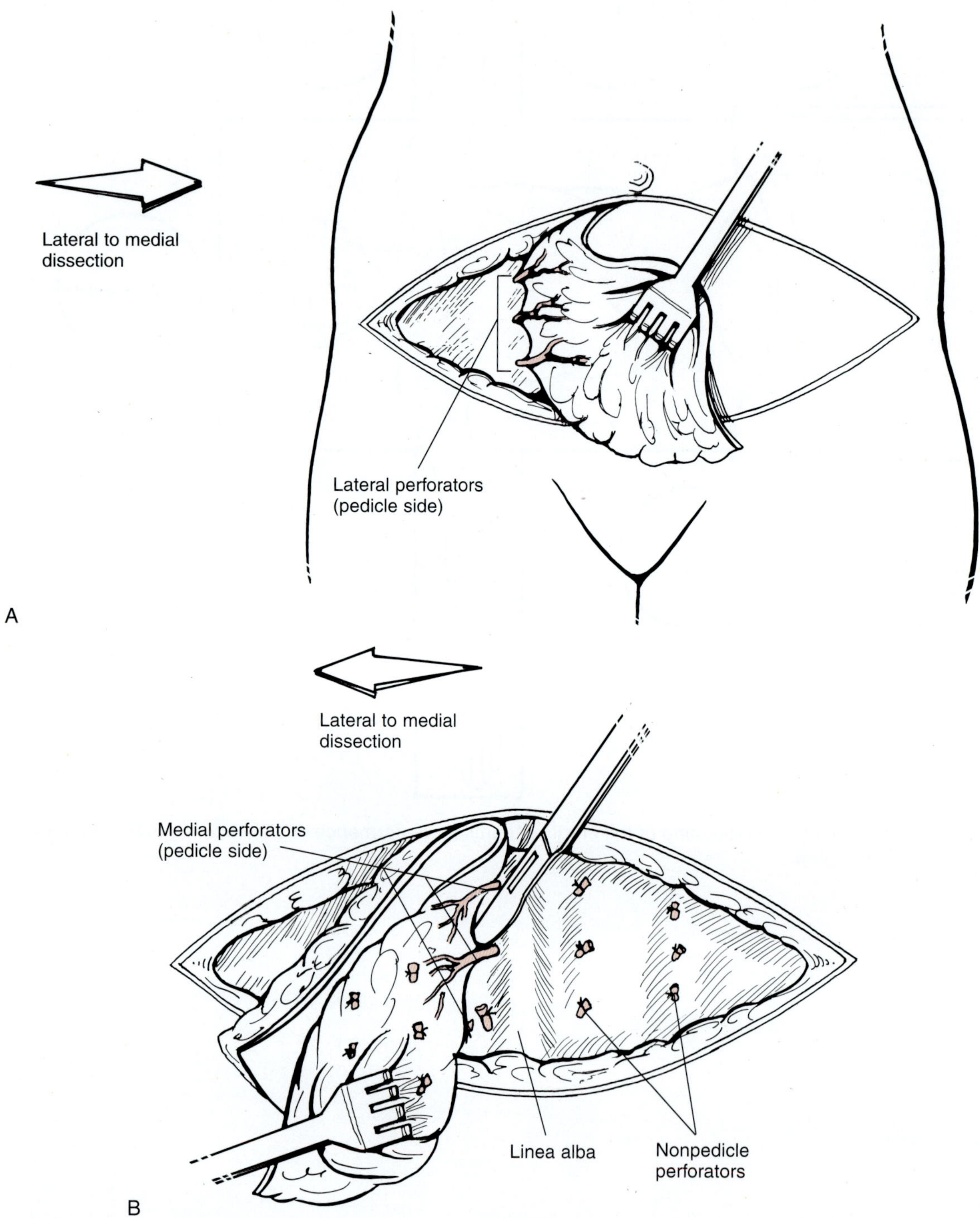

FIG. 5A,B. A: Elevation of the TRAM flap is begun from lateral to medial. When the lateral perforators are encountered these are spared and the dissection is then started on the opposite side. **B:** The perforators on the contralateral side are sacrificed and, in order to spare more fascia, one may also sacrifice the medial perforators on the ipsilateral side.

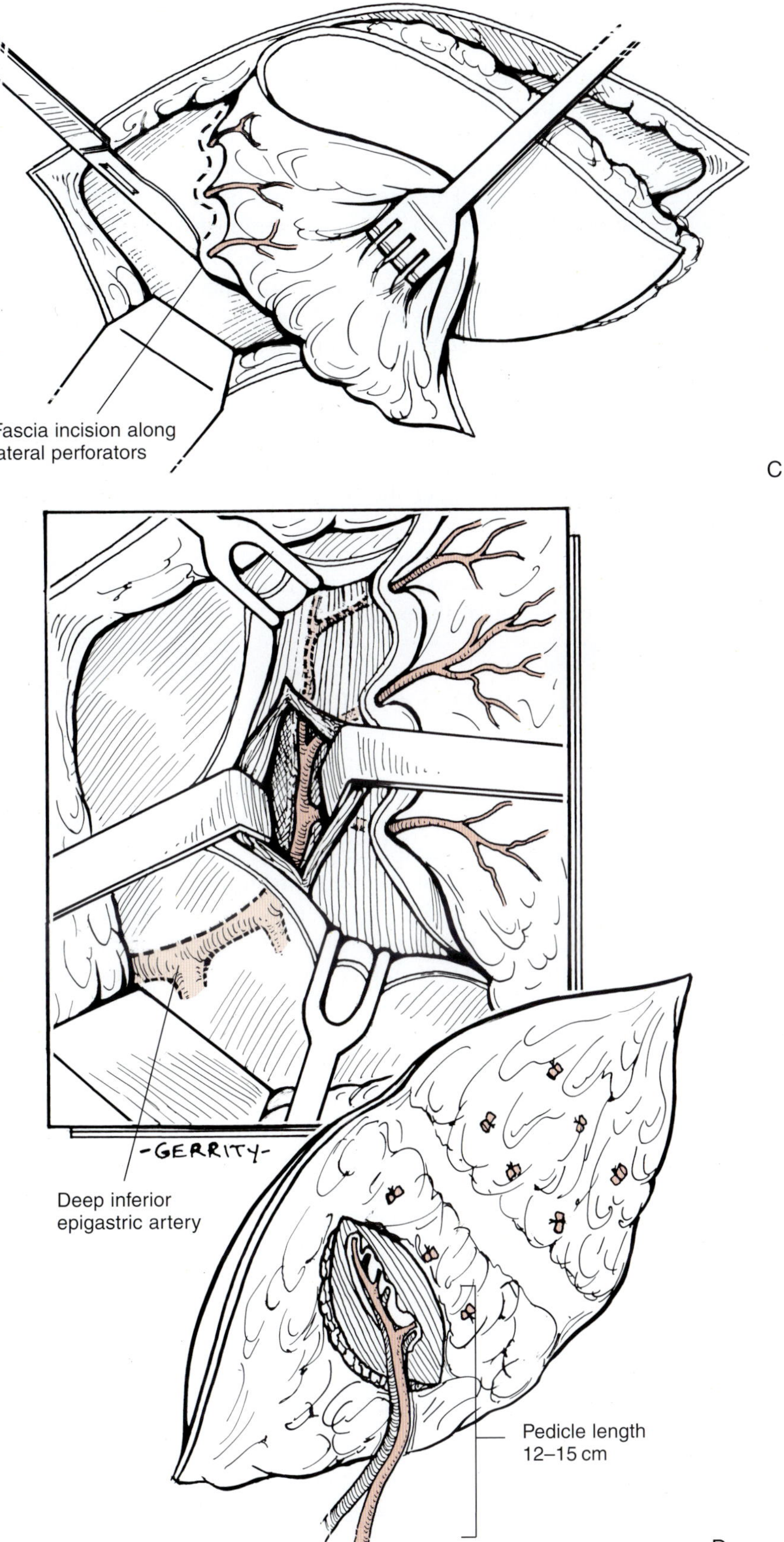

FIG. 5C, D. C: Next the fascia is incised circumferentially around the perforators and the muscle is dissected. **D:** The lateral portion of the muscle is split and the deep inferior epigastric vessel is identified. This is then traced to its origin. By splitting the muscle, one can achieve a pedicle length of 12 to 15 cm with minimal abdominal wall sacrifice.

itself for more projection. One disadvantage of this technique is that it can result in a hollow area in the medial-superior aspect of the reconstructed breast. It is therefore imperative to harvest extra fat on the superior edge of the skin flap, above the umbilicus, to provide extra tissue with which to fill the medial aspect of the reconstructed breast. Again, final flap shape is best determined by gradually excising excess tissue, closing the wound temporarily, and sitting the patient up to note the areas of excess and deficiency. This process should be repeated until the desired size and shape are attained. Once that has been accomplished, the area of the exposed skin paddle is marked and the remaining flap is de-epithelialized. If a skin-sparing mastectomy was done, flap skin will be needed only where the nipple areola complex and any biopsy scar have been removed with the specimen (Fig. 11). Although the excised biopsy scar site may be closed primarily, doing so will alter the skin envelope and change the final shape of the breast. It is often more advantageous to replace the biopsy scar with a patch of skin from the flap. The resulting scar and patchwork look of this maneuver usually fades and is offset by the improved shape of the reconstructed breast.

No matter which orientation is used, the lateral aspect of the breast fold needs to be reconstructed to keep the flap from falling into the axilla. This is done by tacking the flap to the chest wall at the level of the anterior axillary line. When this maneuver is done it is often necessary or desirable to remove a wedge of skin and fat from the area of the umbilicus and suture the flap to itself, thus forming a cone and again enhancing projection of the breast (Fig. 12).

POSTOPERATIVE CARE

The nasogastric tube that is placed after induction of anesthesia is removed prior to the patient's waking up. The patient should be observed in a special care unit for signs of flap ischemia on an hourly basis for at least 3 and preferably 5 days. (Although it is rare, we have had several cases of vessel thrombosis on days 3 to 5.) Devices such as the laser Doppler or the implantable 20 MHz ultrasonic Doppler are used to help assess flap perfusion, but the most important aspect of flap monitoring is clinical assessment by an experienced nurse. Any question of flap viability should be answered by return to the operating room for direct observation of the anastomosis and thrombectomy and revision if required.

In the early postoperative period, it is important to maintain high intravascular volumes with crystalloid solutions and blood as needed. If stable, the patient may start activity and oral intake the day after surgery. Advancement of both with removal of catheters is done gradually, and the patient is normally discharged on the fifth to seventh postoperative day.

Nipple reconstruction is done about 2 months after the TRAM flap. At present, we use either the double-opposing tab flap or the star flap. After the nipple incisions have healed, the areola is created by use of a micropigmentation technique (Fig. 13).

FREE TRAM FLAP FOR BILATERAL RECONSTRUCTION

The TRAM flap is well suited for bilateral breast reconstructions owing to the bilateral nature of the rectus muscles; however, bilateral sacrifice of the rectus muscles diminishes abdominal strength postoperatively and often necessitates the use of plastic mesh to reinforce the abdominal wall. Use of free TRAM flaps rather than pedicled TRAM flaps for bilateral reconstructions limits the abdominal wall sacrifice, facilitates fascial closure, and yields improved postoperative abdominal strength. The technique is the same as the unilateral procedure, except of course that both sides are used and the flaps are transferred ipsilaterally, one at time, with care taken to make sure that the first transfer is stable and the anastomoses patent prior to transfer of the second side (Fig. 14A–E).

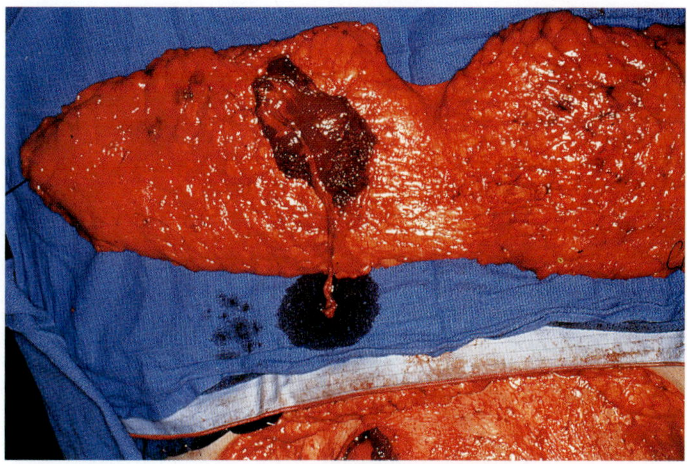

FIG. 6. Example of a free TRAM flap after elevation.

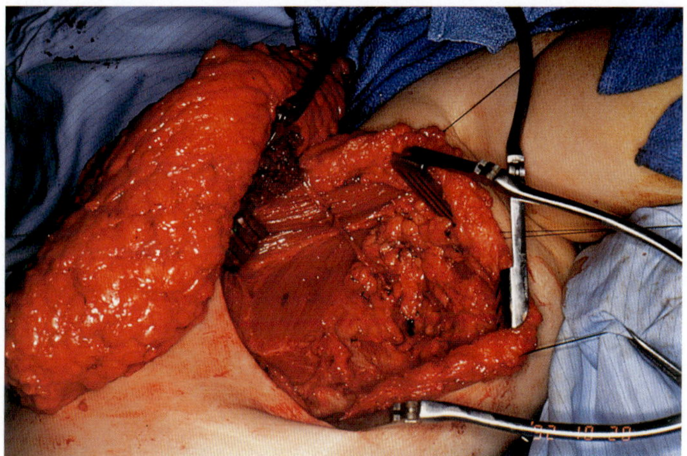

FIG. 7. Once the flap has been elevated it is transferred to the chest wall and the microanastomoses are performed.

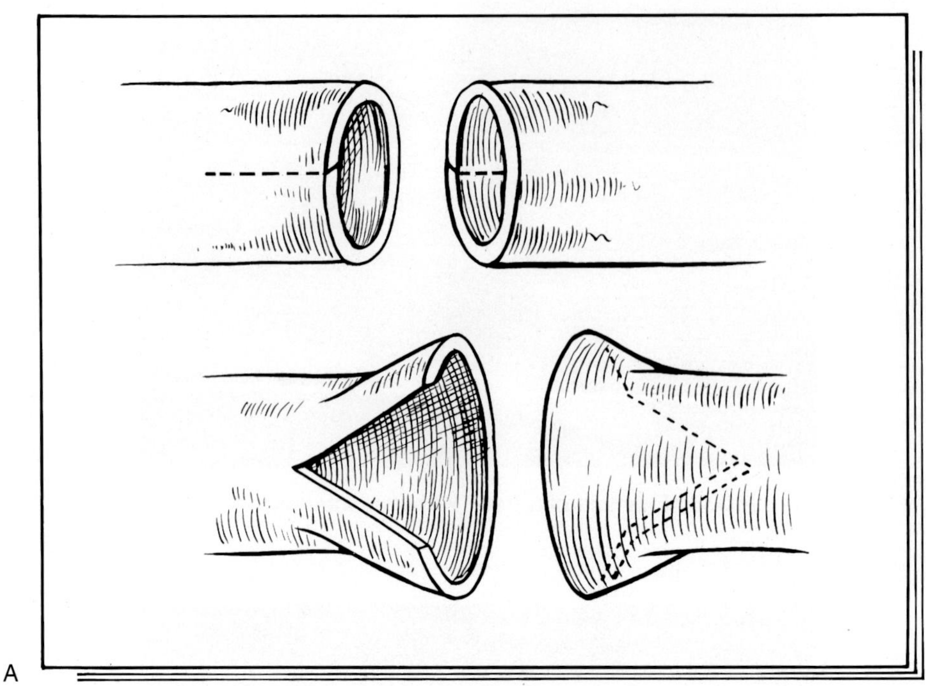

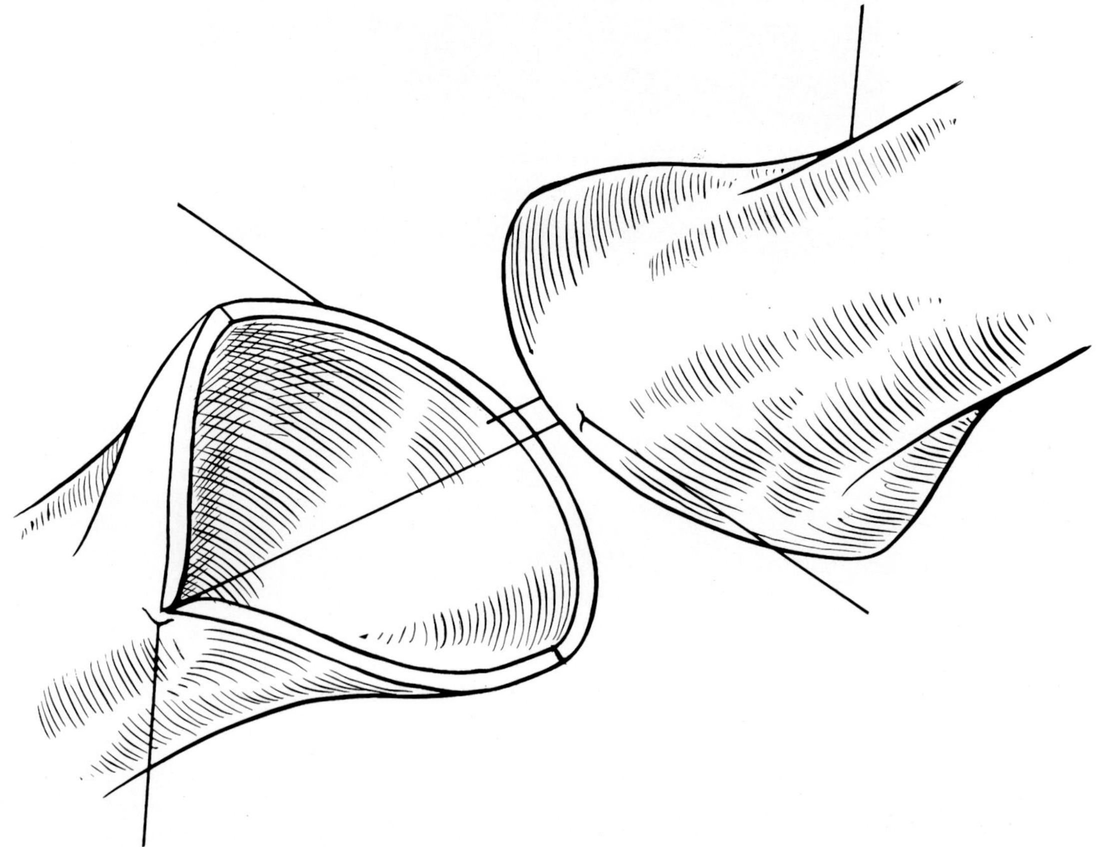

FIG. 8A–D. A: A spatulated end-to-end anastomosis is performed using running 9-0 nylon.

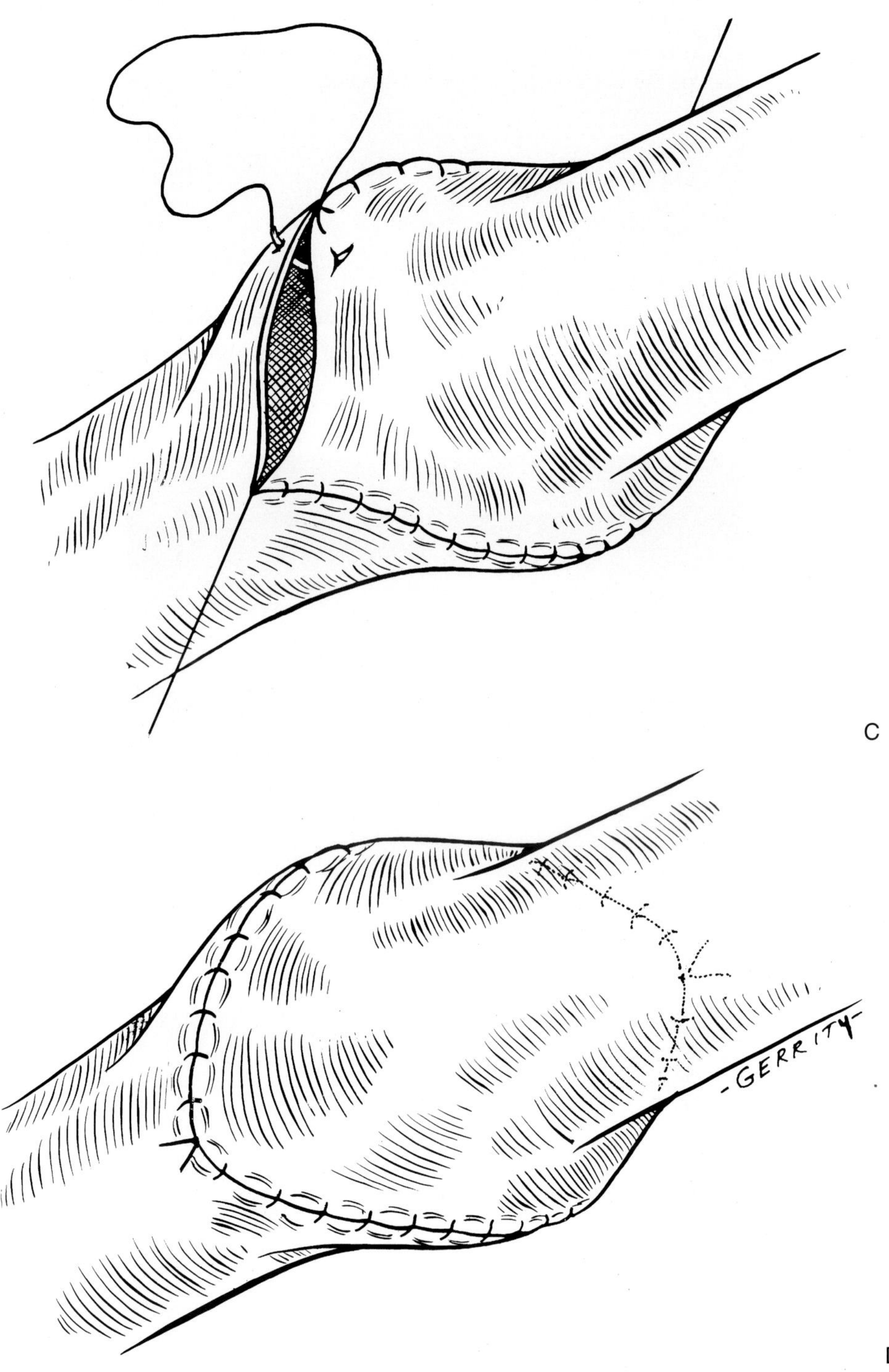

C

D

FIG. 8A–D. *Continued.*

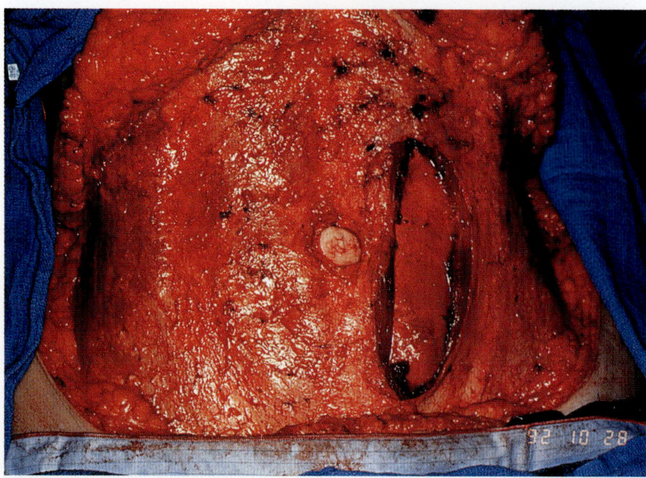

FIG. 9. An example of a typical abdominal wall defect after flap harvest.

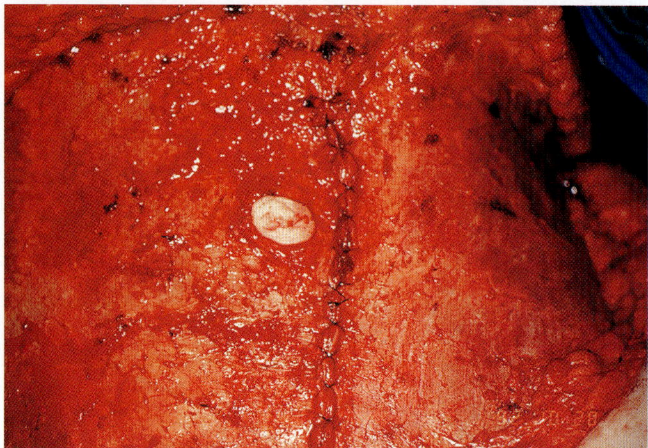

FIG. 10. Closure of this defect is done using a running #1 nonabsorbable suture.

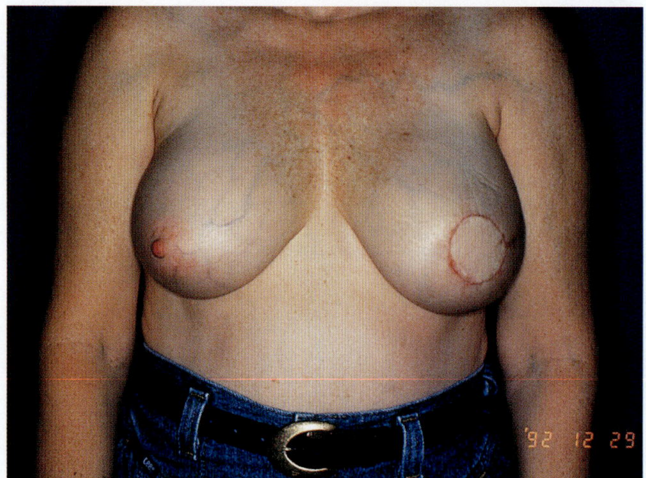

FIG. 11. Postoperative result of patient shown in Figure 2, prior to nipple areola reconstruction. Since a skin-sparing mastectomy has been done, the only portion of the flap skin visible is that where the nipple areola complex has been sacrificed. The rest of the flap has been de-epithelialized and used to replace bulk.

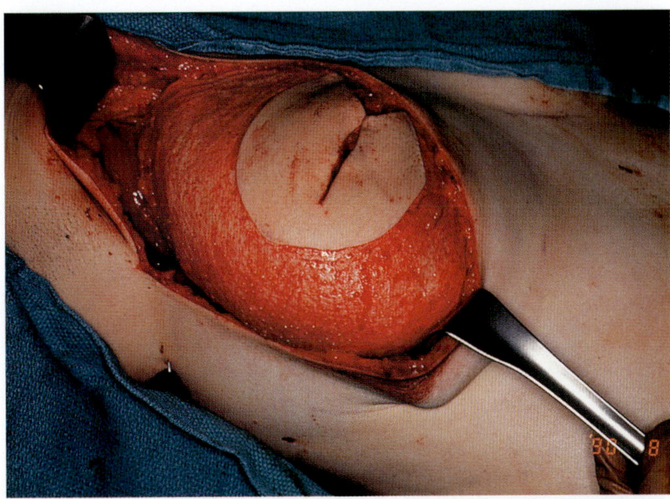

FIG. 12. Photograph illustrating technique of suturing flap to itself in order to achieve more protection.

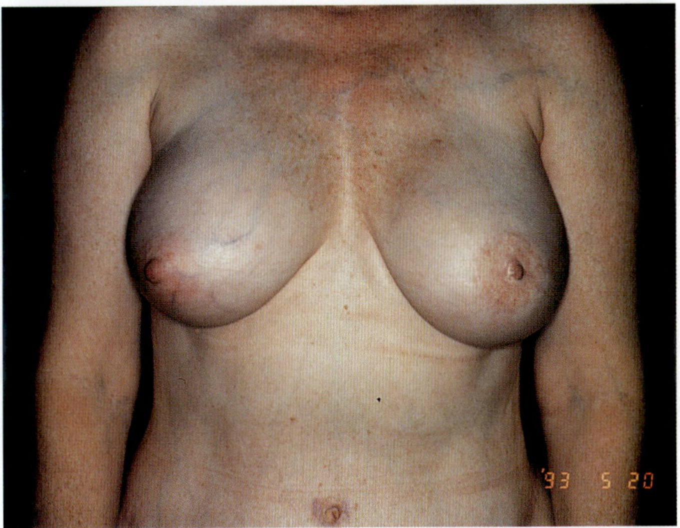

FIG. 13. Postoperative result evident in the immediate free TRAM reconstruction after skin sparing mastectomy and nipple areola reconstruction has been performed.

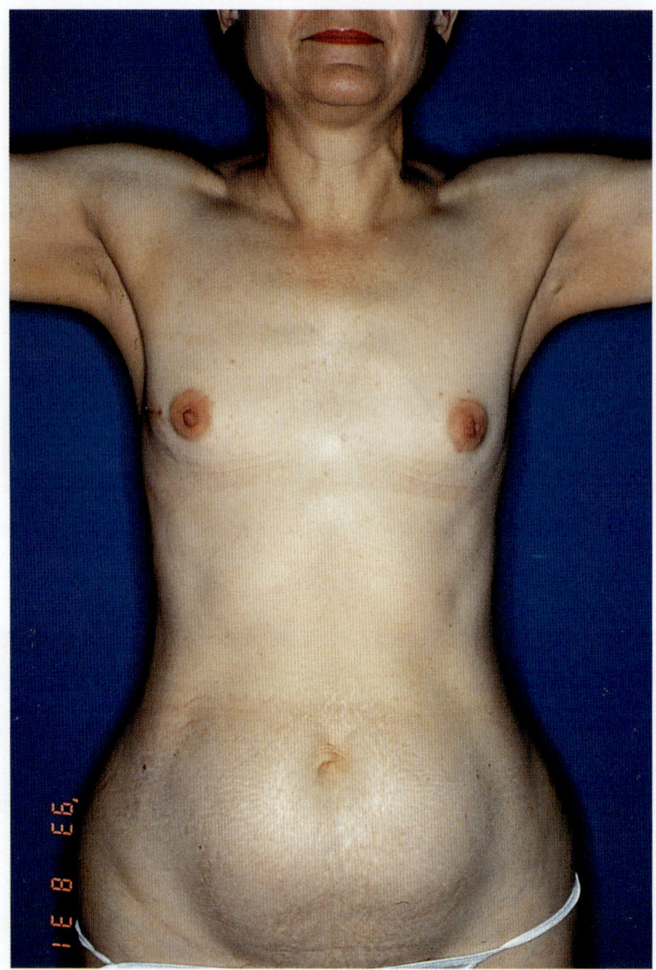

FIG. 14A. An example of bilateral breast reconstruction using the free TRAM flap. Preoperative view of patient.

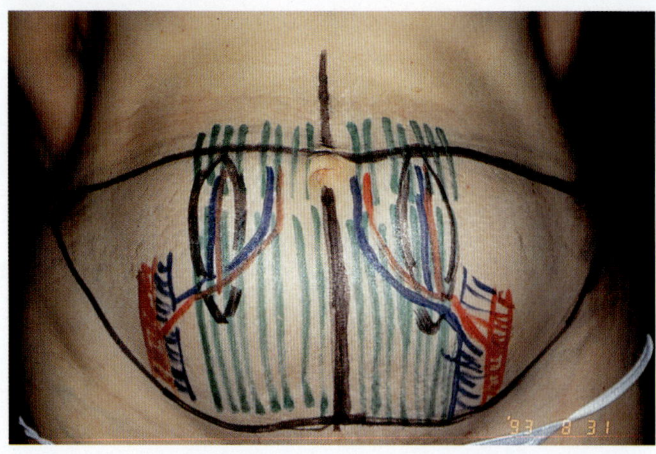

FIG. 14B. Drawing of surgical plan; note the planned utilization of the lateral perforators only, thus limiting the abdominal wall sacrifice.

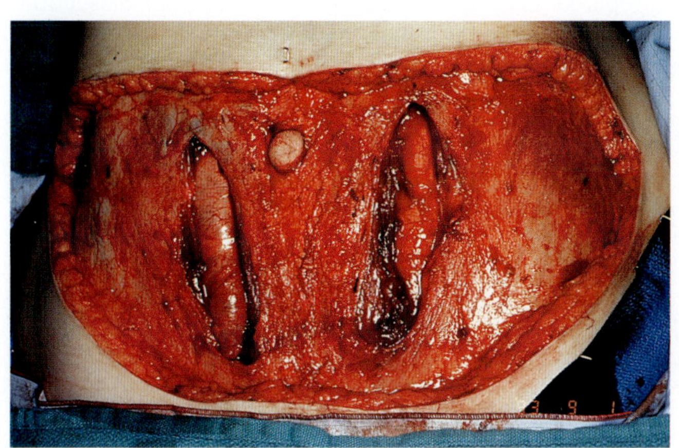

FIG. 14C. The abdominal wall defects are small and can be readily closed primarily.

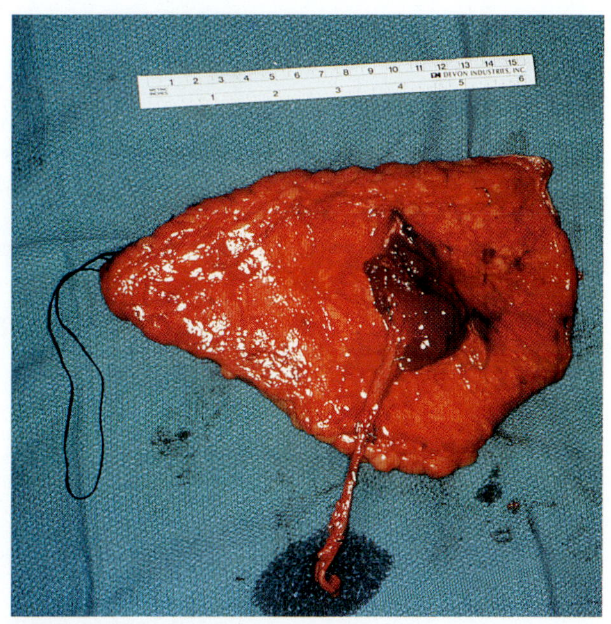

FIG. 14D. The hemiflap with muscle and vascular pedicle. Note the limited amount of muscle and the ample length of the vessels.

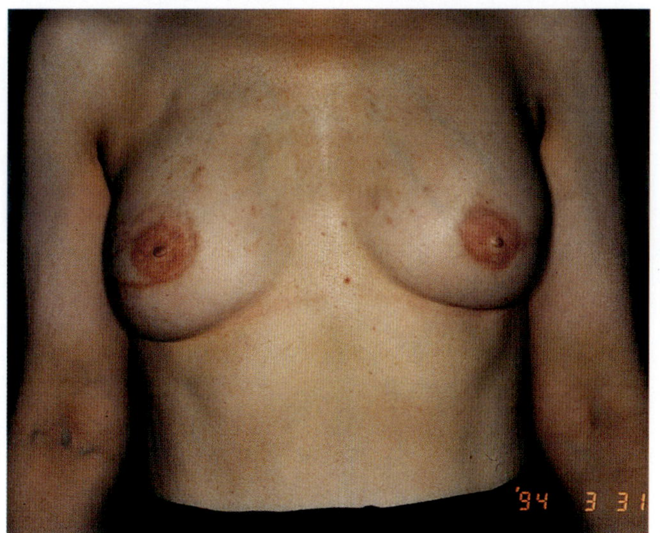

FIG. 14E. Bilateral free TRAM flap, postoperative result.

SUMMARY

The TRAM flap is the standard for autogenous tissue breast reconstruction and the free TRAM flap allows transfer of the flap with improved perfusion and less abdominal wall sacrifice. The free TRAM flap is most useful in the immediate setting, where the thoracodorsal vessels are prepared as recipient vessels by the axillary dissection. The free TRAM flap is also useful for bilateral reconstruction, and use of the fascia sparing technique allows easier closure when both muscles are utilized.

SELECTED READINGS

Anton MA, Hartrampf CR Jr. Nipple reconstruction with the star flap. *Plast Surg Forum* 1990;13:100–103(abstr).

Arnez ZM, Bajec J, Bardsley AF, Scamp T, Webster MH. Experience with 50 free TRAM flap breast reconstructions. *Plast Reconstr Surg* 1991;87:470–478; discussion 479–482.

Arnez ZM, Scamp T. The bipedicled free TRAM flap. *Br J Plast Surg* 1992;45:214–218.

Baldwin BJ, Schusterman MA, Miller MJ, Kroll SS, Wang BG. Bilateral breast reconstruction: conventional versus free TRAM. *Plast Reconstr Surg* 1994;93:1410–1416; discussion 1417.

Banic A, Boeckx W, Greulich M, Guelickx P, Marchi A, Rigotti G, et al. Late results of breast reconstruction with free TRAM flaps: a prospective multicentric study. *Plast Reconstr Surg* 1995;95:1195–1204; discussion 1205.

Blondeel PN, Boeckx WD. Refinements in free flap breast reconstruction: the free bilateral deep inferior epigastric perforator flap anastomosed to the internal mammary artery. *Br J Plast Surg* 1994;47:495–501.

Boyd JB, Taylor GI, Corlett R. The vascular territories of the superior epigastric and the deep inferior epigastric systems. *Plast Reconstr Surg* 1984;73:1–14.

Elliott LF, Eskenazi L, Beegle PH Jr, Podres PE, Drazan L. Immediate TRAM flap breast reconstruction: 128 consecutive cases. *Plast Reconstr Surg* 1993;92:217–227.

Freidman RJ, Argenta LC, Anderson R. Deep inferior epigastric free flap for breast reconstruction after radical mastectomy. *Plast Reconstr Surg* 1985;76:455–458.

Gherardini G, Arnander C, Gylbert L, Wickman M. Pedicled compared with free transverse rectus abdominis myocutaneous flaps in breast reconstruction. *Scand J Plast Reconstr Surg Hand Surg* 1994;28:69–73.

Grotting JC. Immediate breast reconstruction using the free TRAM flap. [Review]. *Clin Plast Surg* 1994;21:207–221.

Grotting JC, Urist MM, Maddox WA. Conventional TRAM versus free microsurgical TRAM flap for immediate breast reconstruction. *Plast Reconstr Surg* 1989;83:828–841.

Hartrampf CR, Jr. Discussion: Conventional TRAM flap versus free microsurgical TRAM flap for immediate breast reconstruction. *Plast Reconstr Surg* 1989;83:842–844.

Holmstrom H. The free abdominoplasty flap and its use in breast reconstruction. *Scand J Plast Reconstr Surg* 1979;13:423.

Kroll SS, Hamilton S. Nipple reconstruction with the double-opposing-tab flap. *Plast Reconstr Surg* 1989;84:520–525.

Schusterman MA, Kroll SS, Miller MJ, Reece GP, Baldwin BJ, Robb GL, et al. The free transverse rectus abdominis musculocutaneous flap for breast reconstruction: one center's experience with 211 consecutive cases. *Ann Plast Surg* 1994;32:234–242.

Schusterman MA, Kroll SS, Weldon ME. Immediate breast reconstruction: Why the free TRAM over the conventional TRAM flap? *Plast Reconstr Surg* 1992;90:255–262.

Shaw WW, Ahn CY. Microvascular free flaps in breast reconstruction. [Review]. *Clin Plast Surg* 1992;19:917–926.

Swartz WM, Jones NF, Cherup L, Klein A. Direct monitoring of microvascular anastomoses with the 20-MHz ultrasonic Doppler probe: an experimental and clinical study. *Plast Reconstr Surg* 1988;81:149–158.

Microsurgical Reconstruction of the Cancer Patient, edited by M.A. Schusterman.
Lippincott-Raven Publishers, Philadelphia © 1997.

9

The Superior Gluteal Free Flap for Breast Reconstruction

Stephen S. Kroll

For patients who are not eligible for a transverse rectus abdominis myocutaneous (TRAM) flap breast reconstruction, the superior gluteal free flap provides a good alternative with which the surgeon can achieve an excellent result without using a prosthetic implant. Unlike the TRAM flap, a superior gluteal free flap can be used to reconstruct two breasts without requiring that both sides be done simultaneously. It is technically more difficult than the TRAM flap, however, and causes more conspicuous alteration of the donor site, so it is used less often. The primary indication for a superior gluteal free flap is a patient who has already had unilateral reconstruction with a TRAM flap who subsequently needs an opposite mastectomy with reconstruction. Other indications would include patients who because of previous abdominoplasty are unable to have TRAM flaps, and those with minimal subcutaneous abdominal fat but an excess of fatty tissue in the upper buttock.

PLANNING THE FLAP

In preparation for a superior gluteal flap operation, the surgeon locates and marks the bony landmarks of the sacrum, including the posterior superior iliac spine (Fig. 1A). A line is drawn from this spine to the greater trochanter of the femur. The superior gluteal artery is usually located on this line, at the junction of the upper and middle third. The skin paddle is designed to include the superior gluteal vascular pedicle and surrounding muscle. Its exact shape will vary depending on how much tissue is needed and the laxity of the buttock. In general, however, the flap is elliptical and

S. S. Kroll: Department of Plastic Surgery, The University of Texas, M. D. Anderson Cancer Center, Houston, Texas 77030.

roughly horizontal (Fig. 1B). To minimize donor site deformity, only enough tissue to form the breast should be excised. The patient's position on the operating table should allow access to both the buttock and the breast. She is therefore placed supine, but the legs and hips are turned crossed so that the donor buttock is exposed (Fig. 2). The table can be banked from side to side to permit surgery on the buttock or breast, whichever requires access at the moment. Both breasts are prepped so that they can be compared during breast shaping after flap transfer.

ELEVATION OF THE FLAP

It is preferable to make the skin incision with a scalpel, but most of the remaining dissection is best performed with electrocautery to reduce bleeding and improve visibility of the anatomy. The dissection is carried down to the muscle, where the superior edge of the gluteus maximus muscle is identified. The plane between the gluteus maximus and medius is then opened and the lateral muscle partially divided approximately 5 cm from the greater trochanter. The branches of the superior gluteal artery are found on the undersurface of the gluteus maximus muscle (Fig. 3). The vessels are followed proximally until the main trunk of the superior gluteal artery is located, just superior to the piriformis muscle. The gluteal muscle is then divided around the pedicle, including with the flap only the minimum amount of muscle required to maintain the flap's blood supply.

In general, the pedicle of the flap consists of vessels of large caliber (2 to 3 mm) but of short length (2 to 3 cm). The pedicle can usually be lengthened to a variable degree by opening the fascia where the vessels exit the pelvis and extending the dissection for a short distance. This additional dissection can make the anastomoses much easier but does entail risk, because any bleeding encountered in the deepest part of the dissection could be difficult or even impossible to control. Consequently, any such dissection should be performed with the most extreme care and under loupe magnification.

Recipient Vessels and Vein Grafts

Because of the very short vascular pedicle of this flap, the internal mammary vessels, which do not require a long pedicle, are often recommended for use as recipients. The internal mammary artery is almost always available and of adequate size. The internal mammary vein, however, is often very small. Because of this, and because in most cases of immediate reconstruction the axilla has already been dissected by the general surgeon, we usually prefer to use the thoracodorsal vessels, which are more dependable. We would not quarrel, however, with those surgeons who prefer to use the internal mammary vessels (Fig. 4).

In most cases, unless the superior gluteal muscle has been completely dissected away from the vessels to provide a longer pedicle, a vein graft is necessary to lengthen the pedicle enough to reach the recipient vessels. This is especially true if the recipient vessels are in the axilla, as is our preference. Vein grafts can be harvested from the leg, using the saphenous vein, or from the forearm, using the cephalic vein. The saphenous vein, having thicker walls, is more suitable for the arterial graft. It is very constant and has some tendency to go into spasm. The cephalic vein is shorter, thinwalled, unlikely to develop spasm, and especially suitable for a venous graft; harvesting it, however, leaves a noticeable scar. In general, we prefer the saphenous graft, but if spasm occurs, we would not hesitate to use a cephalic vein instead.

THE MICROVASCULAR ANASTOMOSES

The recipient vessels are selected and prepared before flap harvest to minimize flap ischemia time. If the internal mammary vessels are selected, and if the flap pedicle is

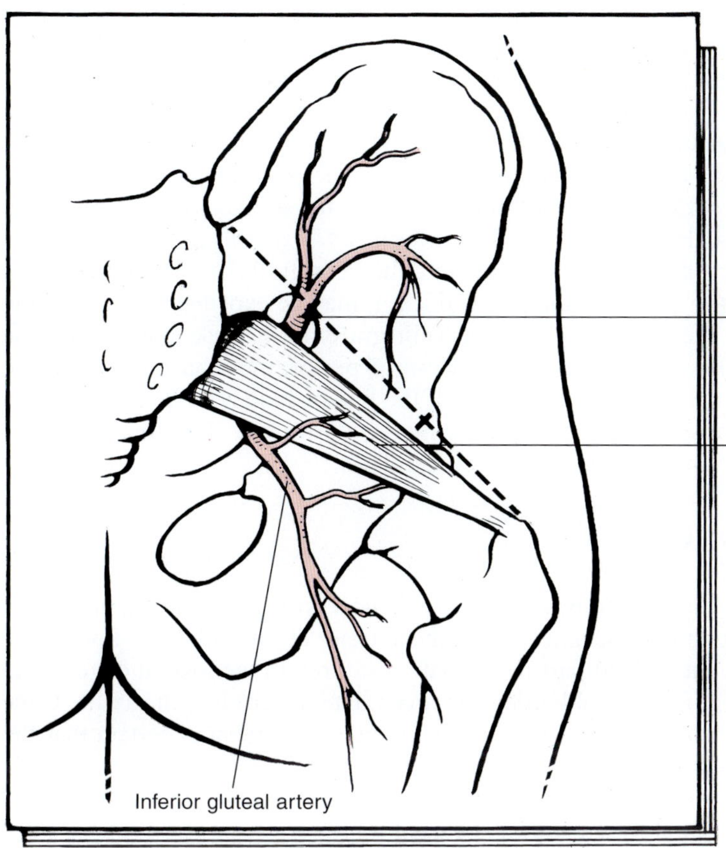

FIG. 1A. Bony landmarks of the sacrum. The superior gluteal artery is located approximately one-third of the way down along a line drawn from the posterior iliac spine to the greater trochanter of the femur.

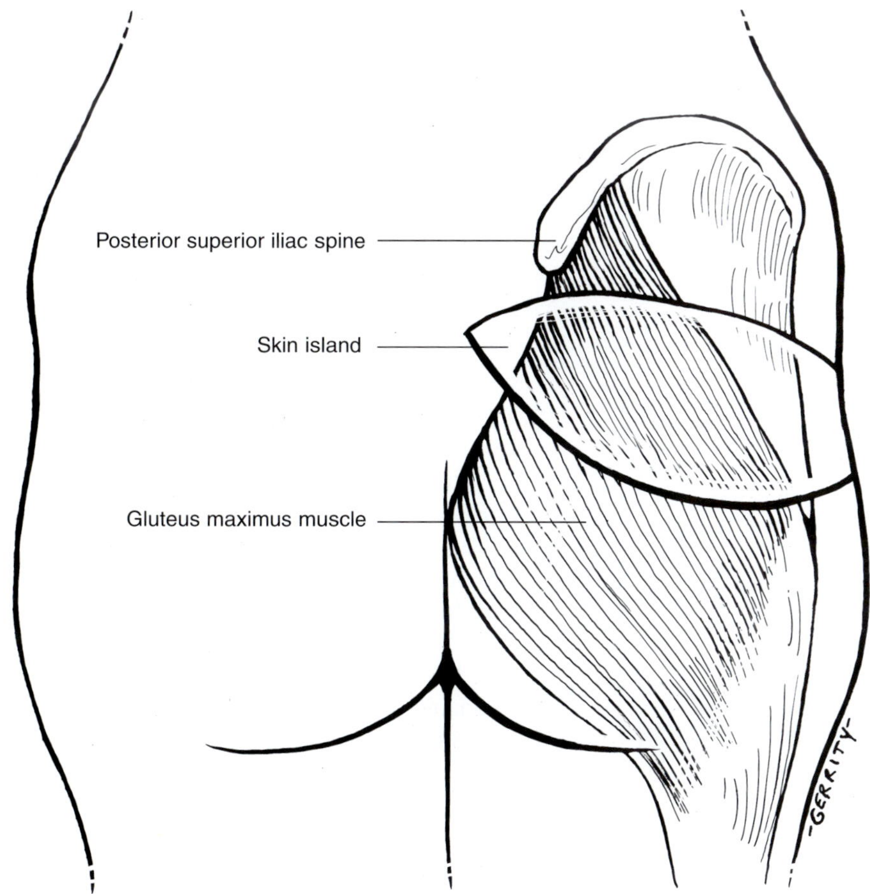

FIG. 1B. The superior gluteal skin paddle is situated transversely over the muscle.

long enough to permit anastomosis without a vein graft, once the vessel ends are prepared the flap can be harvested. If the thoracodorsal vessels will be used, however, harvesting a vein graft will be necessary. First, the axilla is prepared and the thoracodorsal vessels dissected from each other and from the thoracodorsal nerve from the serratus branches to as high in the axilla as possible without dividing the circumflex scapular branch. This allows the vessels to be rotated anteriorly and more superficially, avoiding the need to perform the anastomosis deep in the axilla, where it would be technically more difficult.

After the thoracodorsal vessels are mobilized, the vein grafts are harvested. If the flap pedicle is unusually short and the flap is thick, it may be expedient to harvest the flap and anastomose the flap vessels to the vein grafts on a back table, or on the patient's abdomen. This avoids the awkwardness of performing anastomoses in the axilla to the very short pedicle of a bulky flap. If the flap pedicle is longer, the surgeon may prefer to anastomose the vein grafts to the thoracodorsal vessels before harvest of the flap to minimize flap ischemia time (Figs. 5A, B).

INSETTING THE FLAP

Once the microvascular anastomoses have been successfully completed, the flap is trimmed to the appropriate shape and fixed to the anterior chest wall. In an immediate breast reconstruction, the medial part of the flap is sutured to the medial edge of the mastectomy defect near the sternal border, to prevent lateral drift into the axilla. Once the flap is adequately stabilized on the chest wall and the surgeon is certain that the pedicle is not under tension, care is directed to the donor site. This allows time for release of any vascular spasm in the pedicle and affords the opportunity for any potential thrombosis to occur before the breast is closed.

Closing the donor site is straightforward. The dead space is reduced with deep sutures, and a suction drain is inserted to minimize the risk of seroma. After suturing the skin, the patient's legs and hips are straightened and she is repositioned in the center of the operating table to allow better evaluation of breast symmetry.

The flap is reexamined to be certain that the pedicle is not obstructed. Breast shaping is then completed, sitting the patient upright to better judge breast shape and symmetry. Gluteal subcutaneous tissue tends to retain its original form more than its abdominal counterpart, so the breast must be sculptured into the desired shape instead of merely relying on the skin to support and provide shape as one can often do with a TRAM flap. The axilla and breast are drained (usually with a single drain) and the wound closed. Flap monitoring is by visual inspection of the skin paddle combined with laser or pencil Doppler, depending on the surgeon's preference.

COMPLICATIONS

Breast reconstruction with the superior gluteal free flap is a complex procedure, and patients should be warned that the risk of a complication is significant. Any of the usual complications associated with long, complex operative procedures can occur, including hematoma, wound infection, deep venous thrombosis, and even death. Loss of the flap is naturally one of the risks of greatest concern. Because vein grafts are necessary and two sets of anastomoses are performed, the risk of pedicle thrombosis is higher than in the TRAM flap procedure. Nevertheless, experienced surgeons are capable of obtaining consistently good results with gluteal flaps. Obviously, meticulous technique and careful postoperative flap monitoring reduce the risk of flap loss.

The donor site of a superior gluteal free flap always sustains some contour deformity, which is more noticeable in pants than when the patient wears a dress or skirt. If the reconstruction is bilateral, the deformity becomes symmetrical and is not conspicuous. If unilateral, it can be corrected with surgery on the opposite buttock, but this discards a potential future donor site for the opposite breast. The deformity is reduced,

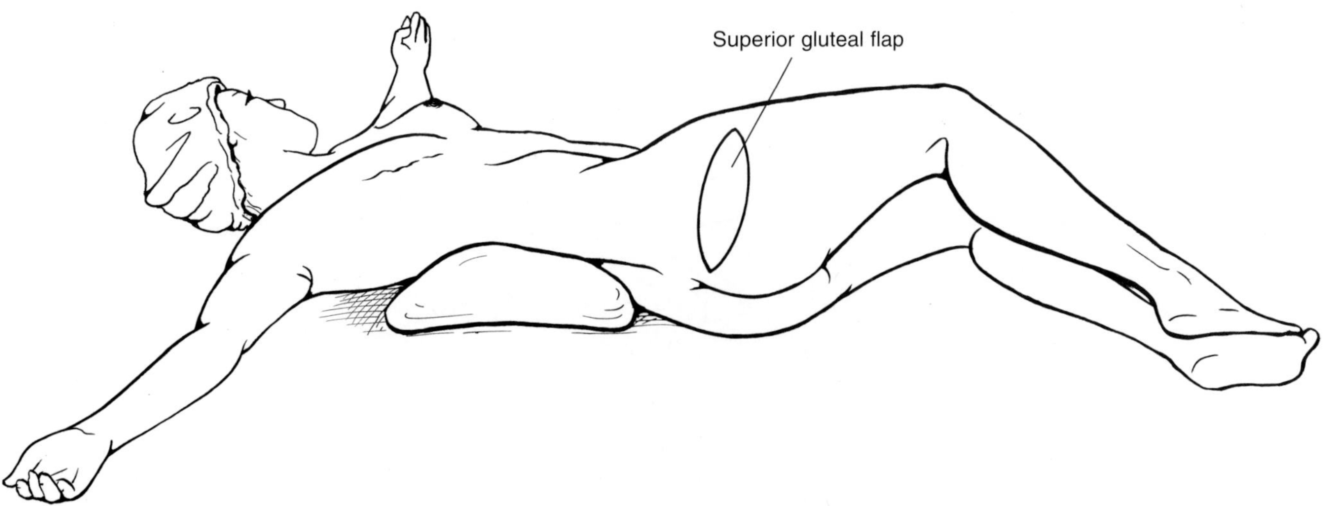

FIG. 2. The patient is positioned so that the recipient and donor site can be accessed simultaneously.

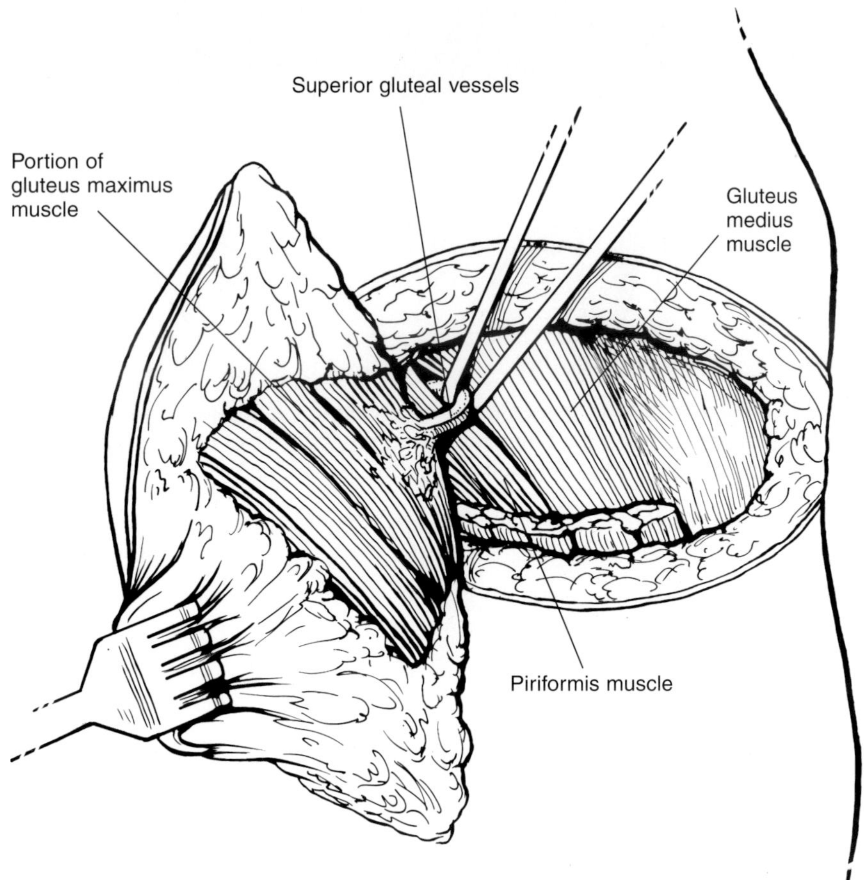

FIG. 3. The flap has been elevated with a portion of the gluteus maximus muscle. The superior gluteal vessels are located on the underside of the muscle and course toward their origin between the piriformis and gluteus medius muscles.

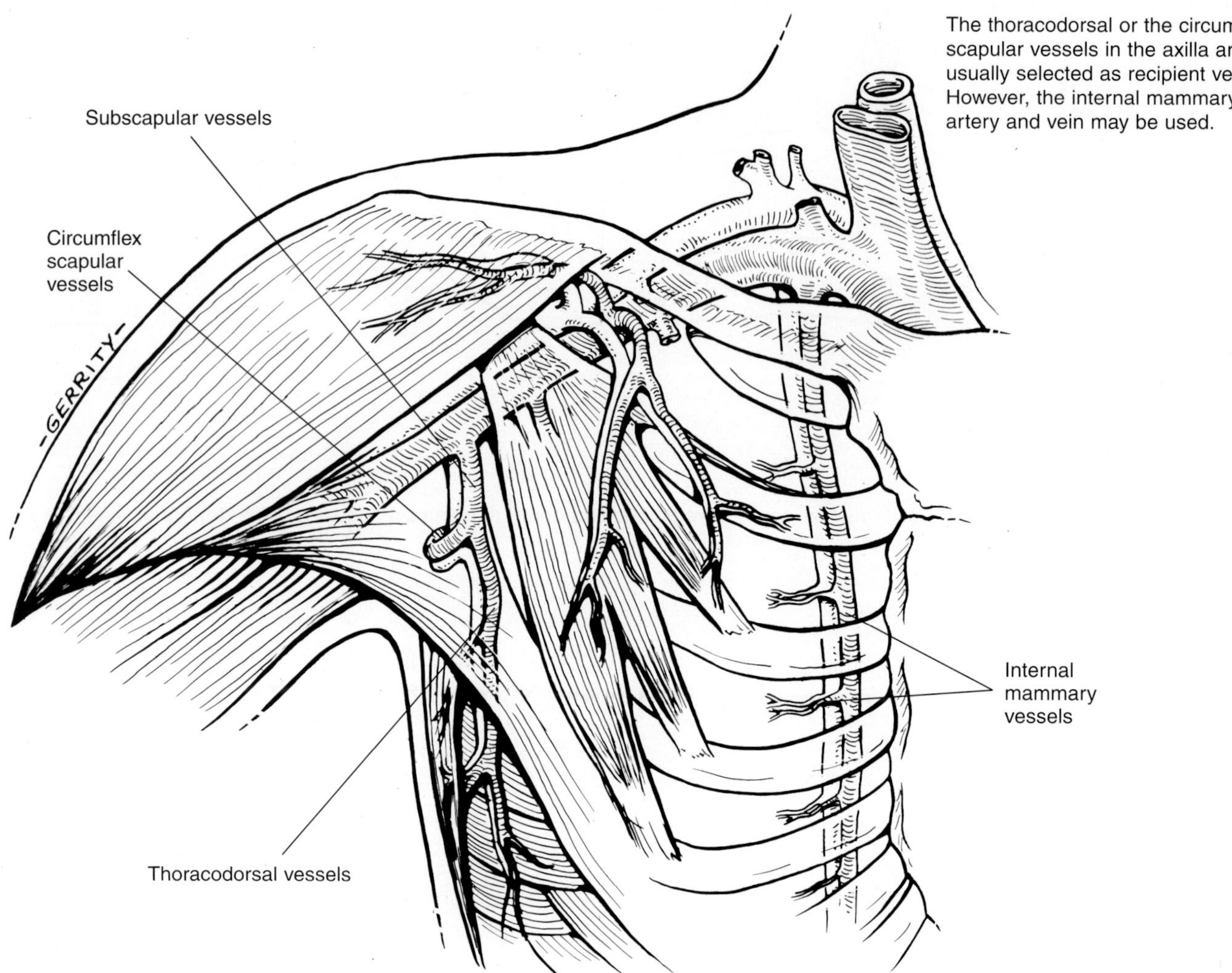

FIG. 4. The primary recipient vessels of choice for immediate reconstruction are the thoracodorsal vessels, with the internal mammary vessels being the secondary vessels of choice. The internal mammary vessels are especially useful in delayed reconstruction when the use of the thoracodorsal vessels is less compelling.

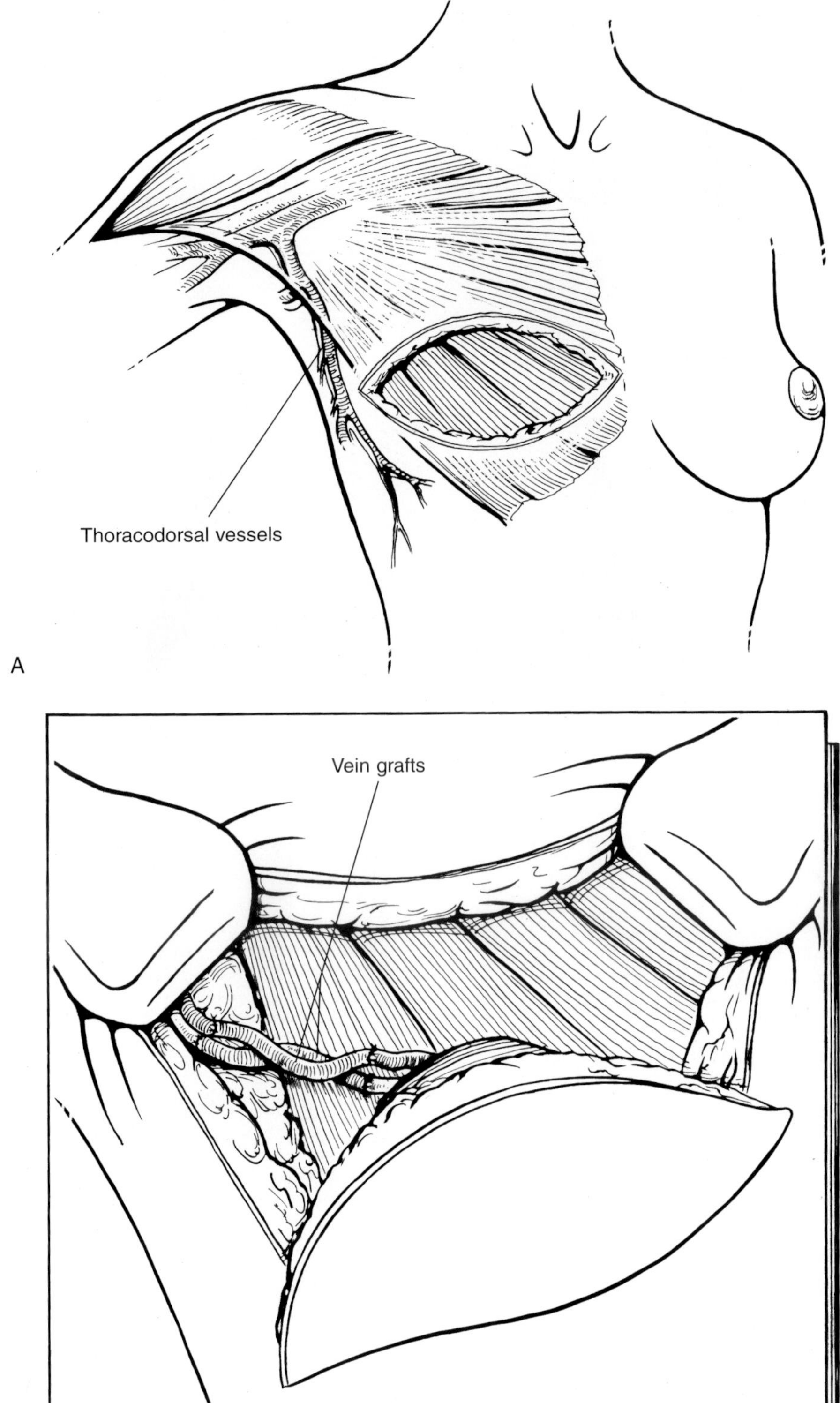

FIG. 5A, B. The flap is inset into the recipient site and vein grafts are used to access the thoracodorsal vessels in an immediate reconstruction.

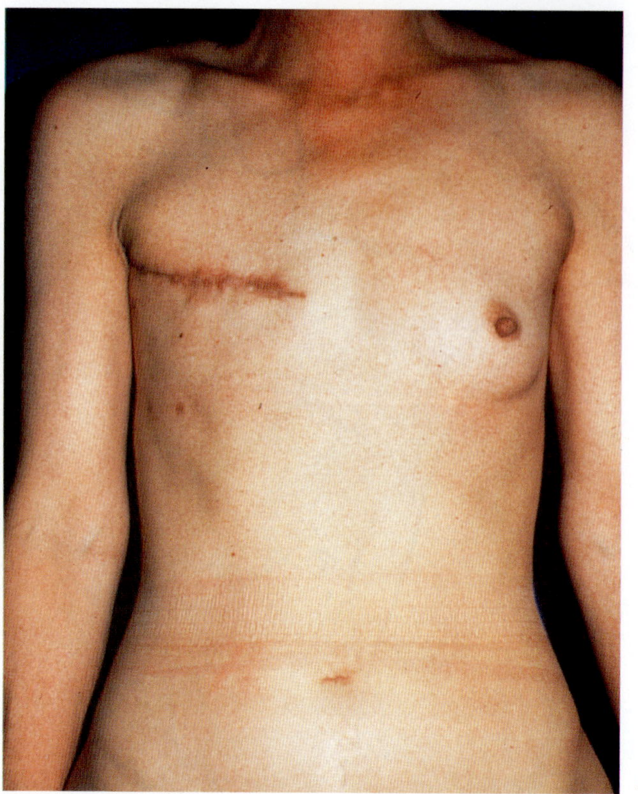

FIG. 6A. A 41-year-old woman after right modified radical mastectomy performed for treatment of cancer.

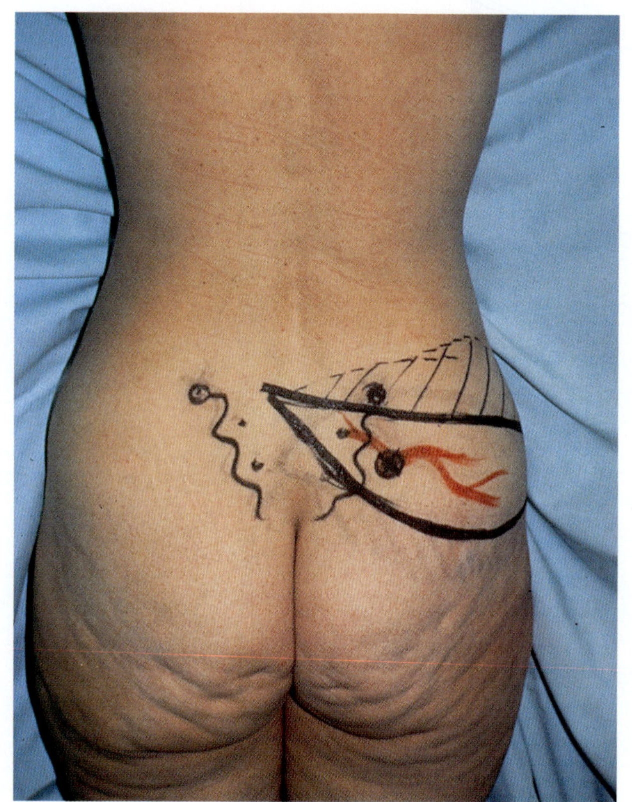

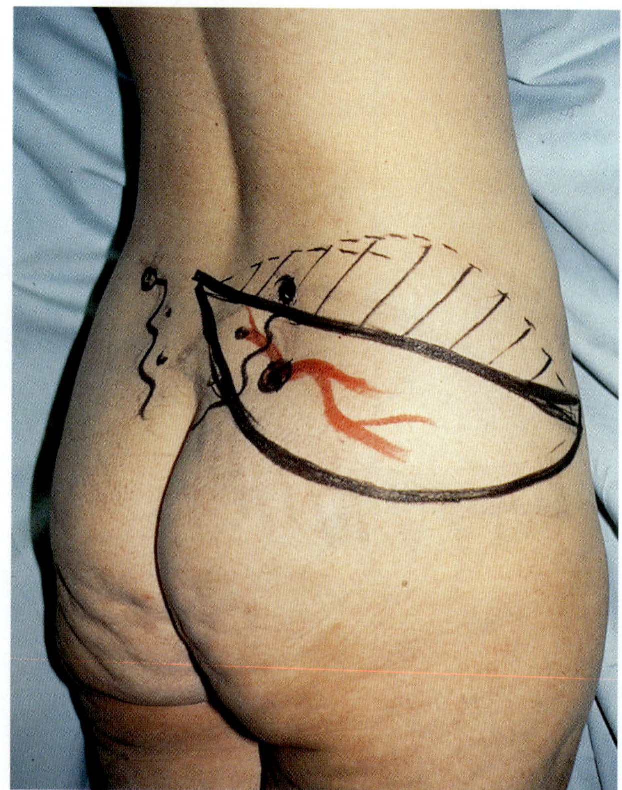

FIG. 6B,C. The plan for reconstruction with a right superior gluteal free flap.

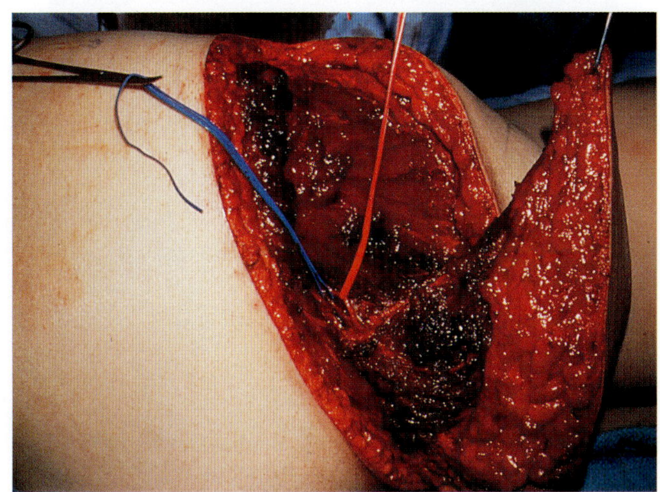

FIG. 6D. The short pedicle after elevation of the gluteal flap.

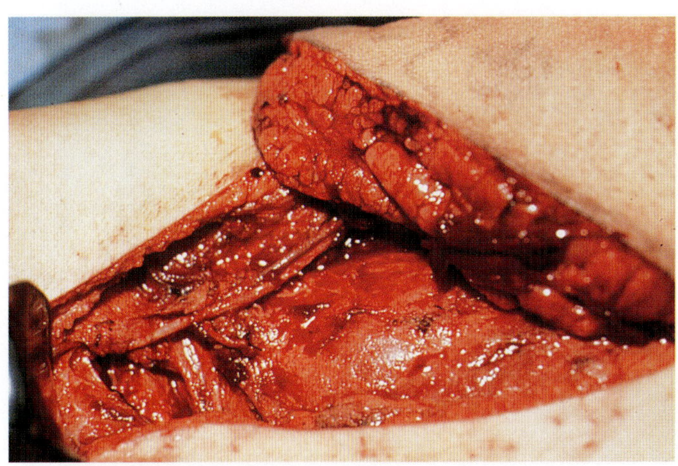

FIG. 6E. The flap after anastomoses to the thoracodorsal vessels using saphenous vein grafts.

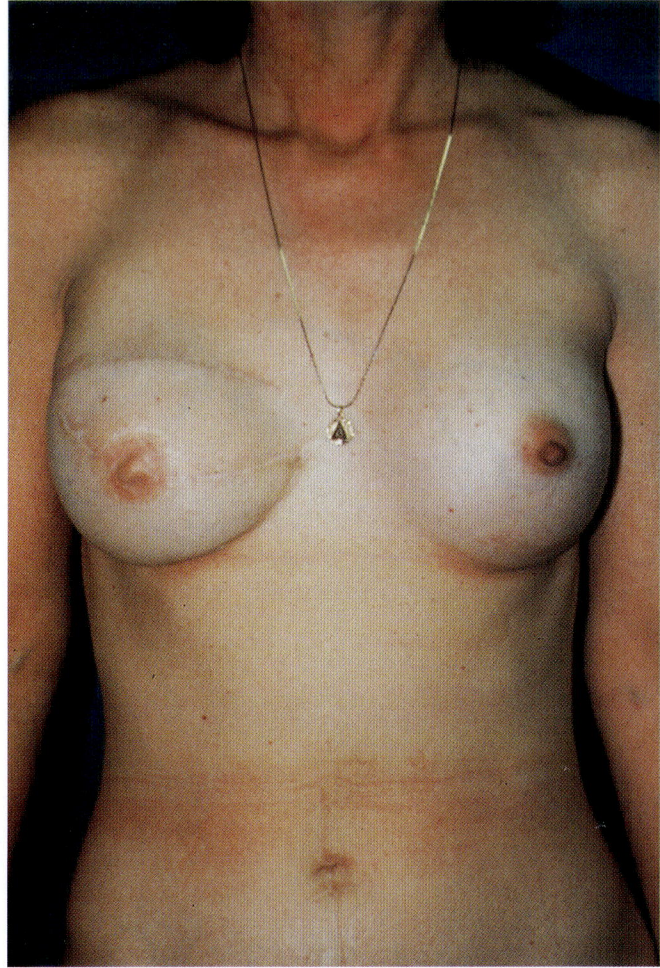

FIG. 6F. The result of right breast reconstruction with a superior gluteal free flap and left breast augmentation.

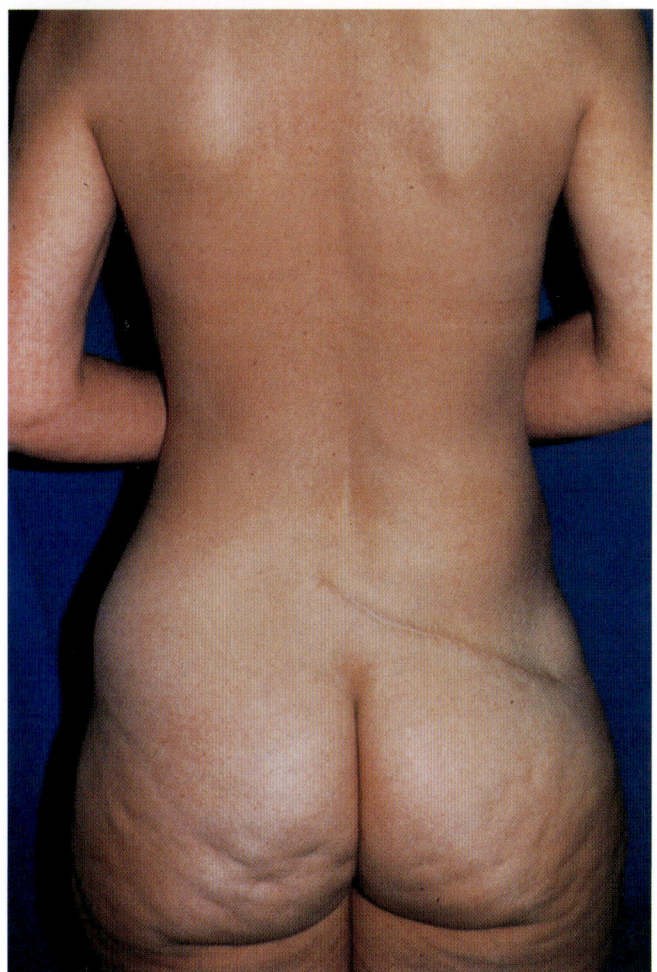

FIG. 6G. The donor site scar.

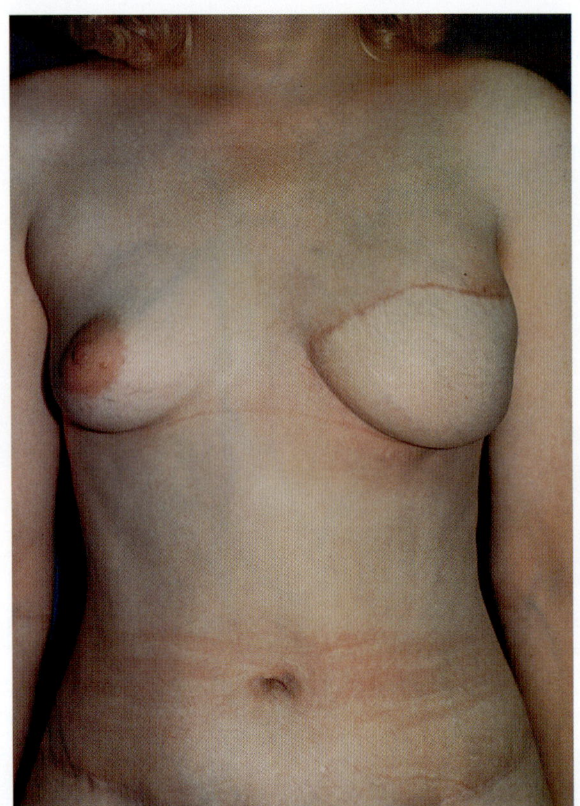

FIG. 7A. A 34-year-old woman (who had previously under-gone delayed TRAM reconstruction of the left breast) with newly diagnosed cancer in the right breast.

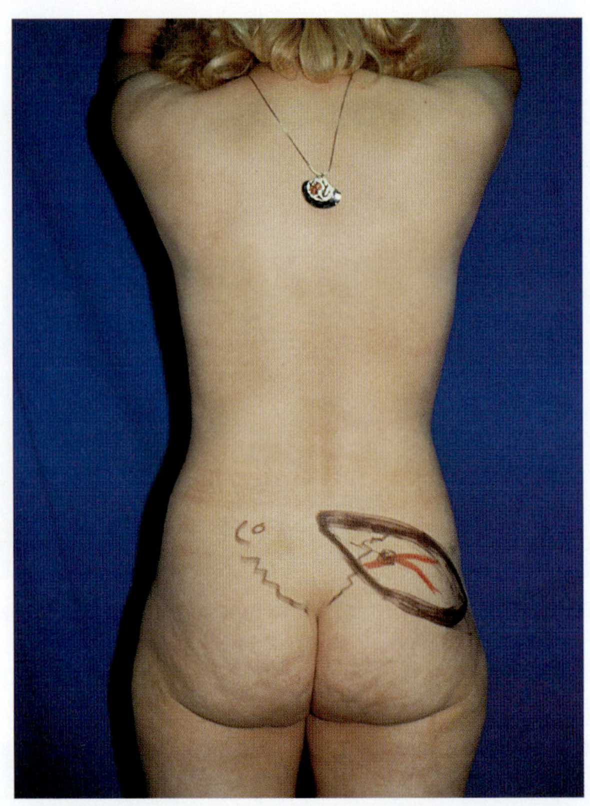

FIG. 7B. Operative plan for a right superior gluteal free flap.

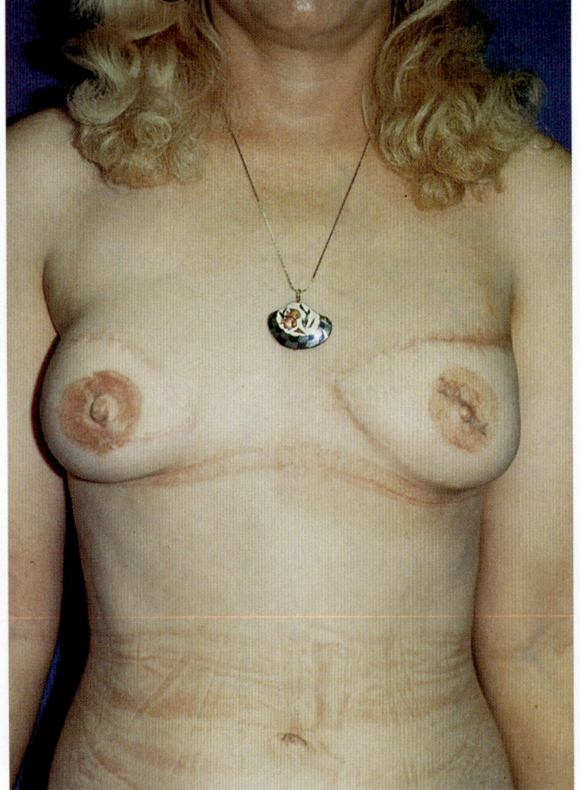

FIG. 7C. The result of breast reconstruction on the left with a TRAM flap and on the right with a superior gluteal flap.

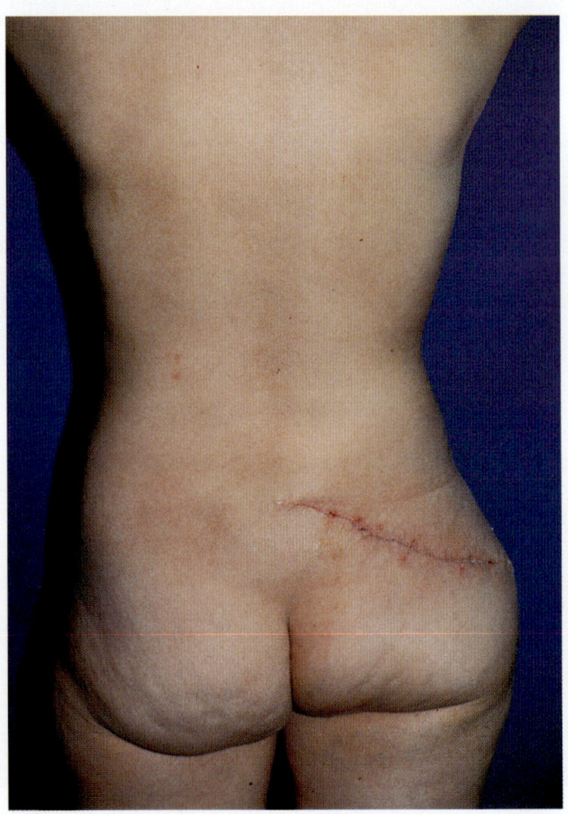

FIG. 7D. The superior gluteal free flap donor site.

but not eliminated, by careful flap planning. This difficulty in concealing the donor deformity is one of the reasons that the superior gluteal has not become as widely used as the free TRAM flap.

The loss of gluteus maximus function can affect walking, but generally only a small part of the muscle is sacrificed, and most patients have little or no postoperative disability.

Results of Reconstruction with the Superior Gluteal Flap

Patient 1 (Fig. 6A) is a 41-year-old woman who requested delayed right breast reconstruction (and augmentation of the left breast) and had rather large buttocks but very little abdominal fat. A right superior gluteal free flap was planned (Fig. 6B,C). The pedicle was very short (Fig. 6D), so vein grafts were used to allow end-to-end anastomoses to the thoracodorsal vessels (Fig. 6E). The final result is shown in Fig. 6F,G.

Patient 2 had previously undergone a delayed left breast restoration with a conventional TRAM flap (Fig. 7A). Subsequently, a second primary cancer was diagnosed in the right breast. A right mastectomy with immediate gluteal free flap reconstruction was planned (Fig. 7B). Following completion of the mastectomy, the flap was harvested and anastomosed to the thoracodorsal vessels using vein grafts. Figures 7C,D shows the final results.

SUMMARY AND CONCLUSION

Excellent results can be achieved with a superior gluteal free flap breast reconstruction. It is more difficult technically than the TRAM or the extended latissimus dorsi flaps, and therefore is not used as often. A superior gluteal unilateral reconstruction also has the disadvantage of causing a contour change in the buttock that may be noticeable when the patient is wearing pants. Vein grafts are usually necessary, especially if the thoracodorsal vessels are used as recipients. For appropriate candidates, however, the superior gluteal flap can be an excellent choice when autogenous reconstruction is required and a TRAM flap is not available.

SELECTED READINGS

Codner MA, Nahai F. The gluteal free flap breast reconstruction: making it work. *Clin Plast Surg* 1994;21: 289–296.

Elliott LF, Beegle PH, Hartrampf CR. The lateral transverse thigh free flap: an alternative for autogenous-tissue breast reconstruction. *Plast Reconstr Surg* 1990;85:169–181.

McCraw JB, Papp C, Edwards A, McMellin A. The autogenous latissimus breast reconstruction. *Clin Plast Surg* 1994;21:279–288.

McCraw JB, Penix JO, Baker JW. Repair of major defects of the chest wall and spine with the latissimus dorsi myocutaneous flap. *Plast Reconstr Surg* 1978;62:197.

Nahai F. Inferior gluteus maximus musculocutaneous flap for breast reconstruction. *Perspect Plast Surg* 1992; 6:65.

Shaw WW. Breast reconstruction by superior gluteal microvascular free flaps without silicone implants. *Plast Reconstr Surg* 1983;72:490.

Shaw WW. Microvascular free flap breast reconstruction. *Clin Plast Surg* 1984;11:333–341.

Webster MHC, Soutar DS. *Practical guide to free tissue transfer*. London: Butterworth, 1986.

Microsurgical Reconstruction of the Cancer Patient, edited by M.A. Schusterman.
Lippincott-Raven Publishers, Philadelphia © 1997.

10

Inferior Gluteal Flap for Breast Reconstruction

Christian E. Paletta and Foad Nahai

The inferior gluteal free flap offers an alternative in autogenous tissue breast reconstruction. The transverse rectus abdominis myocutaneous (TRAM) flap (pedicled or as a free flap) offers an ideal first choice because of its ease of elevation and patient positioning, and because of the normal amount of soft fatty tissue available in the periumbilical and lower abdominal region. There are some patients, however, for whom the free TRAM is not an option. The two most common groups are patients who have had previous abdominal surgery with transection of the lower rectus abdominis muscle and very thin patients with an inadequate amount of fatty abdominal tissue. When the free TRAM is not an option for autogenous breast reconstruction and autogenous tissue is the preferred choice of the patient and the reconstructive surgeon, the inferior gluteal flap offers a good alternative.

The inferior gluteal flap has several advantages:

1. a predictable consistent vascular pedicle,
2. an adequate cutaneous paddle for breast reconstruction,
3. a well-concealed donor site.

ANATOMY

The inferior gluteal artery is the terminal branch of the internal iliac artery. The neurovascular bundle exits the pelvis through the greater sciatic foramen below the piri-

C.E. Paletta: Division of Plastic and Reconstructive Surgery, St. Louis University Medical Center, St. Louis, Missouri 63110.
F. Nahai: Department of Surgery, Emory University School of Medicine, Atlanta, Georgia 30322.

formis muscle (Fig. 1A). The inferior gluteal vascular pedicle is accompanied by the inferior gluteal nerve, which innervates the entire gluteus maximus muscle. The inferior gluteal artery provides a vascular network to the inferior portion of the gluteus maximus muscle. It then continues below the lower portion of the gluteus maximus in the fibrofatty fascia of the biceps femoris and semitendinosus muscles to supply the fasciocutaneous segment of the posterior thigh. It is accompanied in this region by the posterior femoral cutaneous nerve, which also exits the pelvis through the greater sciatic foramen beneath the piriformis. The posterior femoral cutaneous nerve innervates the posterior thigh from just below the inferior gluteal crease to just above the popliteal fossa.

The inferior gluteal artery pedicle can be dissected to a length of 8 to 10 cm and usually has an inner diameter of 3 mm. It can be reliably sacrificed, as the superior gluteal artery provides an adequate collateral circulation to the remaining gluteus maximus muscle. The superior gluteal artery is also a terminal branch of the internal iliac artery. It exits the pelvis through the greater sciatic foramen superior to the piriformis muscle. The superior gluteal artery is accompanied by the superior gluteal nerve, which gives motor innervation to the gluteus medius, gluteus minimus, and tensor fascia lata.

The cutaneous paddle vascularized by the inferior gluteal artery and its corresponding muscle begins at the lower buttock and can extend to within 5 cm of the popliteal fossa as an extended gluteal thigh flap as described by Ramirez. For purposes of autogenous microvascular breast reconstruction, a transverse ellipse of skin is designed, centered just above the inferior gluteal crease and extending approximately 5 to 7 cm below the crease (Fig. 1B). Some of this cutaneous paddle is a true musculocutaneous flap, but the majority represents a fasciocutaneous extension based on the inferior gluteal artery.

PREOPERATIVE MANAGEMENT

The physical examination in the office is an essential part of the preoperative planning. The mastectomy defect is carefully evaluated both to determine the wound healing status of the chest wall region as well as the soft tissue requirements. The axilla is evaluated for any sign of recurrent tumor and lymphedema. Discussion with the surgeon who performed the original mastectomy is helpful especially regarding the status of the thoracodorsal vessels, as they are our first choice of donor vessels. It is also useful to have a copy of the mastectomy operation report. The ipsilateral gluteal region is examined to ensure that the gluteal soft tissue will be adequate for the breast soft tissue requirements. The opposite gluteal region is also inspected to see if there will be significant asymmetry following the inferior gluteal flap. If one anticipates such asymmetry, contralateral liposuction as a secondary procedure is discussed with the patient.

Evaluation of the opposite breast is also an important part of the preoperative evaluation as with any form of breast reconstruction. Each patient is individually assessed for either no surgery, contralateral mastectomy, breast augmentation, mastopexy, or breast reduction. While these ancillary procedures can be performed at the same time as the inferior gluteal free flap, they are usually done 3 to 6 months later on an outpatient basis. They can be combined with other procedures such as contralateral gluteal liposuction and/or nipple-areolar reconstruction.

Finally, the neck and ipsilateral arm are examined to identify an adequate cephalic vein or external jugular vein that may be utilized as a vein graft. The possibility of a vein graft as well as the incisions to harvest a vein graft are discussed with the patient. While the saphenous vein can be used also, its diameter and vessel wall thickness are thought to be less suitable than the cephalic or external jugular veins.

All patients are admitted to the hospital the morning of surgery. Depending on their medical condition, some patients are instructed to donate one to two units of autolo-

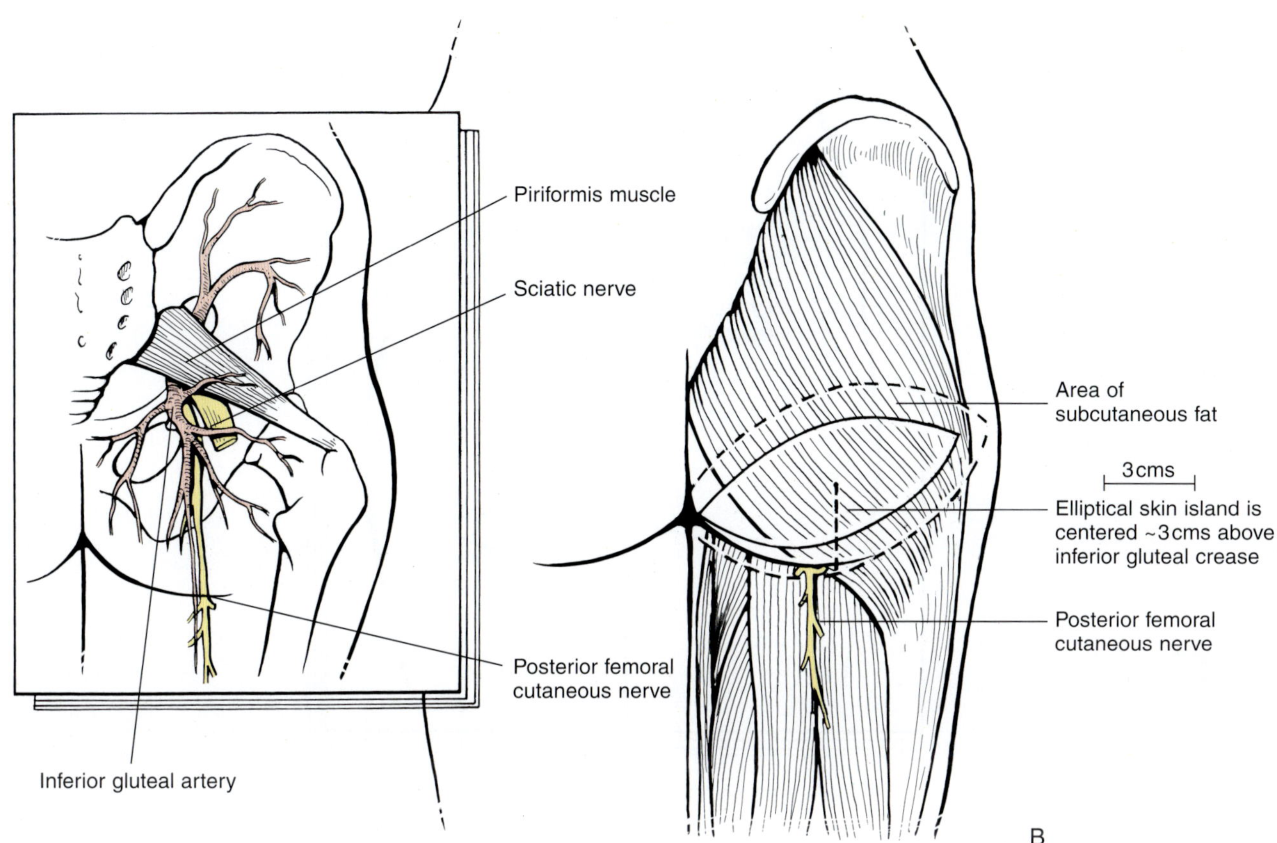

FIG. 1A. Anatomy of the inferior gluteal artery and its relationship to the sciatic nerve and posterior femoral cutaneous nerve of the thigh. The overlying gluteus maximus muscle has been deleted. **B:** The location and orientation of the skin paddle for the inferior gluteal flap.

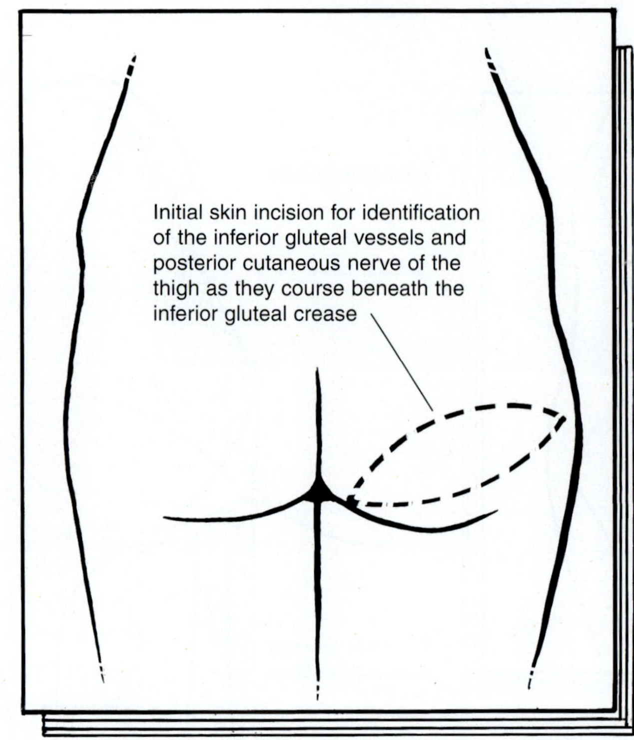

A

FIG. 2A. The skin paddle for the inferior gluteal flap.

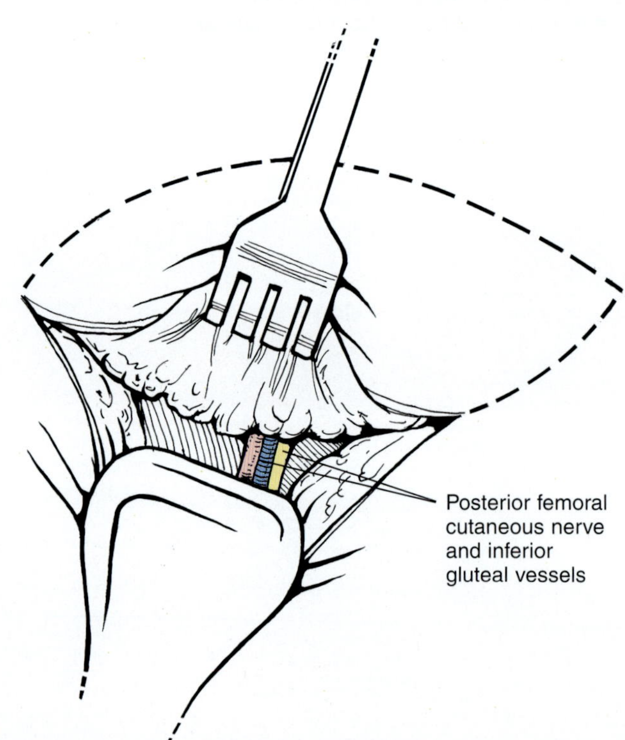

B

FIG. 2B. Inferior dissection to isolate the posterior femoral cutaneous nerve and the accompanying thigh extension of the inferior gluteal pedicle.

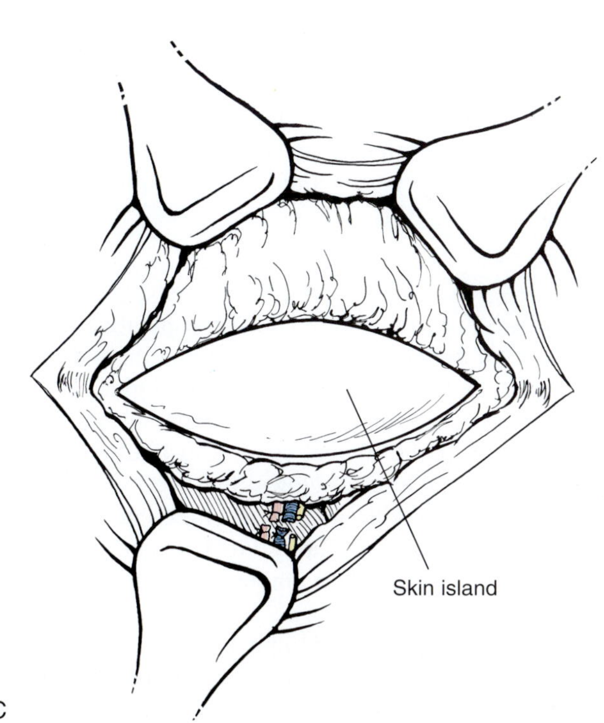

FIG. 2C. The skin island has been dissected and the inferior vessels and cutaneous nerve transected and ligated.

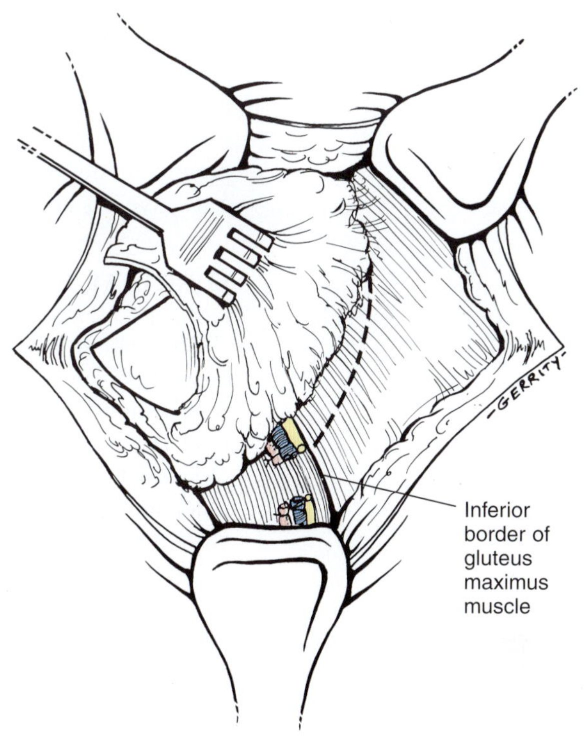

FIG. 2D. Transection of the lower portion of the gluteus maximus muscle adjacent to the skin paddle.

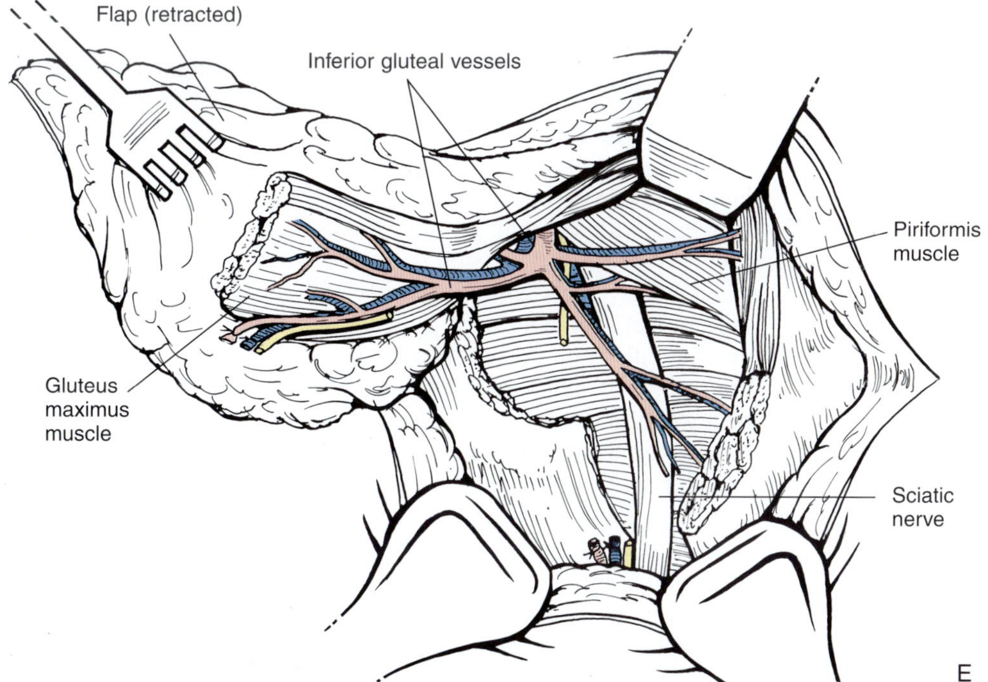

FIG. 2E. Elevation of the flap exposing the inferior gluteal pedicle and its adjacent sciatic nerve.

gous blood 4 to 6 weeks prior to their scheduled surgery. While the inferior gluteal free flap procedure has been done as an immediate form of breast reconstruction, it has been more commonly utilized as a secondary procedure 6 months or more after mastectomy. Smoking, heavy caffeine use, and other habits thought to be detrimental to microsurgical anastomotic patency and flap survival are discussed with the patient preoperatively and should be discontinued 1 month prior to surgery. A hospital stay of 5 to 7 days is anticipated, with a postoperative recovery time of 4 to 8 weeks.

SURGICAL TECHNIQUE

The patient is seen the morning of surgery in the ambulatory preoperative holding area. Preoperative markings are drawn on the chest wall to determine the soft tissue requirements. A transverse skin ellipse is then marked on the ipsilateral gluteal region with the patient in the standing position. If the patient has a moderate amount of redundant skin with gravitational sagging of the gluteal skin, adjustments must be made in the skin markings so as not to base the inferior gluteal flap too low. In such a case, it may be helpful to mark the gluteal flap with the patient in the lateral decubitus position. In either case, the flap is centered approximately 3 to 4 cm above the inferior gluteal crease. Flap width varies between 10 and 15 cm and flap length between 15 and 20 cm.

An intravenous catheter is inserted in the contralateral upper extremity and intravenous fluids are instituted in the preoperative holding area. Intravenous Versed (1 to 2 mg) is usually administered by the anesthesiology staff in order to relax the patient. All attempts are made to keep the patient warm during this preoperative evaluation. Essential before or at the time of preoperative assessment is close communication with the anesthesiologist. Length of procedure (usually 6 to 8 hours), fluid and pharmacologic requirements, avoidance of vasoconstrictor agents (e.g., ephedrine), the possibility of requiring blood transfusion (usually up to two units of packed blood), and the importance of maintaining the body temperature above 36°C should all be discussed preoperatively.

Following anesthetic induction, the patient is positioned on the operating table in the lateral decubitus position. An inflatable beanbag to stabilize this position throughout the procedure may been useful. The ipsilateral arm and neck are prepped in the sterile field in the event that a vein graft is necessary. The ipsilateral arm is prepped in a stockinette in order to allow intraoperative manipulation during dissection of the thoracodorsal vessels. If possible, a two-team approach is used. One team works in the chest and axilla creating the skin flaps on the chest wall into which the gluteal will be inset. The chest wall incision is carried into the axilla to dissect the thoracodorsal and subscapular vessels. Simultaneously with the chest wall and axillary dissection, a second surgical team begins the gluteal dissection. The lower incision is made first beginning laterally (Fig. 2A–C). Dissection is carried down to the gluteus maximus fascia. The fasciocutaneous extension of the inferior gluteal artery can be found just below the lower border of the gluteus maximus muscle just lateral to the ischial tuberosity. If the surgeon desires, the precise location of the inferior gluteal vessels can be identified with a Doppler prior to making the inferior skin incision. Running with this vessel is the posterior femoral cutaneous nerve. Once these are identified and dissected, the medial aspect of the lower gluteal incision is completed. The superior skin incision is then completed and dissection carried down to the fascia of the gluteus maximus muscle. With the skin incision completed and the inferior gluteal vessels identified running beneath the inferior border of the gluteus maximus into the posterior thigh, muscle dissection is begun. It is essential that the patient is fully paralyzed during the muscle dissection so as not to disrupt the vascular pedicle. An approximately 4 cm by 8 cm portion of the gluteus maximus muscle is dissected beginning laterally (Fig. 2D). The flap is elevated superiorly as the muscle is freed. The medial aspect of the inferior gluteus muscle is then incised carefully, observing the inferior gluteal pedicle and

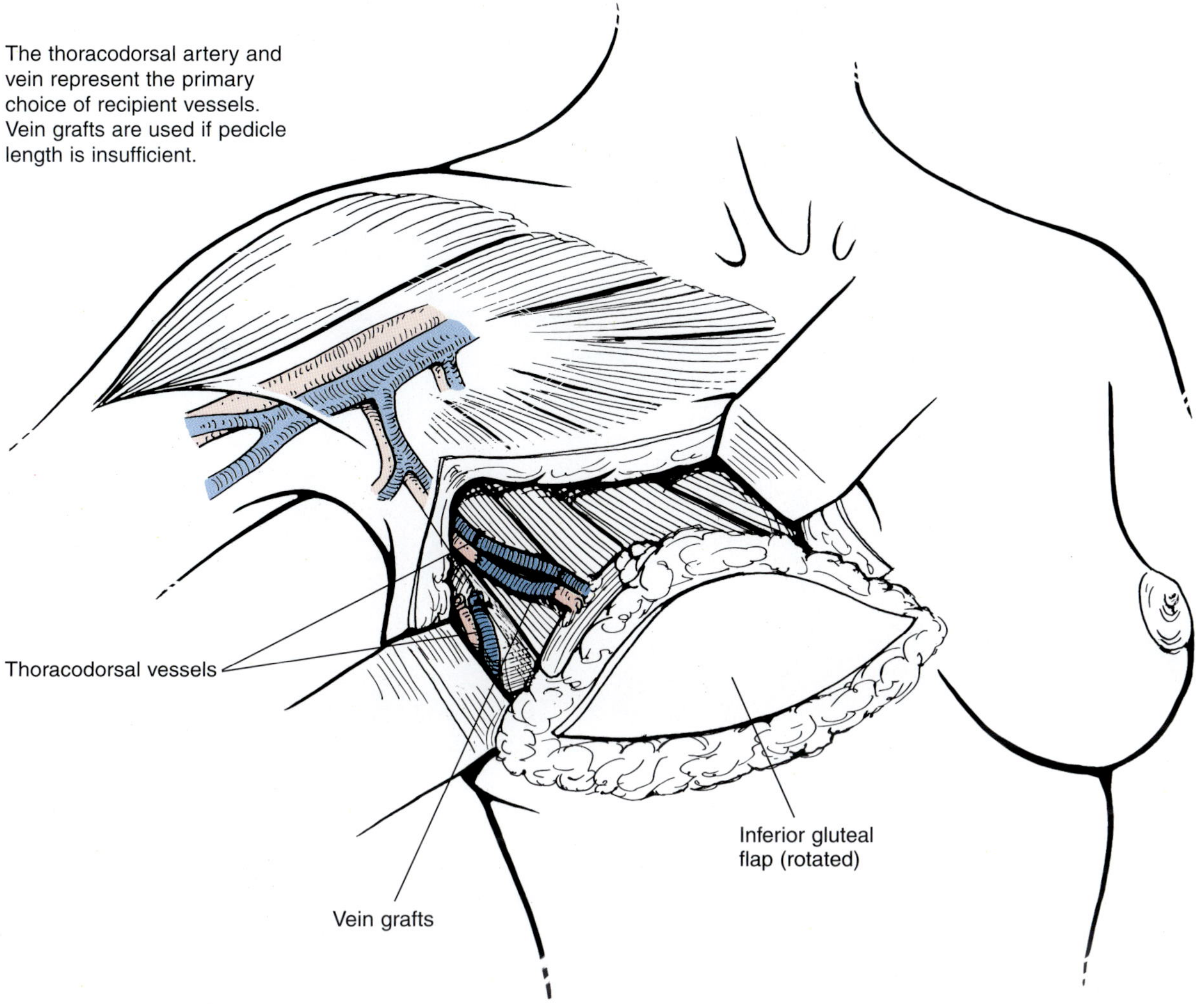

FIG. 3. Microvascular anastomosis to the thoracodorsal vessels prior to insetting of the inferior gluteal flap.

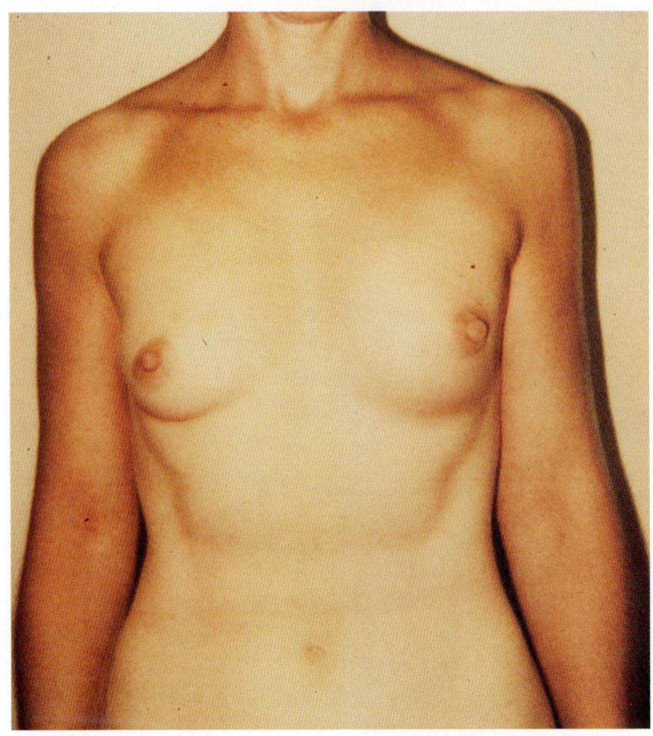

FIG. 4A. Premastectomy frontal view.

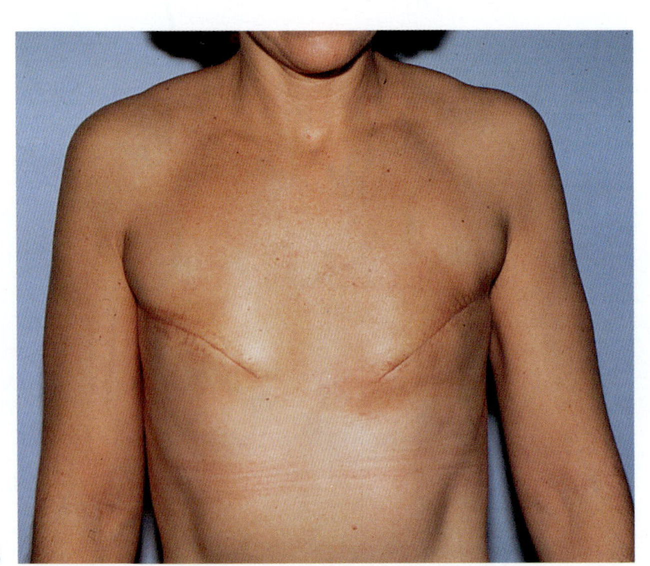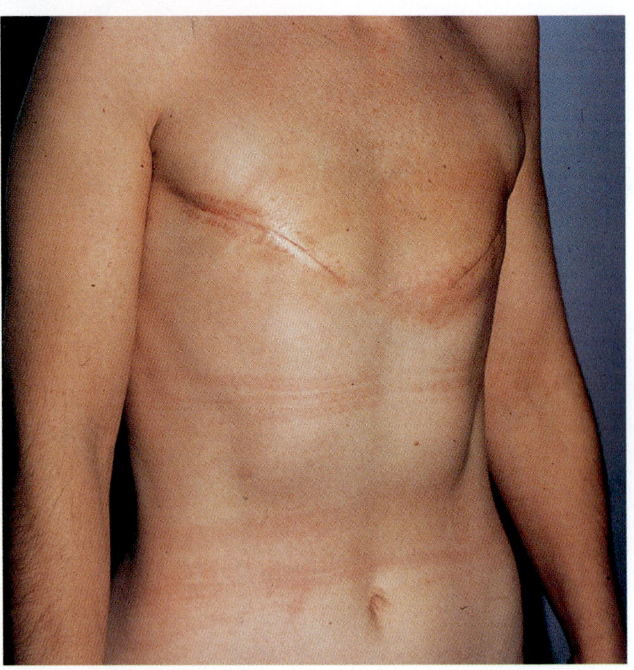

FIG. 4B,C. Postmastectomy, prereconstruction, frontal and oblique views.

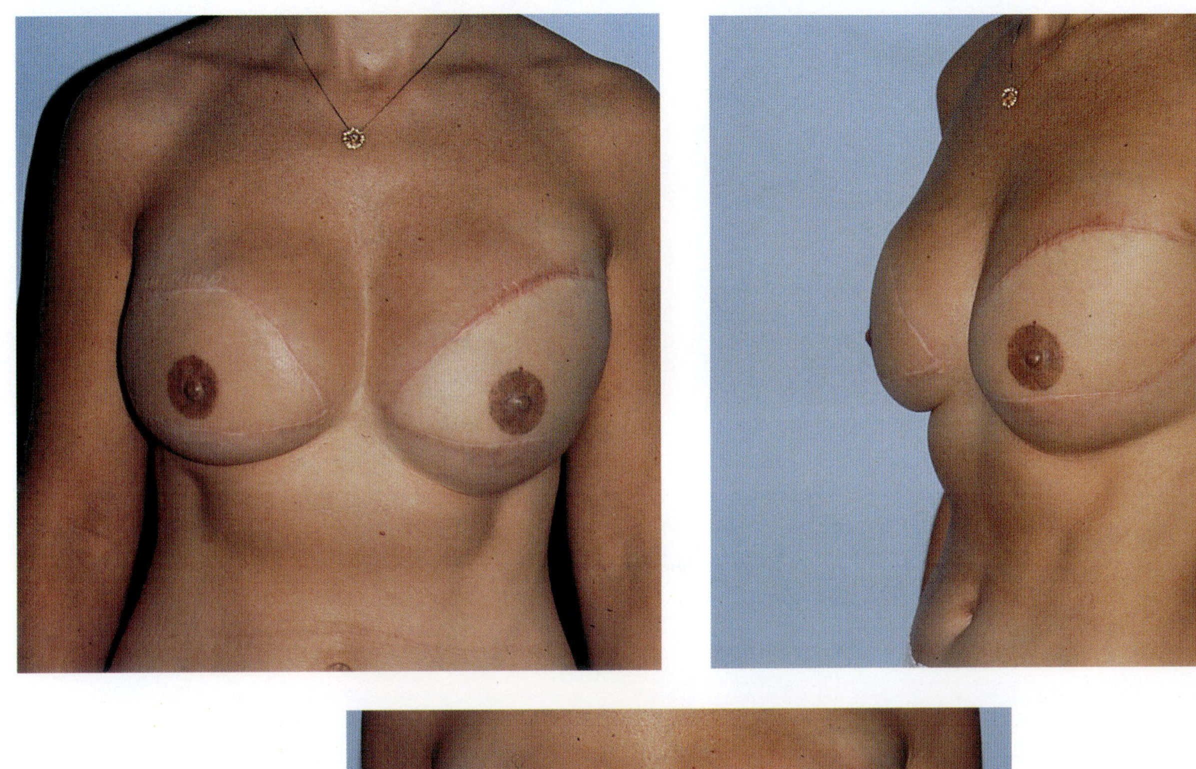

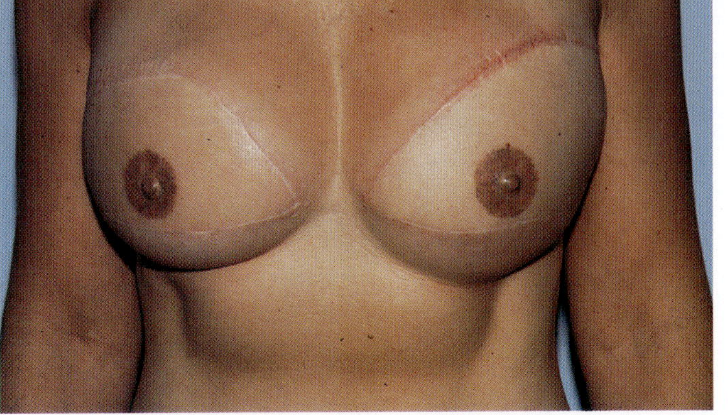

FIG. 4D–F. Early postoperative view after reconstruction with inferior gluteal flap bilaterally.

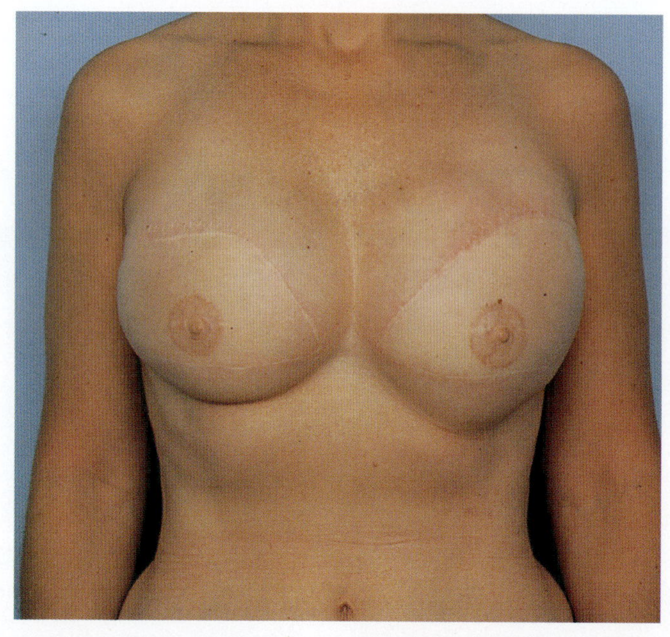

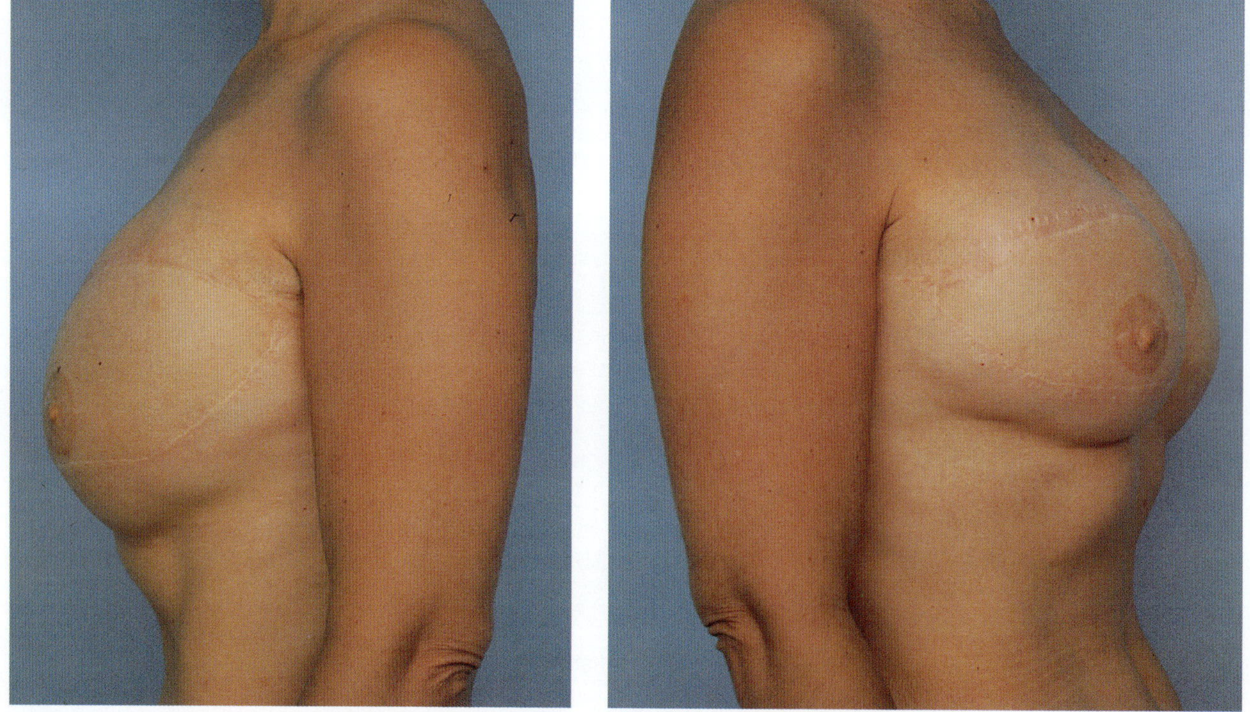

FIG. 4G–I. Appearance at 3 years postreconstruction.

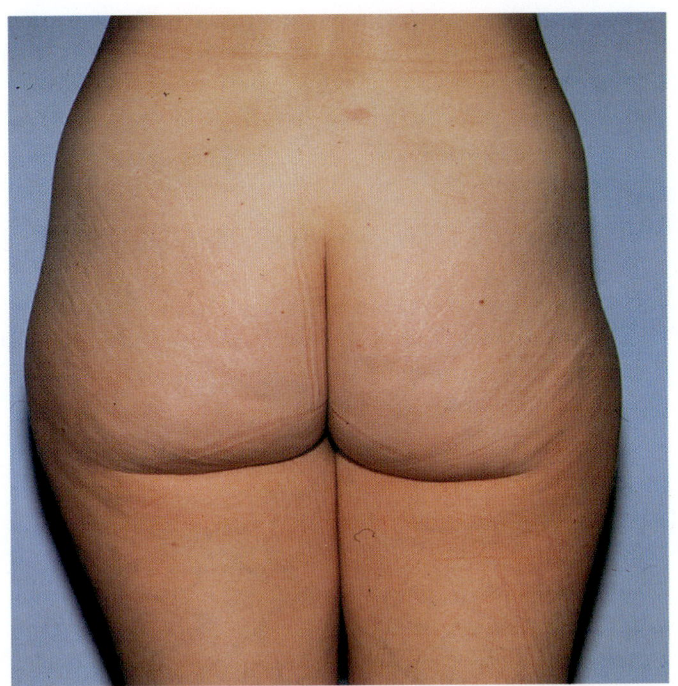

FIG. 4J. Donor site preoperative view.

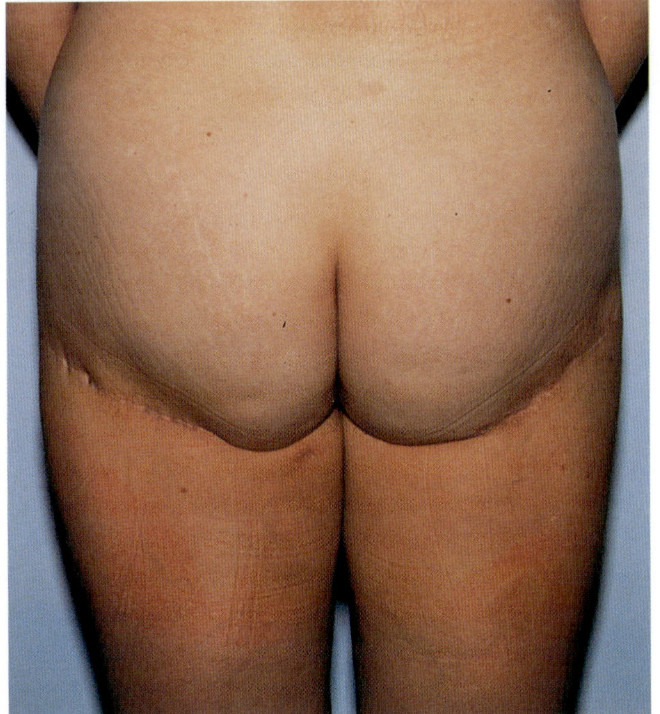

FIG. 4K. Donor site postoperative view.

its muscular attachments as the muscle is dissected. While the posterior femoral cutaneous nerve can be spared, it is usually transected both inferiorly as the flap is being elevated, and superiorly as the superior muscle sleeve is being divided. As one elevates the flap, the inferior gluteal pedicle is noted to emerge inferior to the piriformis muscle. With gentle traction on the muscle, this site of origin can easily be visualized (Fig. 2E). It is safe to divide the muscle superior to the pedicle while the pedicle is under direct visualization. One may choose to leave a small amount of lateral muscle tissue intact until the inferior gluteal pedicle is completely dissected in order to avoid undue tension on the pedicle during its dissection. Care must be taken during pedicle dissection to avoid injury to the inferior gluteal nerve, which emerges through the greater sciatic foramen with the inferior gluteal vessels beneath the piriformis muscle. One should also note and leave undisturbed the sciatic nerve directly beneath the section of muscle included in the flap.

The inferior gluteal artery and vein can usually be dissected for a pedicle length of 8 to 10 cm. The artery diameter is between 2.5 and 3.0 mm, while the vein is 4 to 5 mm. As with any microvascular transfer, the pedicle is not divided until the recipient vessels are prepared for transfer. Once the thoracodorsal vessels are adequately dissected and ready for microsurgical anastomosis, the inferior gluteal vessels are divided and the flap transferred to the chest. Proper insetting of the flap onto the chest wall is critical to ensure adequate location of the breast mound. One must be careful not to inset the flap too far laterally. Once several stay sutures have been placed to secure the flap into its correct position, the microvascular anastomosis is begun (Fig. 3). If there is any tension on the pedicle, then vein grafts are utilized. The cephalic vein from the ipsilateral arm or external jugular vein from the ipsilateral neck is preferred if a vein graft is necessary.

During completion of the microsurgical anastomosis, the gluteal wound is closed. The inferior medial and lateral gluteus muscle segments are approximated to cover the sciatic nerve. It is very important that the sciatic nerve is covered by the overlying gluteus maximus muscle. If necessary, the medial and lateral portions of the inferior aspect of the gluteus maximus can be undermined and mobilized to ensure adequate muscle coverage of the sciatic nerve. A suction drain is placed above this muscle closure. The subcutaneous tissue is then reapproximated. Depending on the amount of soft tissue removed with the inferior gluteal flap, the gluteal closure may be under some tension. It may be necessary to extend the hip in order to relieve tension on this portion of the wound closure. The deep fascia and fatty tissue are closed using a 2-0 braided absorbable suture.

The arterial microanastomosis is usually performed end-to-side to the thoracodorsal artery. The venous anastomosis is usually done in an end-to-end manner; 9-0 or 10-0 monofilament suture is used. Following completion of the microanastomosis, low molecular weight Dextran is begun at 20 to 30 cc/hour.

The inferior gluteal flap is inset into the previously dissected breast pocket and the deep subcutaneous tissue of the flap secured to the pectoralis major muscle with 3-0 or 4-0 absorbable suture. A suction drain is placed between the undersurface of the flap and the chest wall. This usually remains in place for 3 to 6 days following surgery. The skin edges of the flap are then sutured to the mastectomy flaps. A light dressing is placed and held in place with a loosely applied 6-inch Ace bandage. A similar wrap is placed on the inferior gluteal donor site.

POSTOPERATIVE MANAGEMENT

As with all free flaps, the flap is carefully observed hourly for any sign of vascular compromise. The Dextran is continued at 20 to 30 cc/hour until the third postoperative day. It is then decreased to 10 to 15 cc/hour until the fourth postoperative day, when it is discontinued. Most patients are kept on clear liquids for 1 to 2 days postoperatively. Ambulation is allowed on the first postoperative day. Hip flexion is limited depending on the degree of tension of the gluteal closure. Most patients remain hospitalized for 5 to 7 days following surgery. Because of problems with seroma accumulation in the gluteal donor site, the gluteal drain is left in place for 4 to 6 weeks following surgery.

Depending on their degree of activity, few patients return to work before 6 weeks. If flap revision is necessary, this is done as an outpatient 3 to 6 months following the inferior gluteal free flap. At the same time a contralateral mastopexy or breast reduction can be done to achieve breast symmetry. Contralateral inferior gluteal liposuction can also be done at this time.

RESULTS

Our series includes 32 patients who underwent an inferior gluteal free flap for breast reconstruction (Fig. 4A–K). Delayed breast reconstruction was performed in the majority of patients (88%). Ten patients had bilateral breast reconstruction with the inferior gluteal flap. The recipient vessels were the thoracodorsal artery and vein in the majority of cases (75%). Other recipient vessels included the circumflex scapular (9%), the axillary (6.5%), the internal mammary (6.5%), and the subscapular (3%). When the internal mammary vessels were selected (usually due to intense scarring of the axillary vessels), the internal mammary vein was inadequate due to its small caliber compared with the 3- to 4-mm inferior gluteal vein. For this reason, a vein graft is always necessary when the internal mammary vessels are used. Overall, vein grafts were required in 19% of cases.

There were no total flap losses in our series of patients. Some degree of fat necrosis (equal to or greater than 10% of the total flap volume) developed in 6.3%. A seroma developed in the gluteal donor site in 50%. This was successfully treated with aspiration in all but one patient. A mastopexy or reduction mammoplasty of the opposite breast was performed in 6.5% of cases.

SUMMARY

The inferior gluteal free flap is a reliable and dependable source of soft tissue for autogenous breast reconstruction. It is a useful alternative when local tissue with expanders and implants or regional tissue such as a pedicled TRAM is not available. While it can be performed for immediate breast reconstruction, it is generally used in delayed breast reconstruction.

SELECTED READINGS

Codner M, Nahai F. The gluteal free flap breast reconstruction. *Clin Plast Surg* 1994;21:289.

Eaves F, Codner M, Nahai F. The inferior gluteal free flap in breast reconstruction. *Operative Tech Plast Reconstr Surg* 1994;1:58.

Nahai F. Inferior gluteus maximus musculocutaneous flap for breast reconstruction. *Perspect Plast Surg* 1992; 6:65.

Paletta CE, Bostwick J III, Nahai F. The inferior gluteal free flap in breast reconstruction. *Plast Reconstr Surg* 1989;89:875.

Microsurgical Reconstruction of the Cancer Patient, edited by M.A. Schusterman.
Lippincott-Raven Publishers, Philadelphia © 1997.

11

Lateral Transverse Thigh Flap and the Deep Circumflex Iliac Soft Tissue Flap (Rubens Flap)

John M. Shamoun and L. Franklyn Elliott II

LATERAL TRANSVERSE THIGH FLAP

The lateral transverse thigh free flap (LTTF) is a horizontal variant of the more commonly known vertical tensor fascia lata (TFL) myocutaneous free flap. The conventional tensor fascia lata myocutaneous free flap is a type I vascular flap with one predominant vascular pedicle, which is the lateral circumflex femoral artery and vein. The LTTF flap is composed mostly of fat from the prominence of the upper lateral thigh (saddlebags) based on a small plug of underlying TFL muscle (Figs. 1 and 2). The LTTF flap was developed and is primarily utilized as an alternate source of autogenous tissue for breast reconstruction. This alternate source for autogenous tissue breast reconstruction is attractive in that this area is often redundant and excessive in many middle-aged women.

Anatomy

The lateral circumflex femoral vessels reliably supply the saddlebag area of fat extending posteriorly to the gluteal fold. The elevation of the flap is relatively straight-

J.M. Shamoun: Newport Institute of Plastic Surgery, Newport Beach, California 92660.

L.F. Elliott II: Department of Plastic Surgery, Emory University School of Medicine, Atlanta, Georgia 30322; and Atlanta Plastic Surgery, Atlanta, Georgia 30342.

forward. The main concern is balancing the tissue needs in the chest with the resultant residual deformity on the lateral thighs. The distribution of the patient's body fat must be carefully assessed to determine the ideal location of the donor site. It is paramount that the patient accept the position of the scar on the lateral thigh, and this should be discussed in detail with the patient preoperatively.

There are rigid fibrous septa that divide the fat into lobules, thus, providing a supporting framework. As a result, the tissue generally has more internal projection than the same thickness of fatty tissue on the abdomen. This is an important unique characteristic of the LTTF flap.

Surgical Technique

Lateral Thigh Markings

The axis of the flap is determined initially. The patient is marked in the standing position. The anterior superior iliac spine is first located and marked. A second mark is made 10 cm caudal to the anterior superior iliac spine (ASIS), denoting the surface markings of the underlying lateral circumflex femoral vessels. This point also marks the medial border of the flap where the vascular pedicle is found. The next marking is the gluteal fold as it curves anteriorly. A line drawn connecting the lateral extent of the gluteal fold with the point 10 cm caudal to the ASIS creates an oblique line that crosses at or just below the greater trochanter. This delineates the axis of the proposed flap (Fig. 1).

The design of the skin island within the flap axis is then determined. The position varies from patient to patient and is often inferior to the oblique line that has already been drawn. The thighs are viewed from an anteroposterior direction, and the point of maximal lateral projection is chosen as the center of the skin island. By placing the skin island over the point of maximal projection, the new breast will achieve maximal projection, as this is the area of greatest thickness of the lateral thigh (Fig. 2). The skin island can be moved cephalad or caudal to the oblique line, balancing the tissue needs on the chest with the resultant residual deformity on the lateral thigh. The objective is balance between adequate tissue transfer and the resultant contour deformity donor site. The size of the skin island depends on the needs for extra skin on the chest wall. Although a skin island may not be necessary in all patients, it is generally a good idea to retain a small ellipse of skin to monitor the flap postoperatively. The upper limits of the size of the skin island are dictated by the ability to close the elliptical defect primarily. The vertical dimension of the skin island is generally restricted to 6 to 8 cm and varies depending on the patient's body habitus and skin turgor. The horizontal dimension is limited by the girth of the thigh, which is usually 20 to 25 cm in length extending posteriorly from the point already marked below the ASIS to the gluteal fold. Usually, the skin island is designed to precisely replace the amount of skin that has been removed by the ablative surgeon or as a small strip to monitor the flap.

The operative plan takes into account the size and shape of the opposite breast as well as the location of donor vessels for microvascular anastomosis. The flap is harvested from the same side as the mastectomy defect so that the portion of the flap inferior to the skin island is tapered in a wedge-like fashion to simulate the normal superior contour of the breast on the chest wall.

Chest markings are made prior to the ablative surgery if immediate reconstructive surgery is anticipated. With the patient upright, the lateral and superior extension of the mastectomy defect as well as the level of the inframammary fold is marked. If a delayed reconstructive endeavor is planned, the skin deficit is measured in a vertical as well as horizontal dimension. Interaction between the ablative surgeon and the reconstructive surgeon is very important. The mastectomy incision should be positioned to obtain the best result from an oncologic standpoint primarily but with aesthetic considerations secondarily.

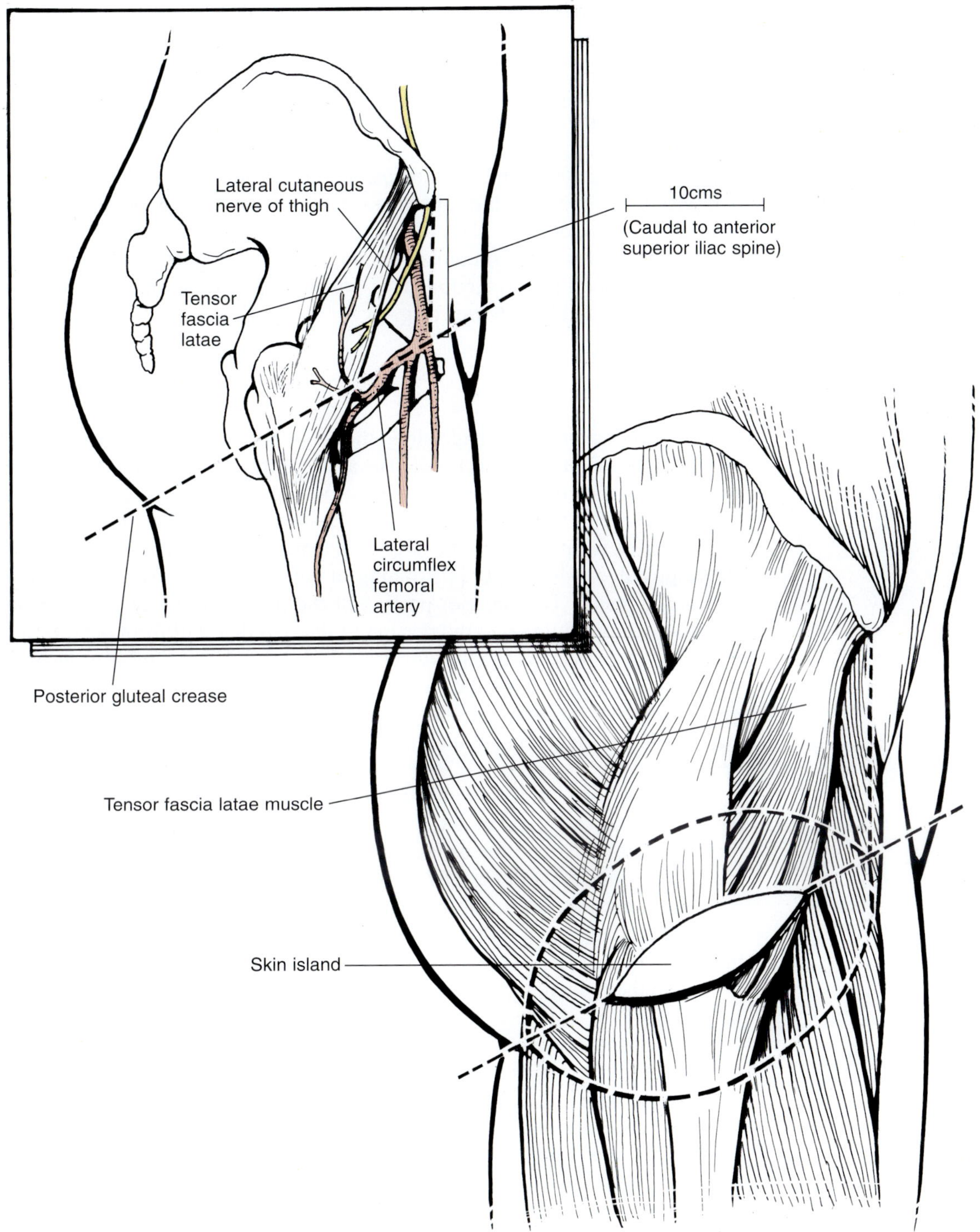

FIG. 1. Vascular anatomy and preoperative planning for LTTF free flap. *Dotted line* denotes fat harvesting. **Inset:** *Dotted line* refers to axis of flap.

No special patient preparation is necessary. Routinely patients are admitted on the day of the operative procedure and are taken directly to the operating room. No angiographic studies of the recipient or donor sites are performed. An estimate of skin and volume requirements for breast reconstruction is made based on the resected weight of the mastectomy specimen, if available for comparison, as well as the size and shape of the patient's opposite breast.

The patient is placed in a supine position on the operative table, and a Foley catheter is inserted. The patient's hips are then rotated 45° and a beanbag is used as a support to maintain this position. The donor site should be elevated to expose the entire area for the flap harvest. The shoulders remain flat on the operating table and all pressure points are padded for protection. This positioning allows simultaneous dissection of the chest and lateral thigh area (Fig. 3).

Flap Elevation

The thigh incisions are made along the previously drawn skin markings. Dissection of the subcutaneous tissue is beveled away from the skin incision to the preoperatively drawn margins of the planned flap. This is usually for a distance of 5 to 8 cm depending on the size of the new breast to be reconstructed. It is best to leave at least 0.5 to 1 cm layer of fat attached to the overlying skin. Inferiorly, the flap is fashioned into a tapering wedge, which after positioning in the chest pocket will fill the superior portion of the breast. The superior portion of the flap is cut to include a thicker bulk of flap giving more fullness to the portion of the flap that will form the inferior aspect of the breast (Fig. 4A). At the inferior limit of the flap, dissection continues through the subcutaneous tissue until the fascia lata is encountered. The fascia lata is incised exposing the vastus lateralis. There is an easily developed plane between the vastus lateralis and fascia lata muscles that is dissected in a superior direction to the level of the vessels.

A superior incision is then made through the subcutaneous tissue and fascia lata at the upper extent of the flap and extended into and through the TFL muscle. Deep to the TFL muscle is the gluteus medius muscle. The bloodless plane between the gluteus medius muscle and the TFL should be followed inferiorly. Dissection continues posteriorly toward the gluteal fold, harvesting a wedge-shaped portion of fat. This will form the medial aspect of the new breast if the thoracodorsal vessels are utilized. It is important not to harvest too much fat in this posterior location because it is usually not needed in the medial portion of the new breast. Furthermore, if the surgeon leaves the fat overlying the gluteus maximus, it will improve the resultant deformity in that area.

The flap is then elevated anteriorly exposing the plane between the TFL and the gluteus medius superiorly and the vastus lateralis inferiorly. An aponeurotic dense intramuscular septum is found that separates the posterior compartment containing the gluteus maximus muscle from the anterior compartment containing the vastus lateralis muscle. This aponeurosis is incised and the flap is elevated off the underlying vastus lateralis muscle revealing the entry of the lateral circumflex femoral vessels into the TFL muscle (Fig. 4B). This point is 10 cm inferior to the ASIS. The incisions through the fascia lata inferiorly and the TFL muscles superiorly are then completed. The rectus femoris and sartorius muscles, which are medial, have not been disturbed at this point.

Dissection of the pedicle can then be approached in one of two ways. The first method is to dissect from superficial to deep in the interval between the rectus femoris and TFL muscles. The second, which is more difficult, is to work from deep to superficial with the posterior portion of the flap retracted anteriorly. The pedicle as it courses medially first lies on the surface of the vastus lateralis muscle. Several large branches are encountered during this dissection to both the vastus lateralis posteriorly as well as the rectus femoris anteriorly (Fig. 2). The pedicle itself generally takes a slightly inferior course as it travels toward its origin on the profundus vessels. With

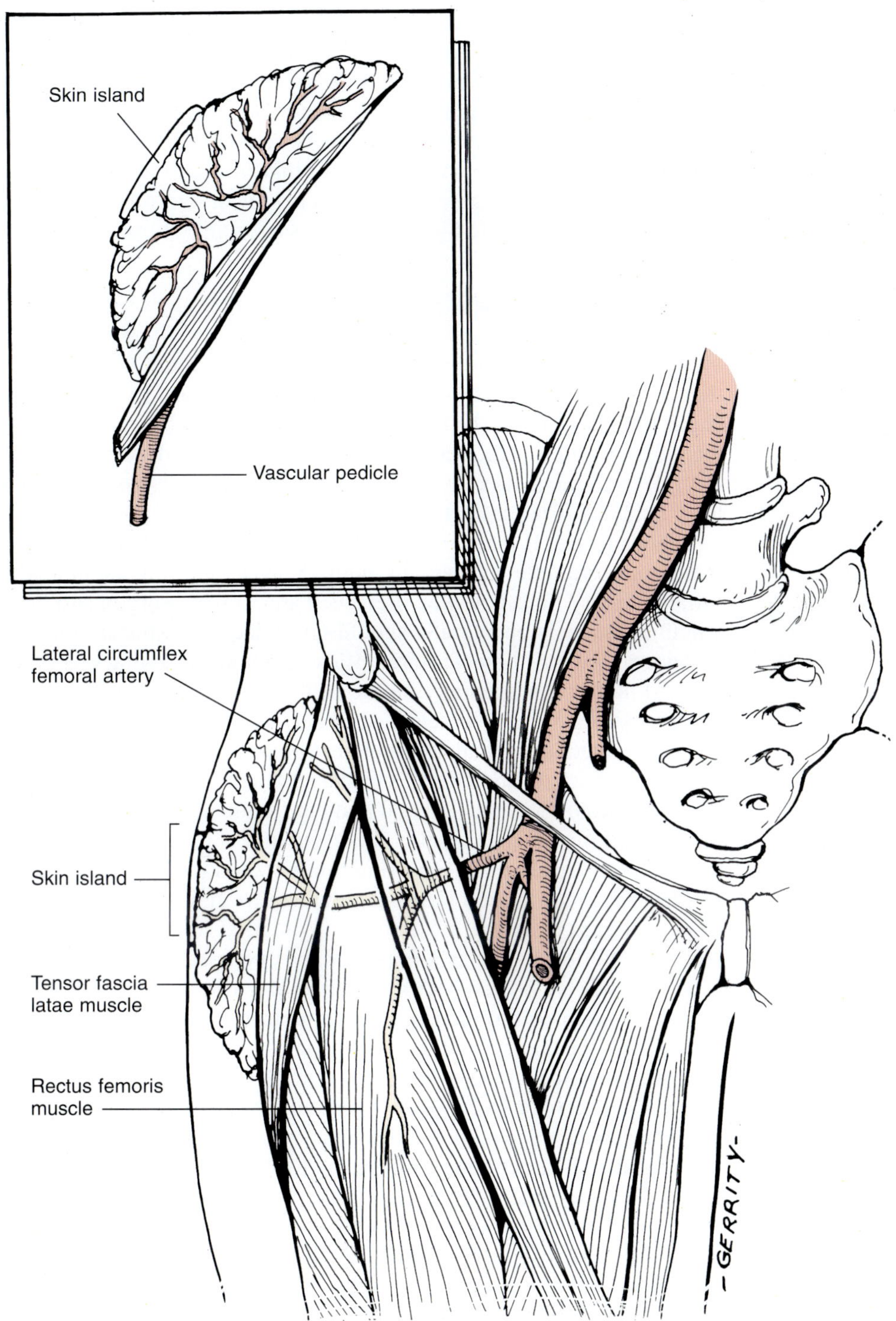

FIG. 2. Vascular anatomy and point of maximum projection of flap. **Inset:** Flap after harvesting.

retraction of the rectus femoris muscle, it is worthwhile to appreciate the course of the main pedicle prior to dividing any of its large branches.

Dissection toward the profundus vessels can increase the length of the pedicle to 6 to 8 cm. At this point, the flap is an island and is ready for transfer. Once isolated, the flap vessels are divided and the flap is removed from the donor site. The flap is weighed and the weight compared with that of the resected specimen for subsequent shaping. The flap is transferred to the chest wall and positioned so that the flap vessels closely approximate the recipient vessels without tension.

Preparation of Recipient Site

The resecting surgeon may perform the mastectomy while dissection of the LTTF flap begins. If the mastectomy has already been performed, two microsurgeons can begin simultaneously. The team on the chest dissects the recipient vessels and prepares the recipient site for the flap, while the second team dissects the LTTF.

In delayed reconstruction, the mastectomy scar is excised and submitted for histologic analysis. The mastectomy defect is re-created by undermining the skin and subcutaneous tissue. If the weight of the mastectomy is known, it is very helpful in anticipating the volume needed, in both delayed as well as immediate settings. The inframammary line should be preserved and, if necessary, it should be re-created. The length of the incision laterally should give adequate exposure for use of either the thoracodorsal, lateral thoracic, circumflex scapular, or axillary vessels for anastomoses (Fig. 5). Retraction medially on the skin flap can allow adequate exposure for use of the internal mammary vessels if need be.

The thoracodorsal and internal mammary vessels have become our choices for anastomosis in an immediate and delayed setting, respectively. In cases of delayed reconstruction, the thoracodorsal pedicle frequently is encased in scar, and, therefore, the internal mammary vessel is preferred and is dissected after removing the third or fourth costal cartilage. When using the thoracodorsal vessels, the anastomosis is performed proximal to the branch to the serratus anterior and latissimus dorsi muscles. This preserves perfusion of the latissimus dorsi muscle via retrograde flow from the serratus anterior branch as a backup flap if necessary.

The vessels are prepared with the aid of magnification and the donor vessels are anastomosed end to end to their respective recipient vessels. We generally use interrupted sutures for the artery and vascular anastomotic device for the vein with standard microvascular technique. The lateral circumflex femoral vessels are of large-caliber width, the artery measuring 3 to 4 mm and the vein measuring 6 to 7 mm in diameter. This may create a 2:1 ratio size discrepancy between the recipient and donor vessels. We would generally accept this discrepancy for an end-to-end anastomosis. If, however, the size discrepancy is greater that 2:1, an end-to-side anastomosis is performed.

Once the anastomoses are completed the microclamps are released and the vessels are bathed in papaverine solution. After excellent blood flow is reestablished, the flap is rotated into an appropriate position on the chest wall, avoiding tension on the anastomosis. The small segment of TFL muscle is sutured to the pectoralis major muscle to prevent any inadvertent tension on the vessels of the flap as the flap is manipulated into an ideal position. The chest wall skin drapes over the flap and is temporarily closed with skin staples. The new breast is shifted around within the pocket to achieve optimal projection and shape with the patient in a sitting position. A drain is placed laterally, near, but not overlying, the anastomosis, and the skin incisions on the chest are closed.

DONOR SITE CLOSURE

Closure of the donor site begins with obliteration of the superior and inferior extent of the subcutaneous pocket using 2-0 Vicryl sutures. After decreasing dead space, two

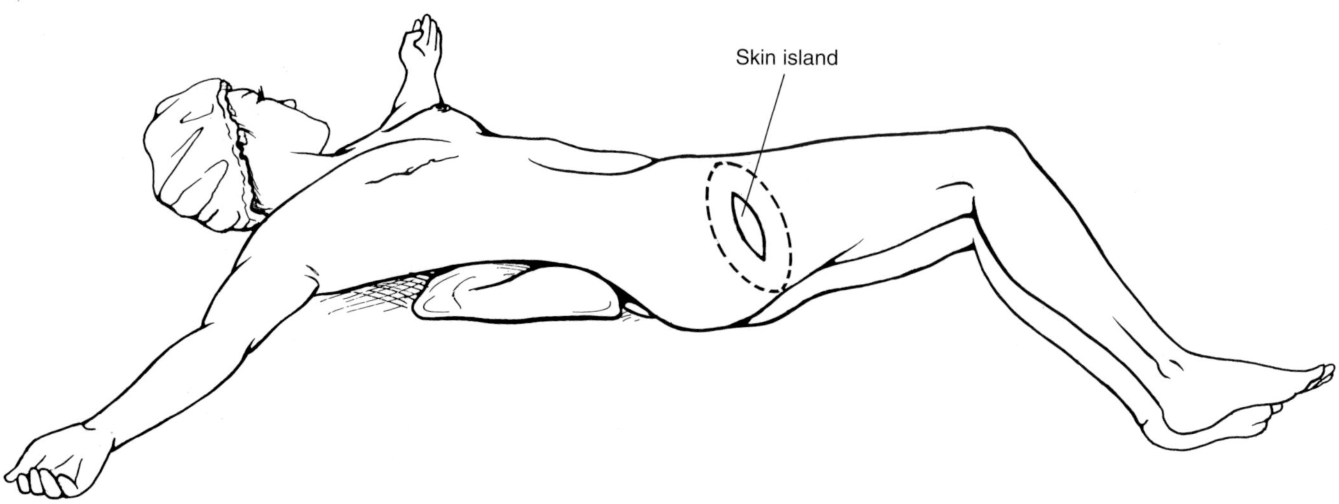

FIG. 3. Positioning of patient enabling simultaneous dissection of chest and lateral thigh.

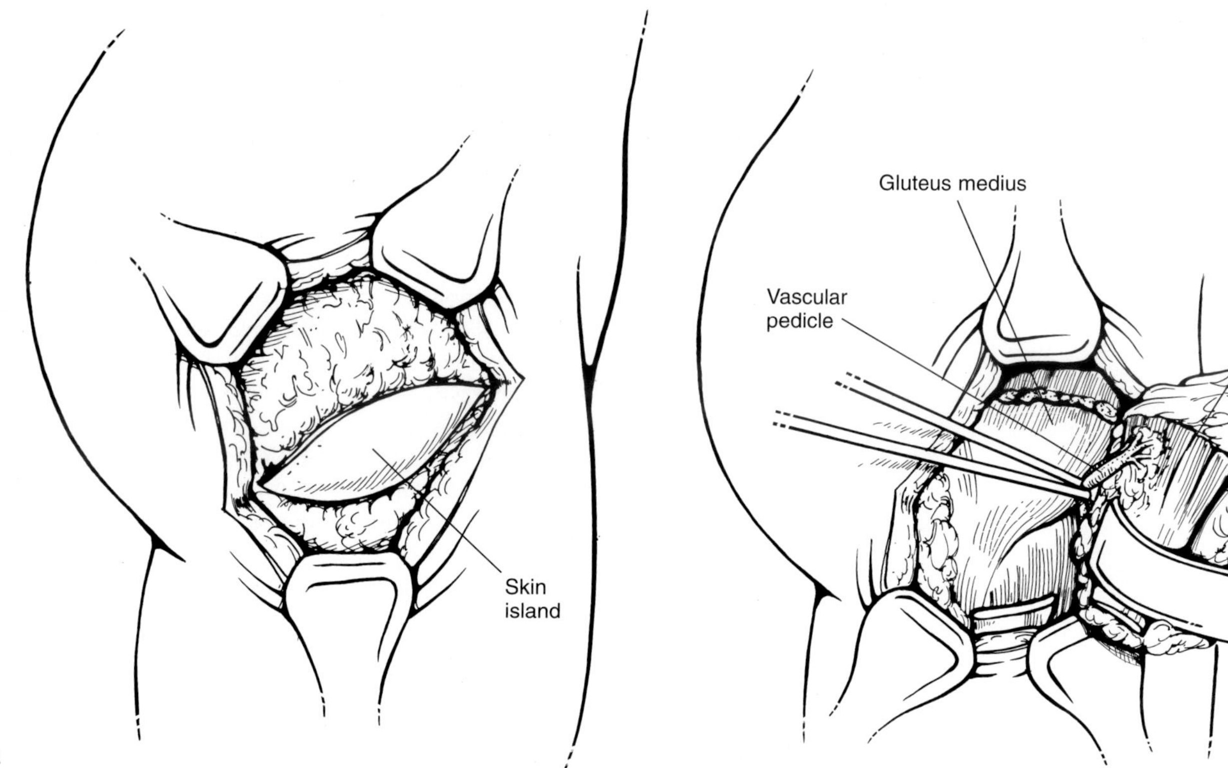

A

B

FIG. 4A. Flap elevation. Note the extra superficial adipose tissue harvested at the superior aspect of the skin island. This extra tissue will help give more fullness to the inferior aspect of the breast.

FIG. 4B. Flap elevation revealing entry of lateral femoral circumflex vessels into TFL muscle. Note vessel loop around lateral femoral circumflex artery and vein.

closed suction drains are placed in the depths of the wound. Overlapping skin is not discarded but is de-epithelialized so that the depression at the skin closure line can be minimized (Fig. 6A,B). Finally, we add an elastic garment prior to hospital discharge to provide continuous external compression to the donor site for 2 to 3 weeks. All incisions are covered with 1-inch sterile paper adhesive tape and each drain is surrounded by a gauze sponge after it has been sutured into place. The flap is observed frequently in the postoperative period and the patient is placed at bed rest for 1 to 2 days. Bilateral reconstruction can be performed either simultaneously or as a staged procedure 2 to 3 days apart during the same hospital admission.

Discussion

The LTTF flap has proved to be a reliable, natural alternative for autogenous tissue breast reconstruction. It has several advantages over other methods of autogenous breast reconstruction: (a) a longer, more peripherally placed pedicle; (b) a straightforward familiar dissection; (c) no need to turn the patient during the procedure; (d) decreased postoperative morbidity and rapid recovery; (e) reduction of an area of excess fat in patients in whom the hips are more prominent than the abdomen (Fig. 7); (f) greater intrinsic internal projection of the flap; and (g) excellent vascularity. The disadvantages: (a) the necessity for microsurgery, (b) the limitations on skin harvest, (c) the scar and contour deformity on the upper lateral thigh (Fig. 8A–F), and (d) the need for a balancing procedure on the opposite thigh.

Our current indications for the LTTF flap are previous transverse rectus abdominis musculocutaneous (TRAM) flap, thigh fat proportions greater than abdominal proportions, and patient preference for this option over the TRAM flap or gluteal flap. Complications have included flap loss, vascular occlusion, fat necrosis, seroma, hematoma, and unsightly scarring and depression.

Scar location should be discussed in detail with each patient. There is almost no bathing suit design that will cover its location because the scar crosses transversely over the greater trochanter. Photographs of previous patients are very useful in helping the patient decide whether the LTTF is the proper choice. Some express little concern with the resultant scar location, whereas others find it totally reprehensible. It is true, though, that with time the scar becomes significantly less visible (Fig. 9).

On the other hand, the contour deformity may be a more long-lasting area of concern for the patient as well as the surgeon. The enthusiasm for using this flap for any given patient should be tempered by considerations of the suitability of the lateral thigh in providing adequate bulk and the aesthetic result of the donor scar primarily. We must keep in mind that a depression in an area that is normally slightly convex becomes quite noticeable when it is concave, and is difficult to correct with liposuction alone (1–3).

To lessen the donor site deformity, it is important to harvest the flap leaving adequate fat underlying the residual skin flaps. It is also important to leave behind fat in a posterior location overlying the gluteus maximus muscle, as fat is usually not needed in the medial portion of the new breast. One must carefully close the residual defect in layers so as to obliterate the dead space and overlap the skin edges whenever possible in a pants-over-vest manner so as to supplement and bolster the incision line to prevent an unnatural depression. Peripheral liposuction at 4 to 6 months has become an important adjunct in lessening the deformity. Recovery after this operation is generally uncomplicated. Early return of activity may be associated with increasing seroma formation, which may necessitate prolonged indwelling drains or frequent aspirations for 6 to 8 weeks postoperatively. Pain syndromes are few and muscle function is essentially normal.

Our experience with the LTTF flap has shown convincingly the advantages of autologous tissue in contouring, softness, warmth, permanency, and patient satisfaction. In this day of a rising demand for reliable and convenient alternatives using autologous

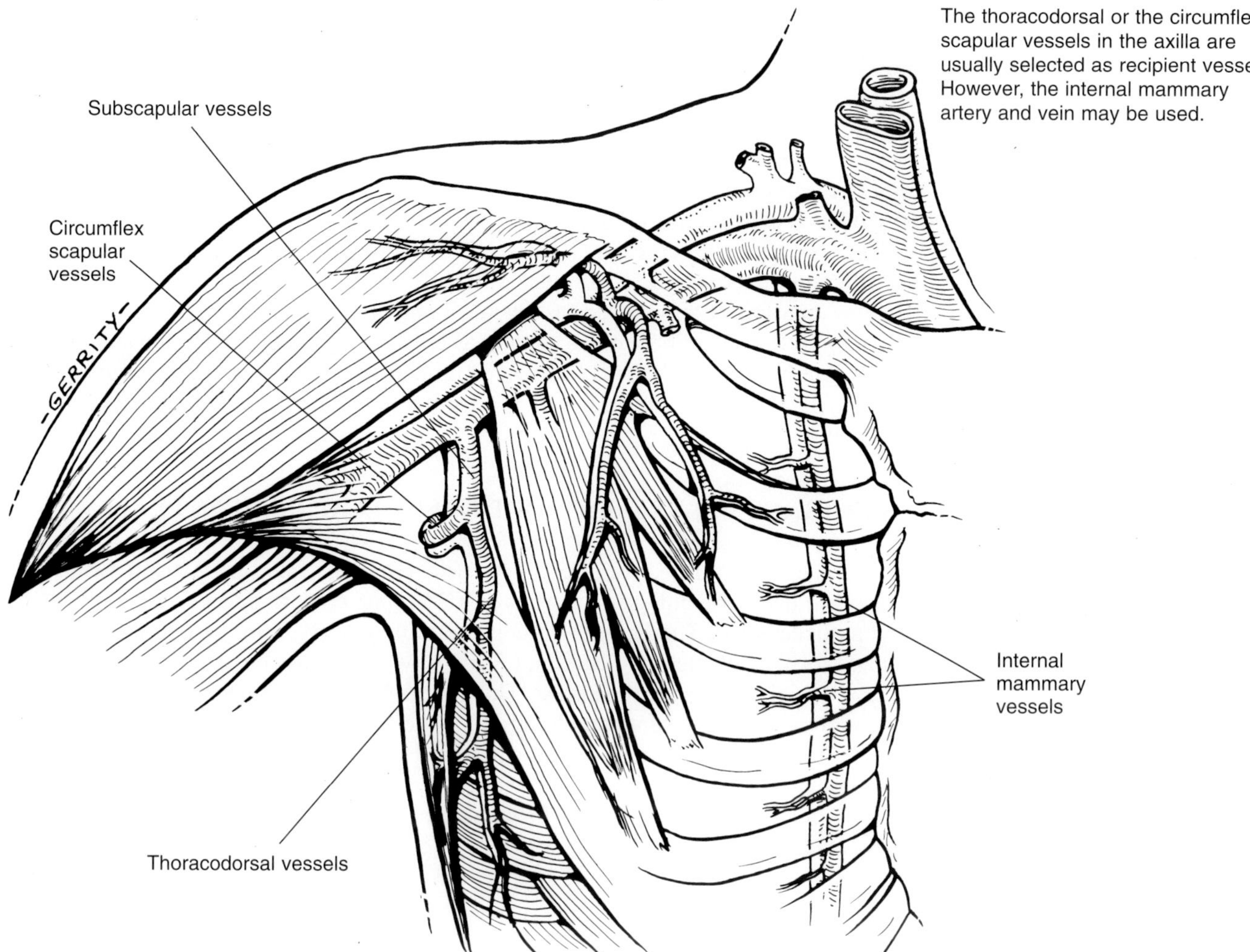

FIG. 5. Possible vessels for anastomosis in chest area. Note pectoralis major has been removed for purposes of drawing.

tissue for breast reconstruction, we believe the LTTF flap is an excellent alternative for autogenous tissue breast reconstruction. However, we believe that the technical advantages of easy dissection, long pedicle, minimal donor discomfort or functional loss, and ease of positioning do not outweigh the donor site morbidity. Therefore, this flap should be reserved for complex and unusual cases in which the TRAM flap is not available, the patient whose fat accumulation in the hips is inordinately greater than that of the abdomen, or the patient who primarily prefers this procedure as opposed to any other reconstructive options.

The conventional vertical TFL myocutaneous free flap has been useful in a number of different scenarios, i.e. abdominal wall, perineal, and chest wall reconstruction (4). We are unaware of any other uses besides breast reconstruction for the lateral transverse thigh flap described in this chapter. It only stands to reason that the lateral transverse modification of the TFL flap can be utilized to fill any soft tissue deficit created by ablative surgery or trauma but must be tempered by its unusual donor site cosmetic deformity.

DEEP CIRCUMFLEX ILIAC SOFT TISSUE FLAP (RUBENS FLAP)

The deep circumflex iliac artery soft tissue (Rubens) free flap is a soft tissue variant of the deep circumflex iliac artery (DCIA) iliac crest flap as described by Taylor and associates (5). The Rubens nomenclature is derived from the observance of the female form as painted by Peter Paul Rubens, which shows an area of particular fullness at or just above the iliac crest. This myocutaneous free flap is a type I vascular flap with one predominant pedicle, which is the deep circumflex iliac artery and vein.

The Rubens flap is composed mostly of fat from the flank and hip. Like the LTTF and gluteal free flap, it was originally developed, and is primarily utilized, as an alternate source of autogenous tissue for breast reconstruction. Not unlike the LTTF, this flap is taken from an area that is a source of extra tissue in the middle-aged woman.

Anatomy

The deep circumflex iliac vessels reliably supply a sizable fat deposit in the flank overlying the iliac crest. The dominant branches of the deep circumflex iliac vessels pass over the iliac crest and enter the subcutaneous tissue over or just lateral to the iliac crest. A subperiosteal iliac crest dissection protects these dominant perforators (Fig. 10).

Like the LTTF flap, the elevation of this flap is relatively straightforward, and the main concern is balancing the tissue needs on the chest with the resultant residual deformity on the flank. The distribution of the patient's body fat must be carefully assessed to determine the ideal location of the donor site. Also like the LTTF flap, the consistency of the fat in the flank is similar to that of the hip, in that rigid fibrous septa divide the fat into lobules providing a supporting framework. The shaping of the breast follows the guidelines as mentioned previously for the LTTF flap. The flap is shaped as it is harvested so that shaping on the chest wall is minimized. A small muscular cuff of the abdominal wall musculature is prudent to include with the flap in order to protect any perforators arising just medial to the iliac crest. The muscular cuff consists of the external oblique, internal oblique, and transverse abdominis musculature. The vessels lie just deep to the internal oblique, 0.5 cm cephalad to the iliac crest.

Surgical Technique

Flank Markings

The axis of the flap is determined initially. The patient is marked in a standing position and the anterior superior iliac spine, along with the iliac crest, is located and

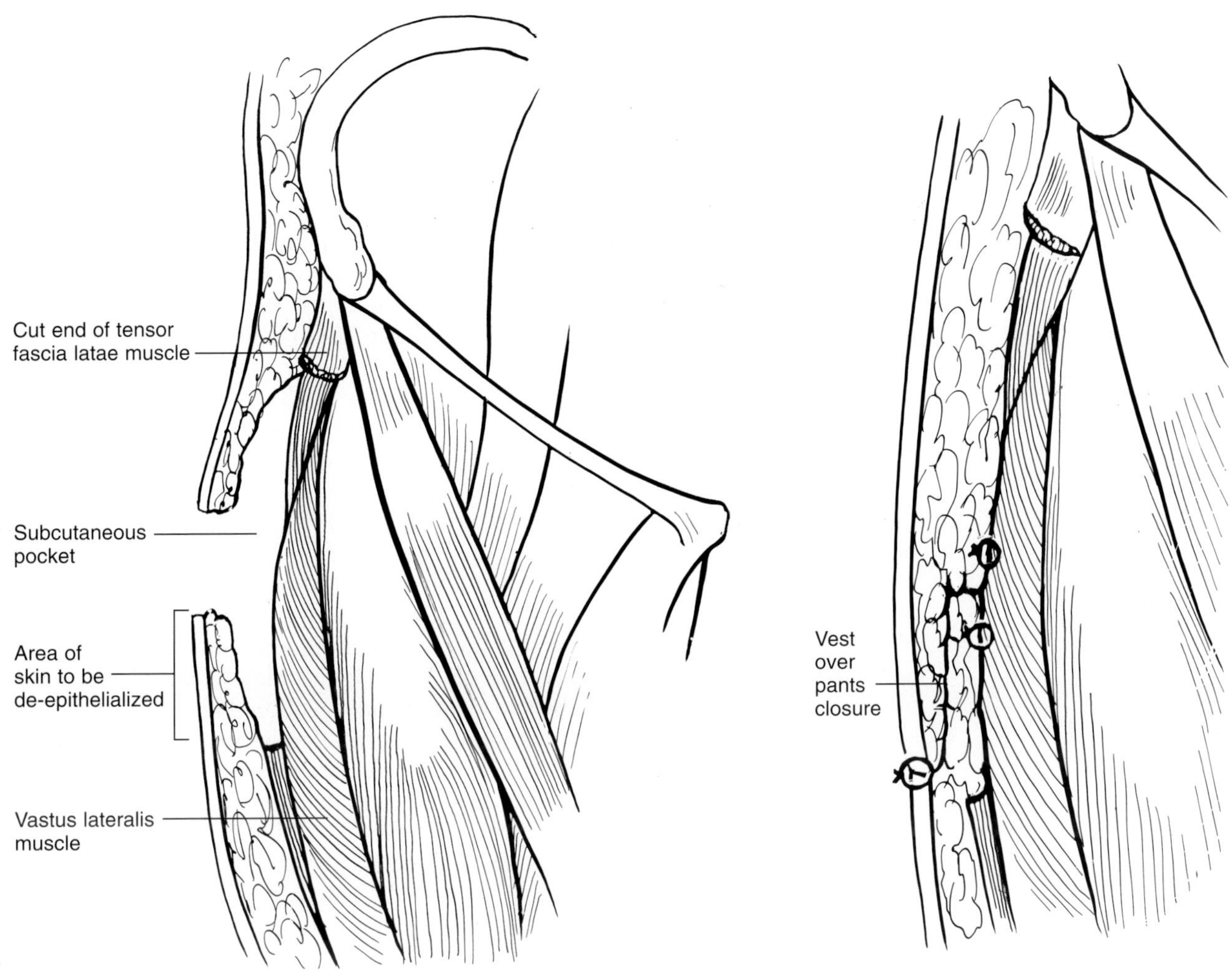

FIG. 6A,B. Donor site closure. Note vest over pants closure, which helps minimize donor site morbidity.

marked. The flank is viewed from an anterior posterior direction, and the point of maximal lateral projection is chosen as the center of the skin island. By placing the skin island over the point of maximum projection overlying the iliac crest, the new breast will achieve maximal projection, as this is the area of greatest thickness of the flank. The skin island can be moved cephalad or caudad to the iliac crest axis, balancing the tissue needs on the chest with the resultant residual deformity on flank. The size of the skin island depends on the thickness of the peri-iliac soft tissue redundancy and the needs for extra skin on the chest wall. The upper limits to the size of the skin island are dictated by the ability to close the fusiform defect primarily. The vertical dimension of the skin island is generally limited to 12 to 15 cm and varies depending on the patient's body habitus and size. The horizontal dimension is limited by the girth of the abdomen and flank, which is usually 25 to 30 cm in length extending posteriorly from the anterior superior iliac crest (Fig. 10). The flap is usually harvested from the same side as the mastectomy defect, therefore allowing simultaneous dissection of the chest and flank as well as obviating the need for repositioning the patient.

Preoperative preparation and patient positioning are commensurate with the LTTF flap previously discussed. No angiographic studies of the recipient or donor sites are performed. An estimate of skin and volume requirements for breast reconstruction is made based on the resected weight of the mastectomy specimen, as well as the size and shape of the patient's opposite breast, if available for comparison. The patient is placed in a supine position, general endotracheal anesthesia is induced, and a Foley catheter is inserted using sterile technique. The patient's hips are then rotated 45° to 50° and a beanbag is used as support to maintain this position (Fig. 11). The donor site should be elevated to expose the entire area for the flap harvest. The shoulders are allowed to lie flat on the operating table and all pressure points are padded for protection. This positioning enables simultaneous dissection of the flank and chest. The inferior medial portion of the peri-iliac flap outline is incised initially.

A transinguinal approach through the floor of the inguinal canal above the inguinal ligament is performed. After incising through the external oblique, internal oblique, and transversus abdominis, the deep circumflex iliac artery and vein are isolated. After inspection of the pedicle for vessel size and length, the superior and inferior portions of the flap are elevated. Dissection is carried down to include a generous amount of subcutaneous fat. A 3 cm wide by 10 cm long cuff of external and internal oblique as well as transverse abdominis muscle and transversalis fascia is left attached to the flap so that the perforators from the deep circumflex iliac artery can be included (Fig. 12). The myocutaneous flap is then elevated from the iliac crest in a subperiosteal plane to protect the deep circumflex iliac artery and vein and residual perforators. No iliac bone is taken. It is important to harvest the flap leaving adequate fat overlying the gluteal muscles. One must carefully harvest only the amount of fat needed to fill the residual defect. The free flap is then weighed and compared with the mastectomy specimen. An end-to-end or side-to-side microsurgical anastomoses is then performed to the thoracodorsal or internal mammary vessels (Fig. 13). Preference is given to the thoracodorsal vessels in immediate reconstruction. The internal mammary vessels are utilized in delayed reconstruction when scarring in the axilla is anticipated.

Closure of the donor site (Fig. 14) is performed in layers with an initial closure of the transversalis fascia to the iliacus muscle and fascia with a heavy 2-0 Vicryl suture. The abdominal wall muscles and fascia are then closed to the iliac crest utilizing 2-mm drill holes in the iliac crest with a continuous or interrupted double suture of 0-nylon. The external oblique muscle is closed over the iliac crest to the fascia, lata, and gluteal fascia. The skin is then closed over two closed suction drains.

The free tissue transfer is positioned and shaped to match the contralateral breast (Fig. 15A–C). A minimum of dressings are used after the operation. The flap is observed frequently in the postoperative period and the patient is placed at bed rest overnight. If bilateral reconstruction is anticipated, it is performed either simultaneously or as a staged procedure 2 to 3 days apart during the same hospital admission (Fig. 16A–D).

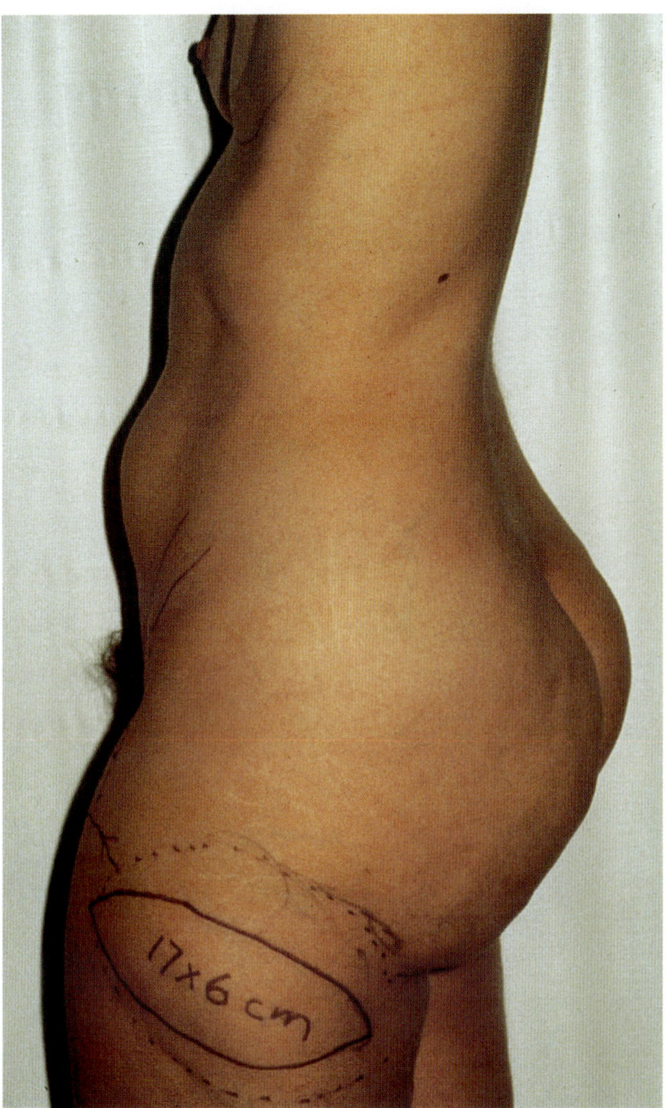

FIG. 7. Patient with body habitus of large hips and small abdomen, which lends itself well to use of lateral thigh flap.

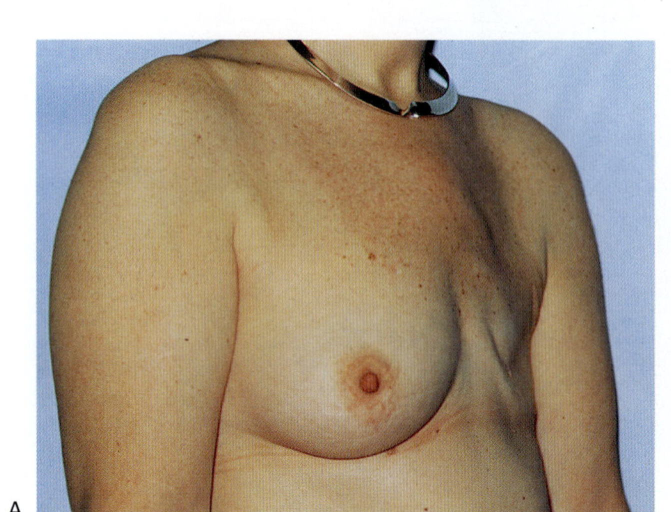
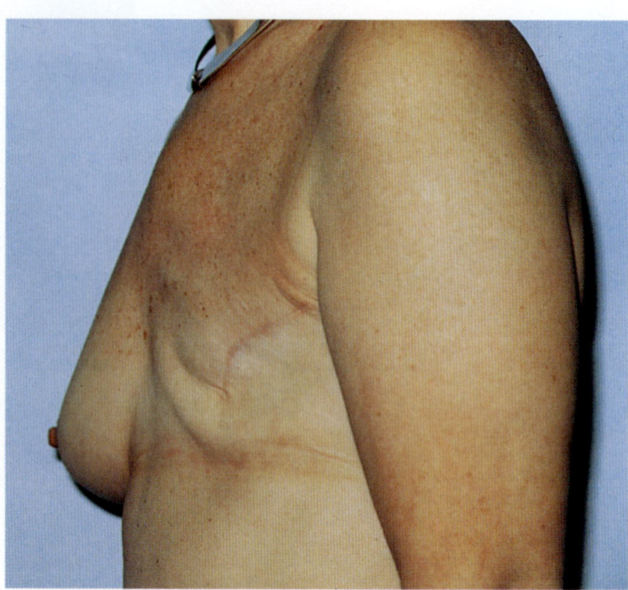

FIG. 8A,B. Preoperative views of patient requiring left breast reconstruction.

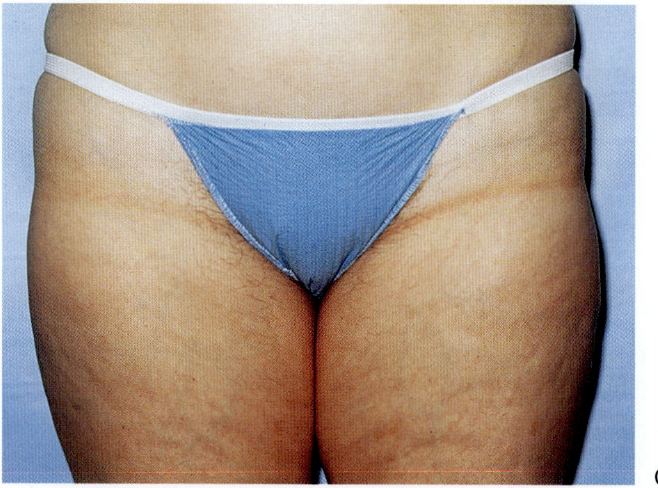

FIG. 8C. Preoperative view of donor site.

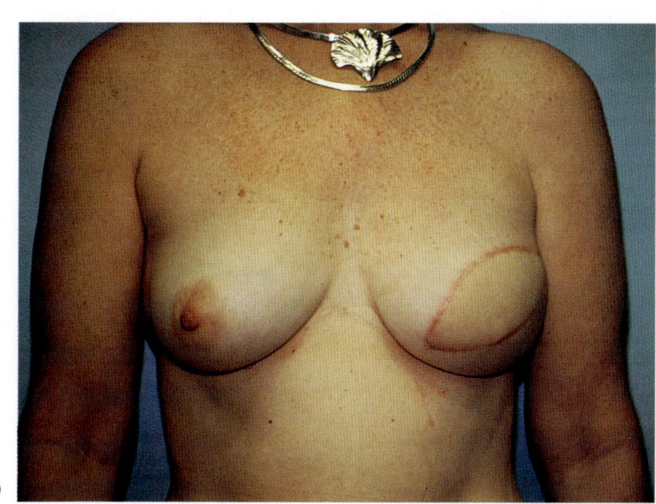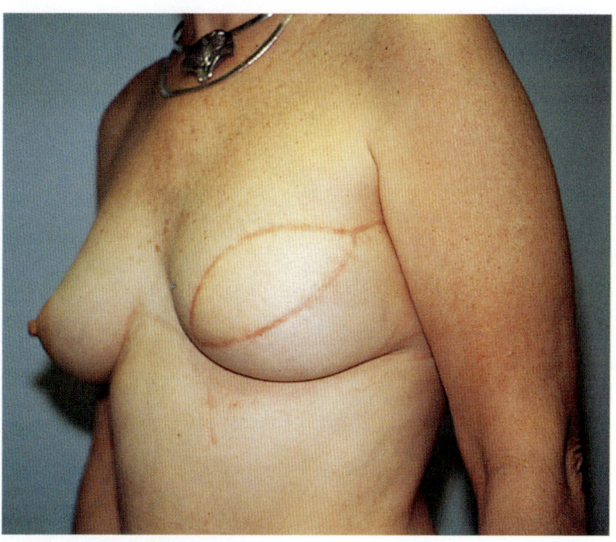

FIG. 8D,E. Postoperative view of reconstructed breast.

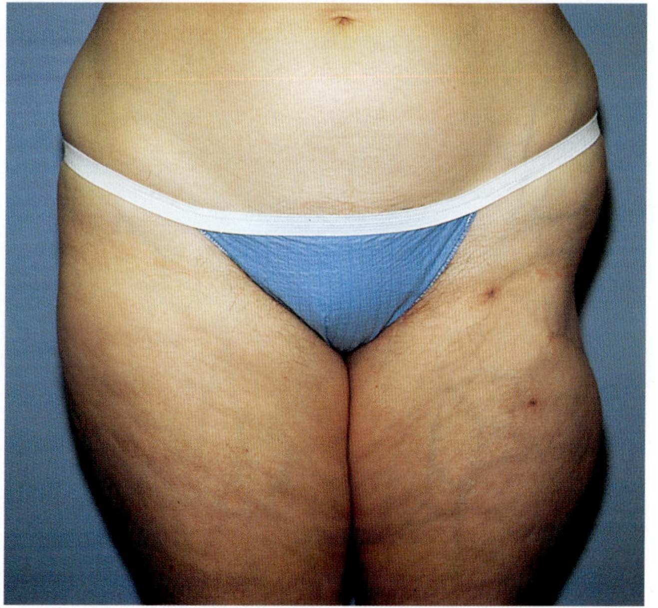

FIG. 8F. Postoperative view of donor site. Note the contour deformity.

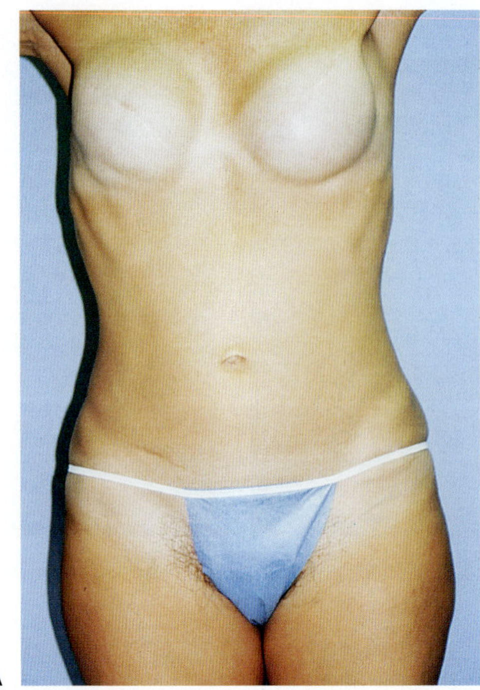

FIG. 9A. Preoperative view of patient with previous reconstruction of both breasts with implants.

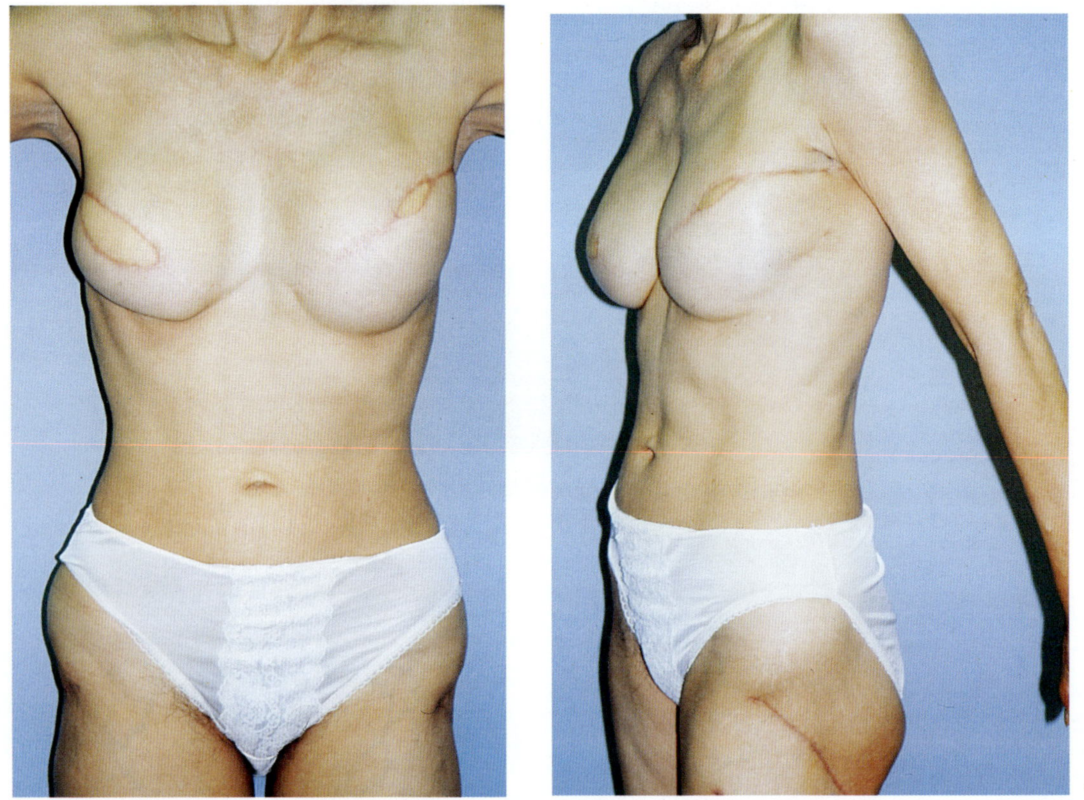

FIG. 9B,C. Postoperative view of both breasts reconstructed with LTTF flaps.

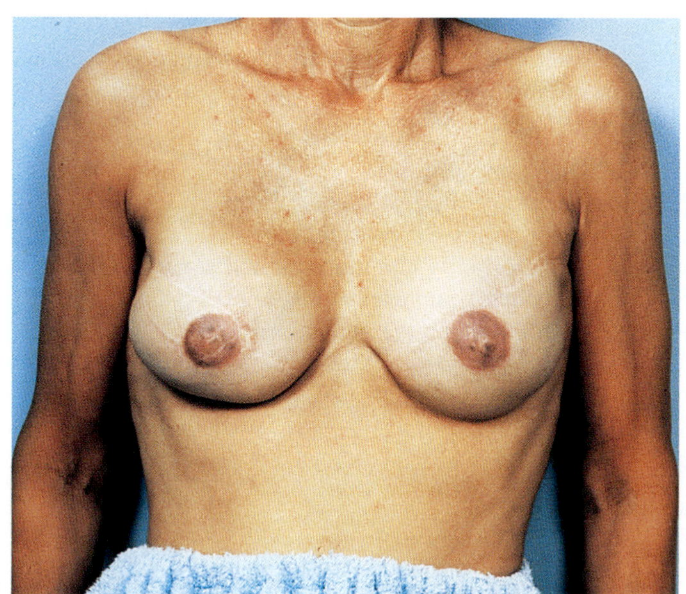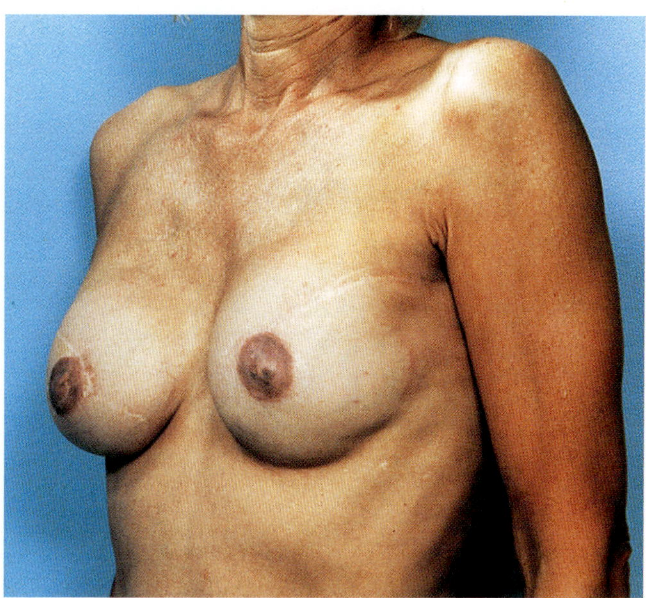

FIG. 9D,E. Postoperative view after nipple-areola reconstruction.

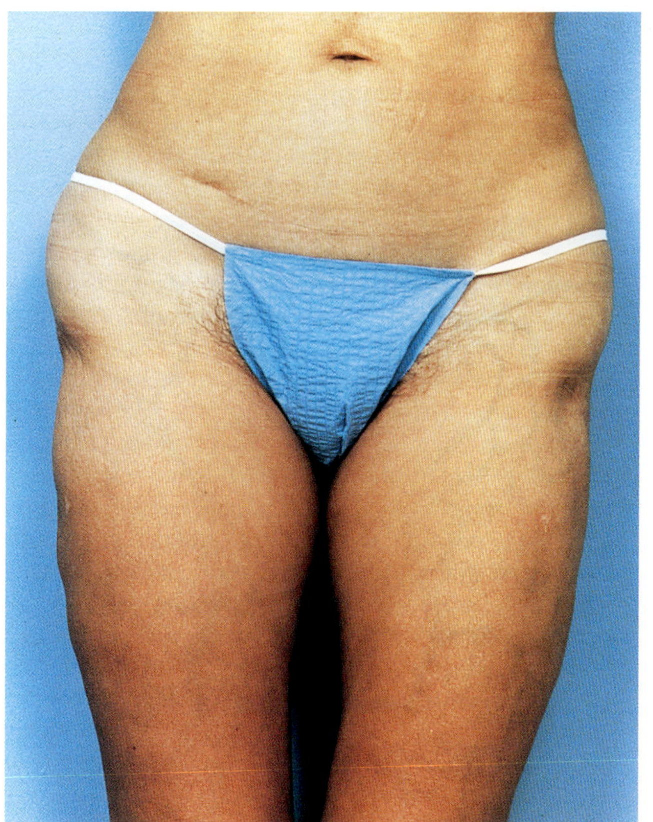

FIG. 9F. Postoperative view of bilateral donor sites.

The Peri-Iliac Soft Tissue Flap (Rubens Flap)

The peri-iliac soft tissue flap (Rubens Flap) is a new modification of an old flap (DCIA flap). It has proven to be a reliable natural alternative for autogenous tissue breast reconstruction. It has several advantages over other methods of alternative autogenous breast reconstruction:

1. It involves a relatively easy dissection.
2. It has a long constant pedicle.
3. There is no need to turn the patient during the procedure.
4. It entails decreased postoperative morbidity and more rapid recovery.
5. It results in improved abdominal contour, with reduction of excess fat in patients in whom the flanks are more prominent than the abdomen.
6. It results in greater intrinsic internal projection of the flap.
7. It results in excellent vascularity.
8. This flap can be used in patients with previous TRAM, failed TRAM, or abdominoplasty.

The disadvantages of the Rubens flap:

1. Microsurgery is required.
2. The amount of skin available is usually not as great as that with a standard transverse rectus abdominis musculocutaneous flap.
3. The scar is long and more visible along the flank region.
4. A balancing procedure on the opposite flank is usually necessary.
5. Donor site morbidity of abdominal wall weakness, hernias, and gait disturbances are potential problems if not closed properly.

Our current indications for the Rubens Flap are unavailable transverse rectus abdominis musculocutaneous flap, previous abdominoplasty precluding transverse rectus abdominis musculocutaneous flap, flank fat proportions greater than abdominal portions, and patient prefers this option to all other available flaps.

It is important to note that this is a flap that has added a critical option to one particular type of patient seeking breast reconstruction: the patient who has previously had an abdominoplasty or TRAM flap and desires autogenous tissue breast reconstruction. This may be a patient who has not had previous breast reconstruction as in an abdominoplasty, or a patient who has previously had a TRAM breast reconstruction and who subsequently requires a second mastectomy. Patients have been very satisfied with sacrificing the lateral hip fat to reconstruct a new breast and obtain improved contour along the waist line. This is a relatively new free flap used for autogenous breast reconstruction, but it is reliable and has clear indications for clinical usefulness. In some patients it may even provide more tissue than the standard TRAM flap. The Rubens flap has a large-caliber long pedicle, and involves straightforward dissection and simple positioning. The donor site defect appears to be more acceptable than the gluteal free flap or lateral transverse thigh free flap. The only drawbacks involve a technically more demanding dissection, a more challenging shaping of the flap because of its fusiform shape, and the potential need to treat the contralateral Rubens fat pad to achieve symmetry.

Early return of activity is noted with this technique. Pain syndromes are few and muscle function is essentially normal. As with all aspects of free flap breast reconstruction, the harvest of the Rubens flap dictates the resultant shape of the new breast. The experience with the Rubens flap has shown convincingly the advantages of autogenous tissue in contouring, softness, warmth, permanency, and patient satisfaction. We reserve this flap for complex and unusual cases, where the TRAM flap has already been harvested, or is not available for use. We also reserve this flap for patients in whom fat accumulation in the flanks is inordinately greater than that of the abdomen, and for patients who primarily prefer this procedure to any other reconstructive options.

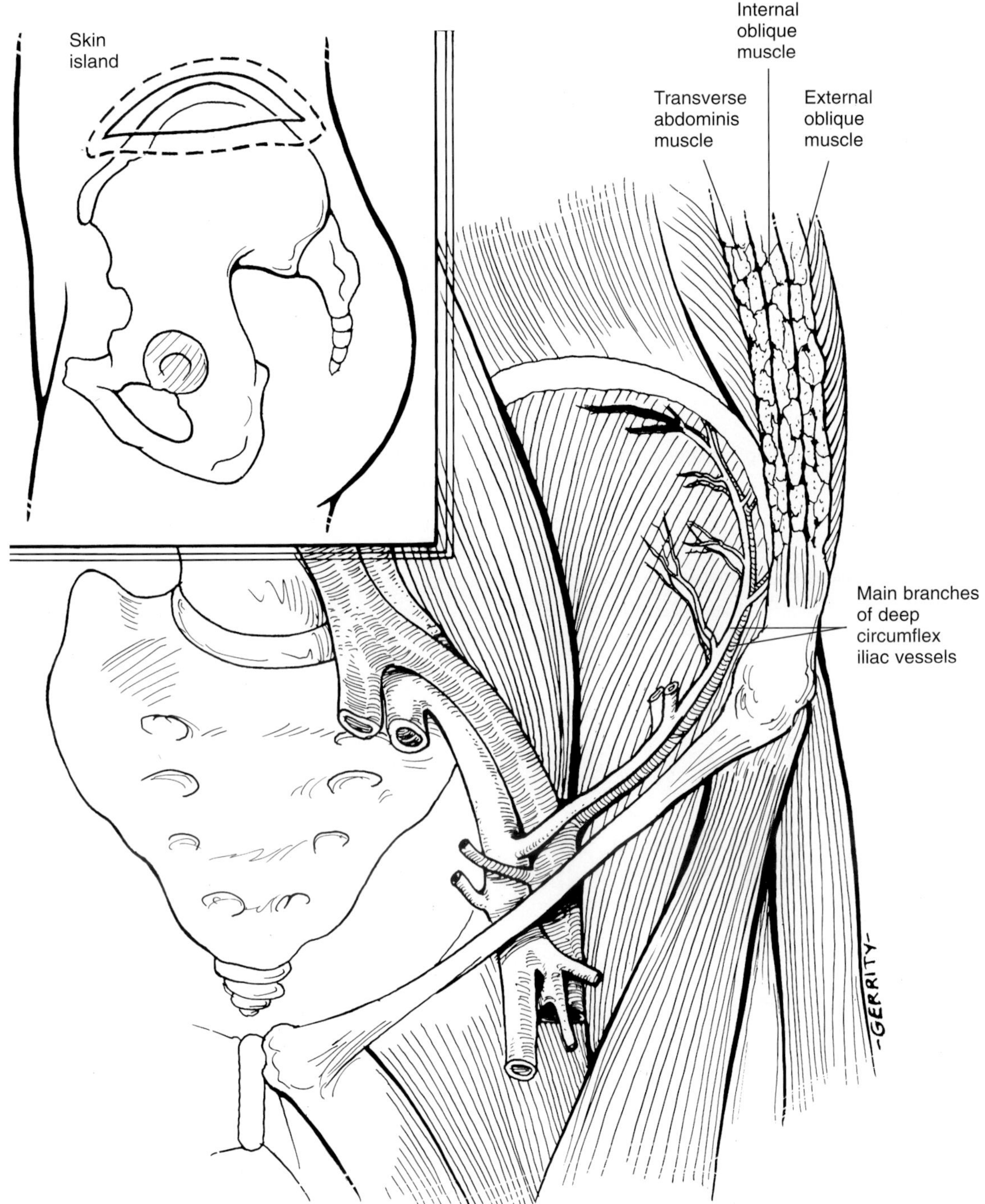

FIG. 10. Vascular anatomy and preoperative planning of Rubens flap. Takeoff of deep circumflex iliac artery with perforators is shown. **Inset:** Typical design of skin island with *dotted line* representing fat excision.

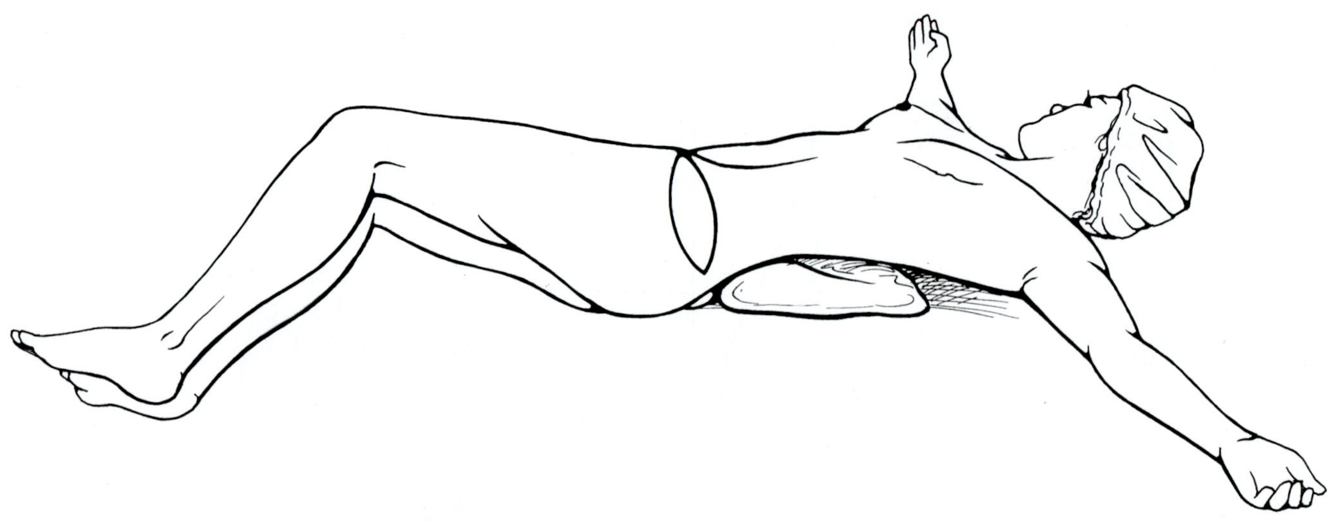

FIG. 11. Positioning of patient for Rubens flap elevation and transfer.

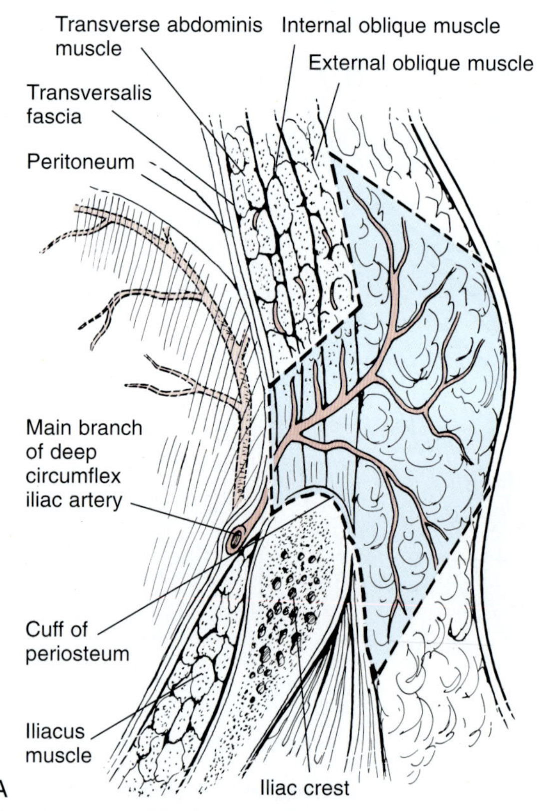

FIG. 12A. Dissection of Rubens flap. *Dotted line* denotes dissection borders of Rubens flap.

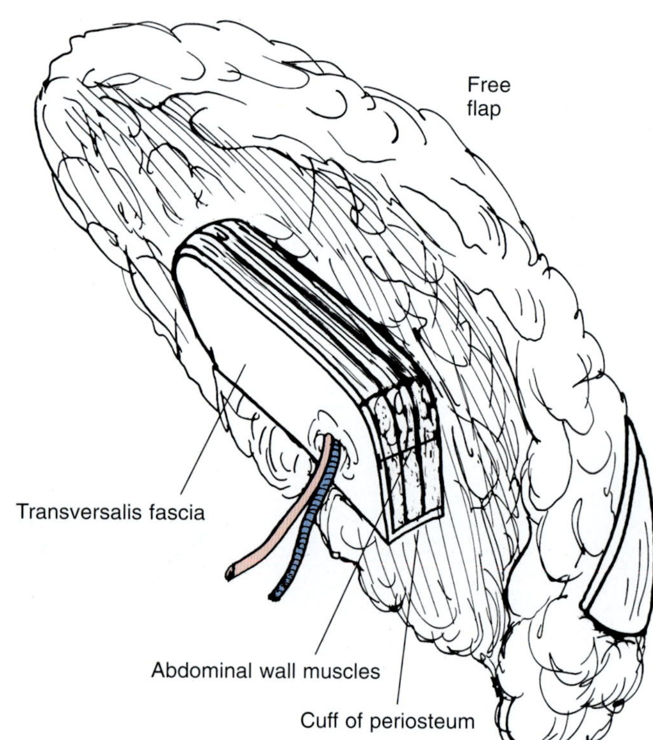

FIG. 12B. Rubens flap after harvest. Note small cuff of underlying muscle.

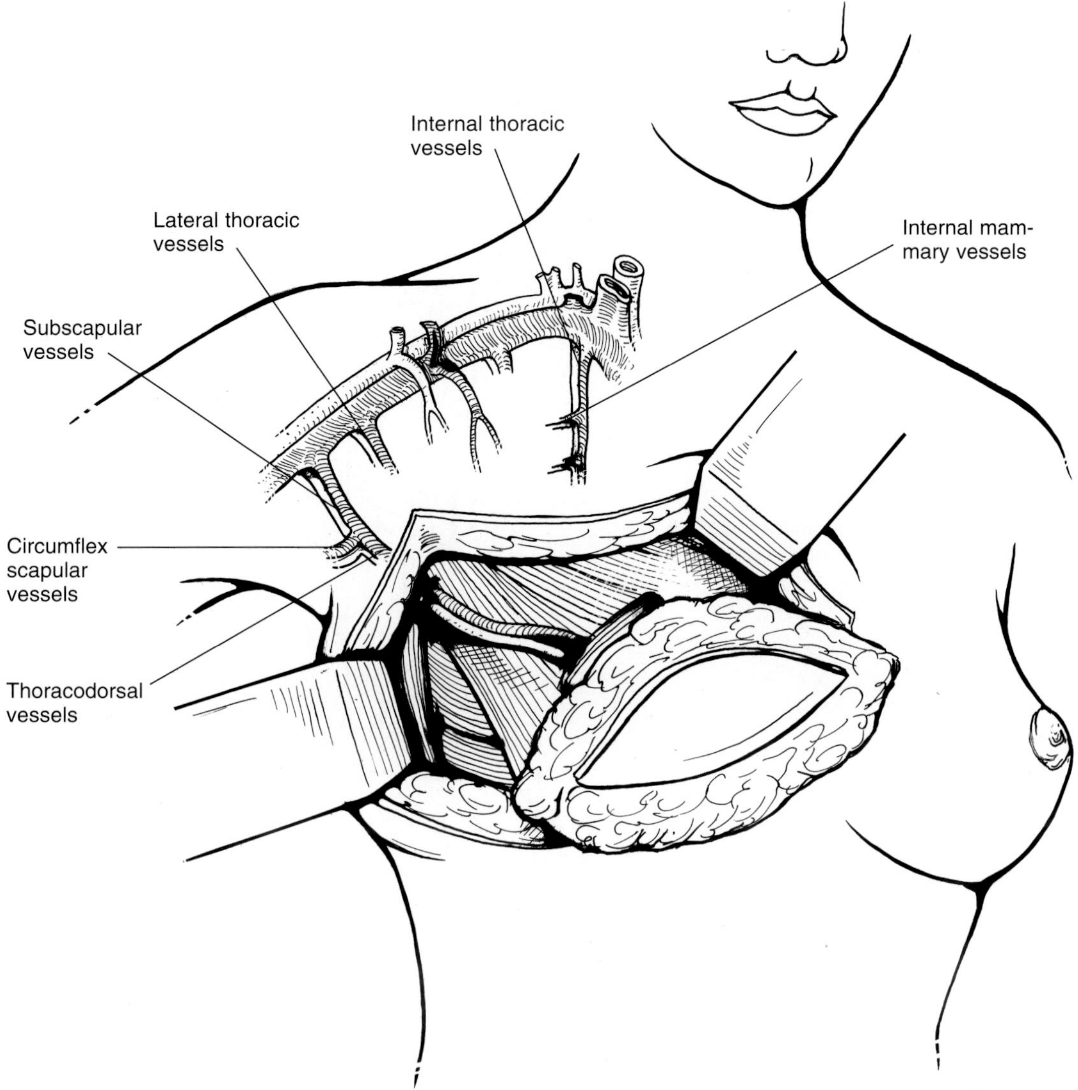

FIG. 13. The flap is revascularized to the thoracodorsal vessels. The internal mammary vessels are available if the thoracodorsal vessels are unsuitable.

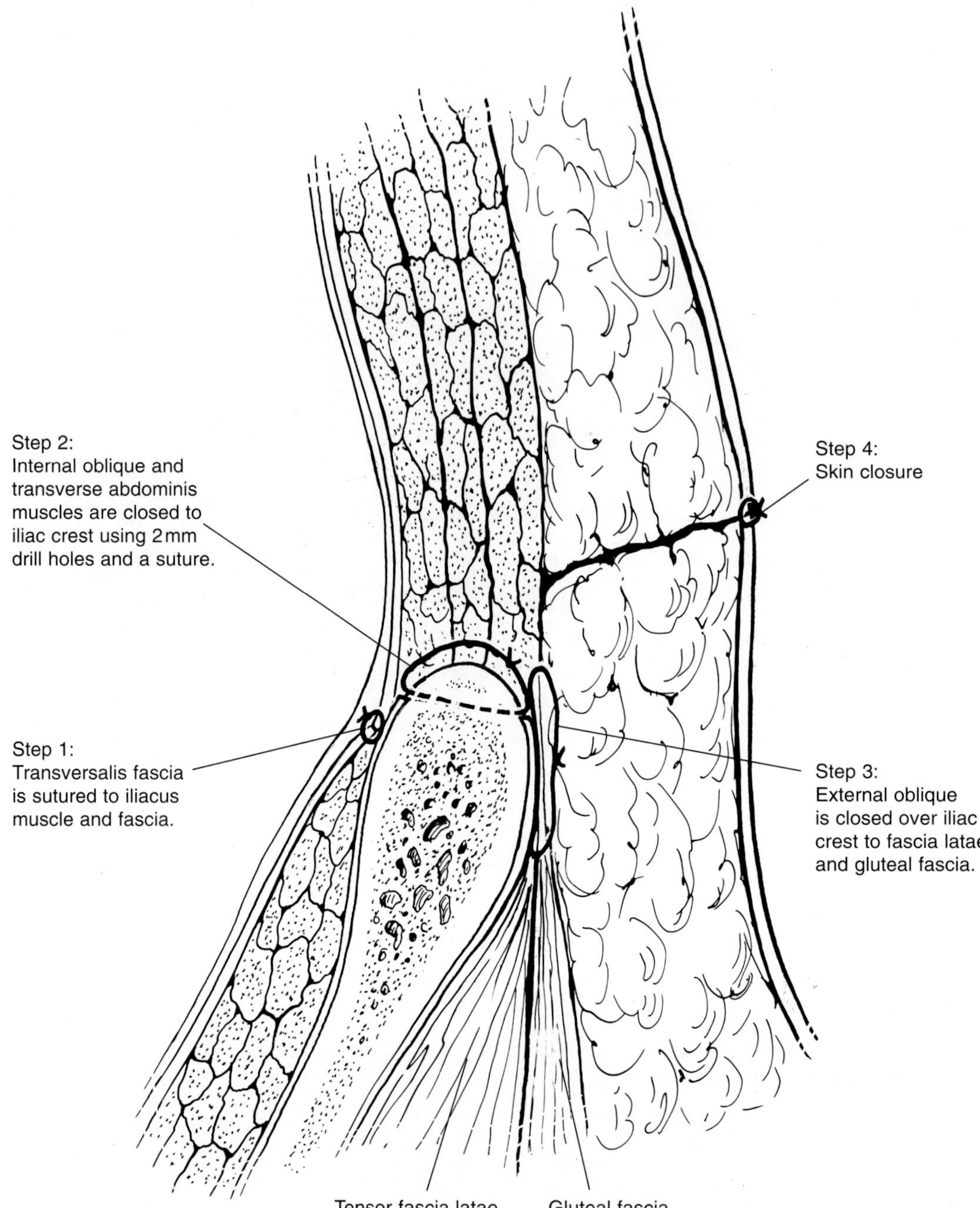

FIG. 14. Closure of donor defect in sequence steps 1–4. Step 1: Transversalis fascia sutured to iliacus muscle and fascia. Step 2: Internal oblique and transversus abdominis muscle closure to iliac crest using 2-mm drill holes and suture. Step 3: External oblique closed over iliac crest to fascia lata and gluteal fascia. Step 4: Skin closure.

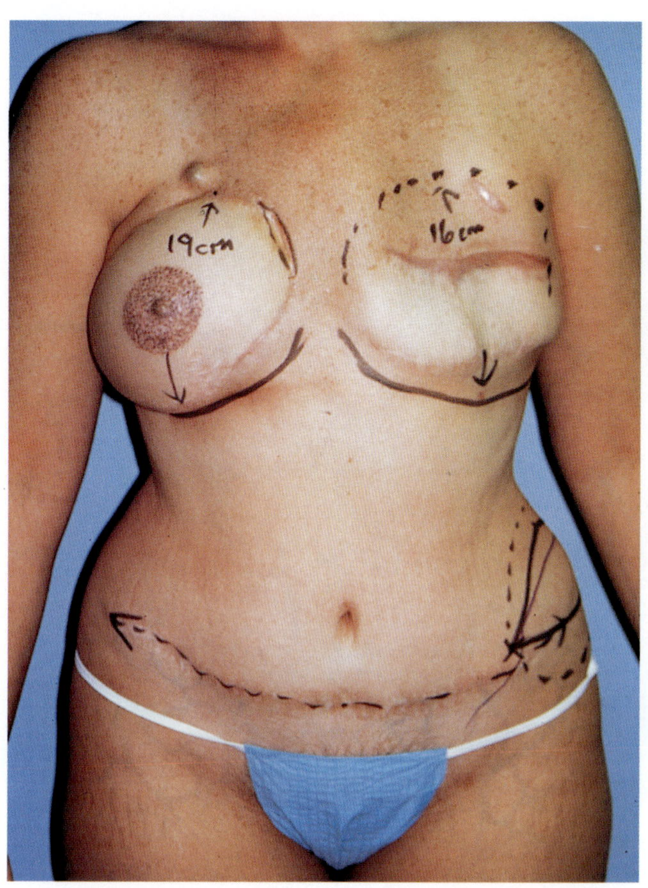

FIG. 15A. Delayed unilateral reconstruction using the Rubens flap. Preoperative view.

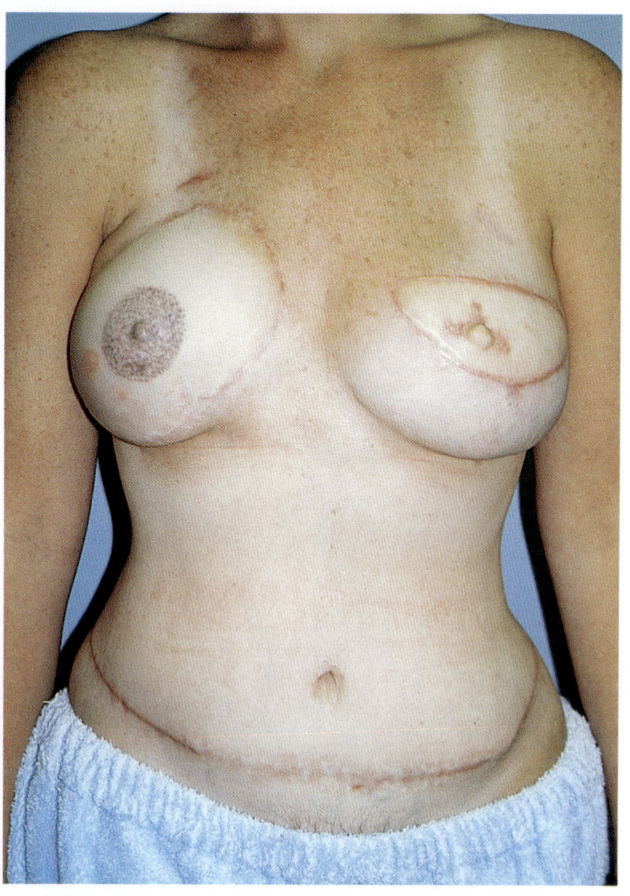

FIG. 15C. Final result after nipple reconstruction and excision of contralateral hip tissue.

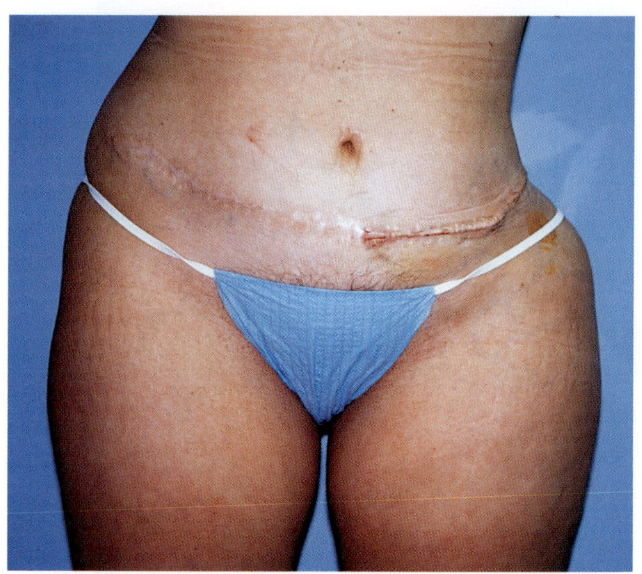

FIG. 15B. Postoperative appearance of donor site prior to excisional procedure of contralateral flank to achieve symmetry.

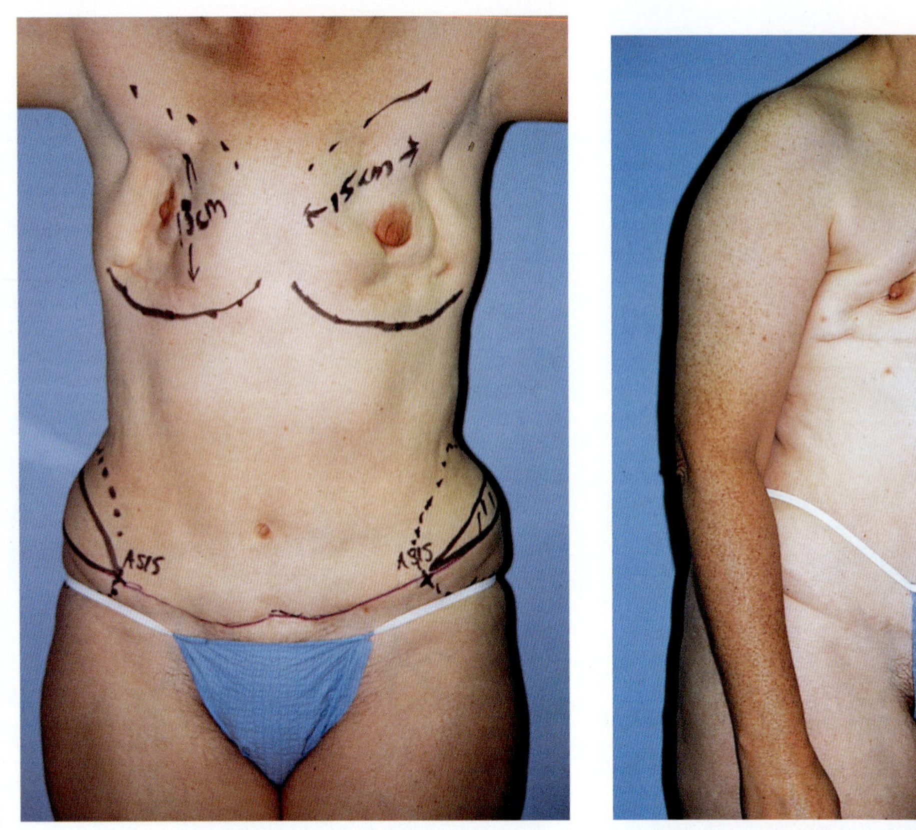

FIG. 16A,B. Preoperative view of bilateral reconstruction using Rubens flap.

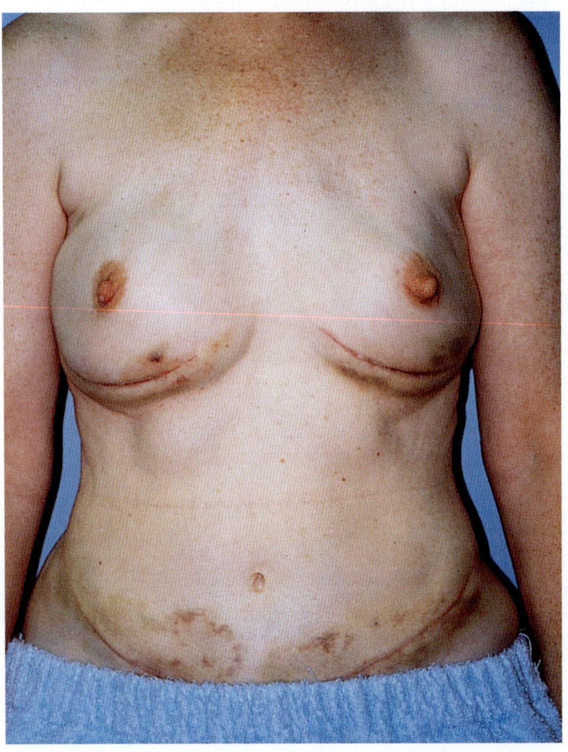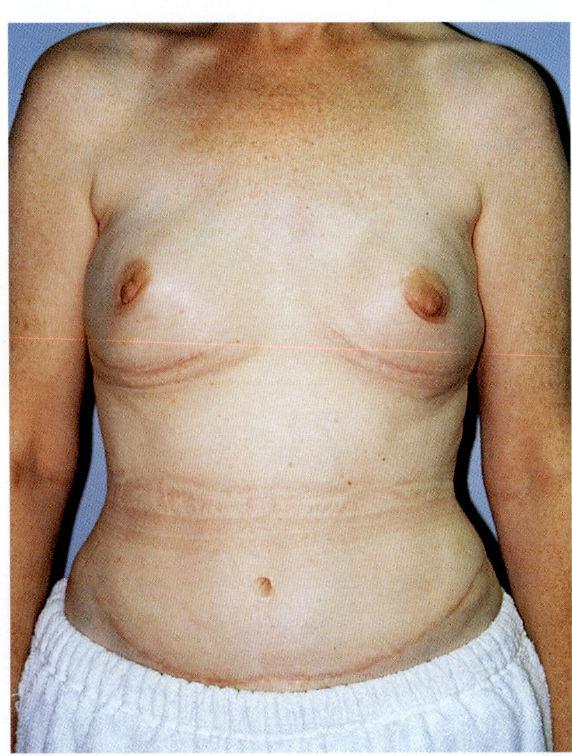

FIG. 16C,D. Postoperative view.

REFERENCES

1. Elliott LF. The lateral transverse thigh free flap for autogenous breast reconstruction. *Perspect Plast Surg* 1989;3:80.
2. Elliott LF. Options for donor site for autogenous breast reconstruction. *Clin Plast Surg* 1994;21:177–189.
3. Elliott LF, Beegle PH, Hartrampf CR. The LTTF: an alternative for autogenous tissue breast reconstruction. *Plast Reconstr Surg* 1990;85:169–176.
4. Hartrampf CR Jr, Noel RT, Elliott LF, Bennett GK, Beegle PH, Drazan L. Rubens fat pad for breast reconstruction. *Plast Reconstr Surg* 1993;93:402–407.
5. Taylor GI, Corlett R, Boyd JB. The extended deep inferior epigastric flap: a clinical technique. *Plast Reconstr Surg* 1983;72:751.

SELECTED READING

Shaw WW, Fenner GC, Ahn CY. *Alternatives to TRAM flap for breast reconstruction: experience with 121 flaps.* Presented at American Association of Plastic Surgery Annual Meeting, Hilton Head, SC, May 1996.

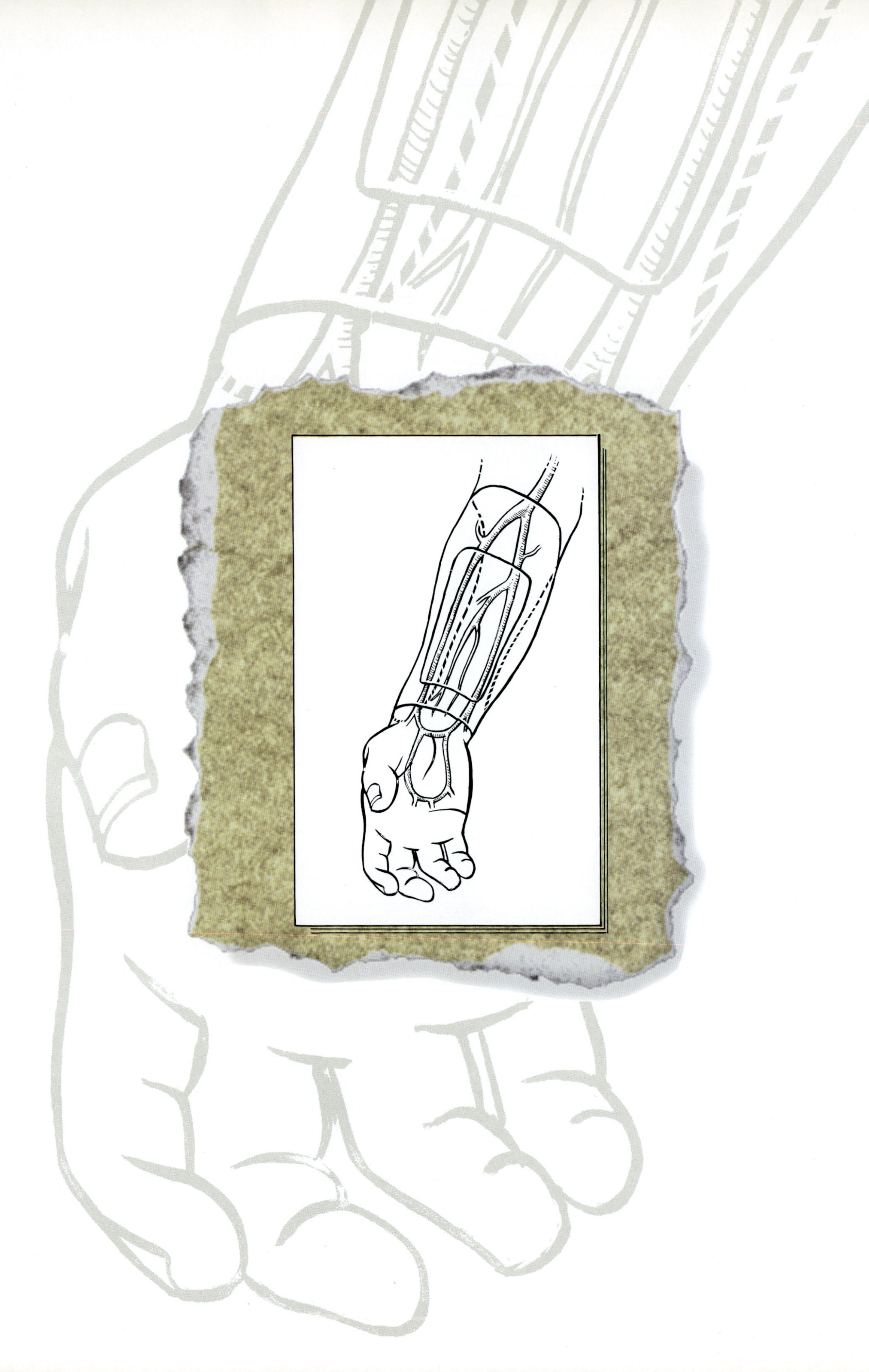

Extremities

Microsurgical Reconstruction of the Cancer Patient, edited by M.A. Schusterman.
Lippincott-Raven Publishers, Philadelphia © 1997.

12

Principles of Extremity Microvascular Reconstruction

Gregory R.D. Evans and Daniel P. Goldberg

Most of our knowledge concerning extremity reconstruction has been gained from reconstructive defects due to trauma. The utilization of these techniques has been extrapolated to reconstruction following resection of extremity tumors. Limb salvage, rather than amputation, has become a dominant goal in the care of the patient with cancer of the extremity. To ensure function, preservation or reconstruction of bone, blood vessels, soft tissue, and nerves is vital.

This chapter discusses an approach to the extremity cancer patient who requires reconstructive microsurgery, and identifies those patients for whom limb salvage may not be the most appropriate therapeutic decision and who may be better served by primary amputation.

THE DISEASE

A variety of malignant tumors can involve the extremities. Malignant melanoma, basal cell carcinoma, and squamous cell carcinoma are the most common extremity neoplasms and, despite their frequency, they are generally confined to the cutaneous structures. Consequently, reconstructive options involve primary closure, skin grafting, and local cutaneous and myocutaneous flaps. Conversely, soft tissue and bony sarcomas, although constituting only about 1% of adult malignant neoplasms, are the most frequent neoplastic extremity wounds encountered by the microvascular surgeon. Despite differences in biologic behavior attributable to various tissue types of each

G.R.D. Evans: Department of Plastic Surgery, The University of Texas, M.D. Anderson Cancer Center, Houston, Texas 77030.

D.P. Goldberg: Division of Plastic and Reconstructive Surgery, Case Western Reserve University, Cleveland Ohio 44106-5044.

sarcoma, all sarcomas pose similar clinical management problems. Local recurrence is common after inadequate excision. Bony invasion may occur, but invasion of major arteries, veins, and nerves is relatively uncommon. Distant metastases develop in a high frequency of patients (30-50% hematogenous metastasis to the lung with high-grade sarcomas) despite adequate local control.

Adjuvant therapy (e.g., radio- and chemotherapy) has achieved better local control of extremity sarcomas, fostering the expansion of limb-sparing therapeutic options. The utilization of these modalities, however, has a negative impact on wound healing, thus necessitating microvascular transfer of nonirradiated tissue to facilitate healing.

PATIENT EVALUATION

Reconstructive demands in the cancer patient create a new level of complexity for the issues of extremity defects. A thorough history and physical examination is critical in deciding on the type of reconstruction. The most important factor in determining the reconstructive plan is tumor size. Larger-size tumors increase the demands for flap size, and additionally may involve vital structures such as nerves, blood vessels, bones, or joints. These complex defects may then require a more involved reconstructive approach. Adjunctive radiation and chemotherapy is used routinely. The use of either or both of these therapies, either pre- or postoperatively, may have an impact on the reconstructive plan. A detailed history of prior therapy, including surgery, and the planned postoperative therapeutic regimen should be obtained during the initial patient evaluation.

Ancillary diagnostic tests are important in planning the resection and reconstruction. Computed tomography and magnetic resonance imaging are important to determine extent of tumor and involvement of vital structures. In addition, angiography and electrical muscular stimulation and nerve conduction studies may be of assistance.

The most important structural component of the extremity is the bone, and if bone is involved, the anticipated size of the defect should be assessed. Although autogenous bone grafts, both vascularized and nonvascularized, have been used, freeze-dried cadaver allograft has been the replacement tissue of choice for the orthopedic oncologists with whom we practice. Smaller noncompromised wounds may only require nonvascularized bone or bony shortening. Occasionally, free tissue transfer can provide not only coverage but functional restoration as well. The gracilis and latissimus dorsi muscle may serve as a functional replacement for resected muscles. Tendon transfers may be required for extremity restoration. Will the weight-bearing surfaces of the foot be resected? Stable coverage is required for future ambulation and flap selection should consider the bulk of the reconstruction and the ability for the foot to fit into specialized shoes. Finally, extremity sarcoma patients are frequently subjected to further postoperative treatment with chemo- and radiotherapy. Closure of the defects with well-vascularized, durable tissue allows early healing and progression of adjuvant therapy.

THE ROLE OF AMPUTATION—CRITERIA FOR LIMB SALVAGE

The principles of limb-sparing surgery are threefold. First, tumor resection with wide surgical margins is necessary. The need for accurate evaluation of frozen sections cannot be overemphasized. Delayed reconstruction does have a lower rate of functional restoration. Second, skeletal reconstruction should be addressed. Third, muscle and soft tissue defects must be addressed. Soft tissue coverage is mandatory, because it decreases postoperative wound complications.

Although the following criteria are relative contraindications for limb-sparing surgery individually, a combination of these may indicate the need for amputation:

1. Major neurovascular involvement.
2. Pathologic fractures: It is often difficult to determine the extent of local spread of the disease with direct bony involvement and pathologic fractures secondary to hematogenous spread of the disease within the bone marrow. Realistic appraisal of reconstructive options is required.
3. Contaminated biopsy sites or poorly executed biopsies leading to tumor spread.
4. Infection: Infection may alter reconstructive options, delay adjuvant therapy, and increase the risk of further compromise to the patient's medical condition.
5. Age: Immature skeletal age has traditionally been a relative contraindication to limb-sparing procedures; however, with the advent and use of Ilizarov techniques and microvascular bony transfer, this may not persist as a relative contraindication. Consideration must be given to the additional procedures a child must endure. Children adapt well, and amputation with resumption of their active lifestyle may be preferred.
6. Extensive muscle involvement not permitting functional restoration.
7. Poor nutrition associated medical conditions.
8. Lack of patient motivation for rehabilitation and multiple surgeries.

In summary, management options for limb preservation for the surgeon and patient revolve around three basic issues: First, the chance of local recurrence after local resection should not be greater than after amputation. Second, overall survival should not be jeopardized. Third, the reconstructive options should maximize the functional outcome, produce limited morbidity, minimize the need for additional surgery, and not force the patient to endure an unreasonable rehabilitative period. Although controversial, preservation of the extremity as a biologic prosthesis with high sciatic and brachial plexus injuries is currently considered for selected patients. Nerve reconstruction is required in these patients and protective sensation may take up to 2 to 3 years for reinnervation. With aggressive rehabilitation, some patients are able to function quite well with this bioprosthesis. Patients should consider, however, that their extremity is on loan. Significant wound complications or infections may ultimately lead to amputation.

NERVE RECONSTRUCTION

Goals for Extremity Nerve Reconstruction

The approach to the patient with nerve injury/resection requiring repair can be defined by the following criteria:

1. Quantitative preoperative and postoperative clinical assessment is required for both motor and sensory systems. If the brachial plexus is involved, or if multiple nerve injuries are present, the minimal goal of upper extremity reconstruction is restoration of a stable shoulder joint, with maintenance of the humeral head and glenoid fossa, and restoration of elbow flexion and median nerve sensibility. Repair of the medial, radial, and ulnar nerves should proceed if proximal nerve injury is not present. For the lower extremity, the reestablishment of plantar sensation is critical. This may avoid the ulcerations and injury that may lead to infection and possible amputation.
2. Microsurgical repair should be performed. Our common method of nerve repair includes the use of the operative microscope and 9-0 and/or 10-0 nylon suture with epineural repair. Nerve ends should be approximated and not tied so tight that axonal material is extruded on the contralateral side. Epineural and interfascicular repair are useful and should be available depending on the extent of the injury. Complete nerve transection may require epineural repair. If, however, partial transection of a nerve occurs, or if a group motor or sensory fascicle can be identified, interfascicular repair may be more appropriate.

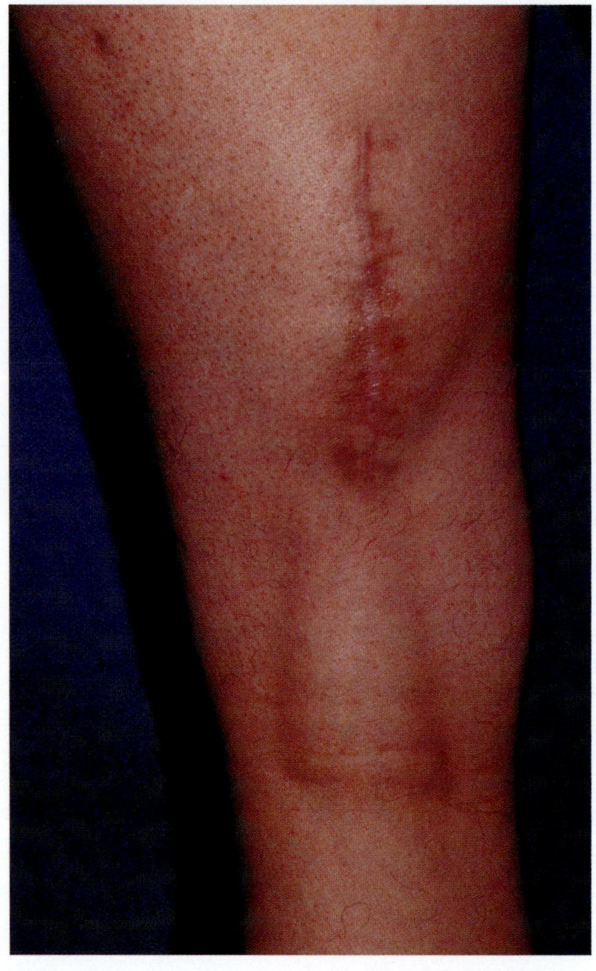

A

FIG. 1A. A 23-year-old man with a recurrent malignant fibrous histiocytoma of the left posterior thigh. The patient was noted to have foot drop on preoperative evaluation.

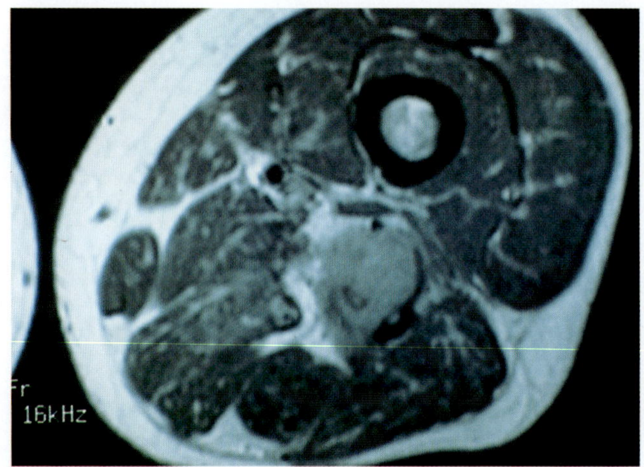

B

FIG. 1B. A magnetic resonance image confirmed tumor involvement of the sciatic nerve.

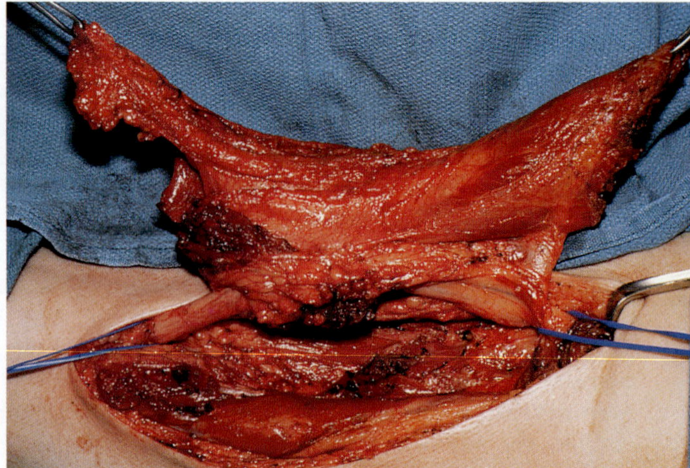

C

FIG. 1C. The tumor has been partially resected isolating the involved portion of the sciatic nerve.

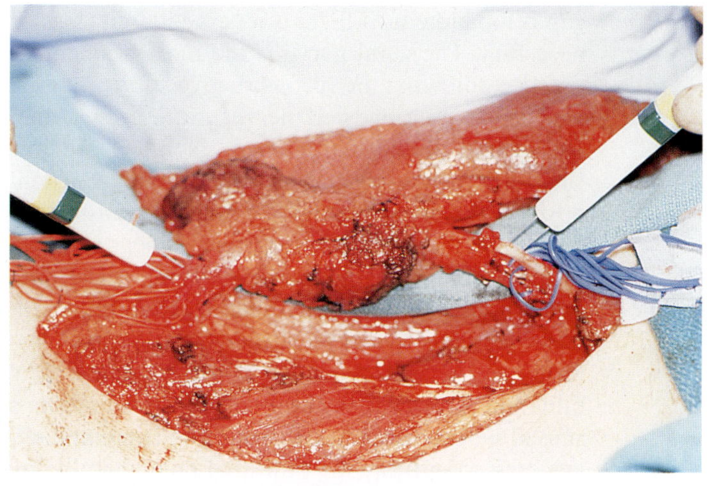

FIG. 1D. Intraoperative stimulation of the sciatic nerve is used for mapping purposes to aid in the reconstruction.

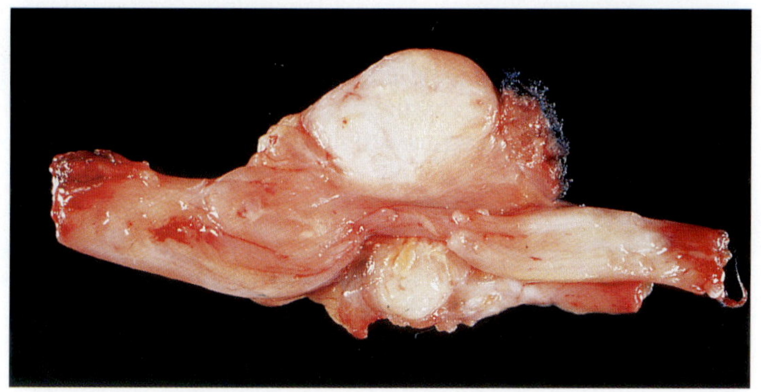

FIG. 1E. The specimen after final resection.

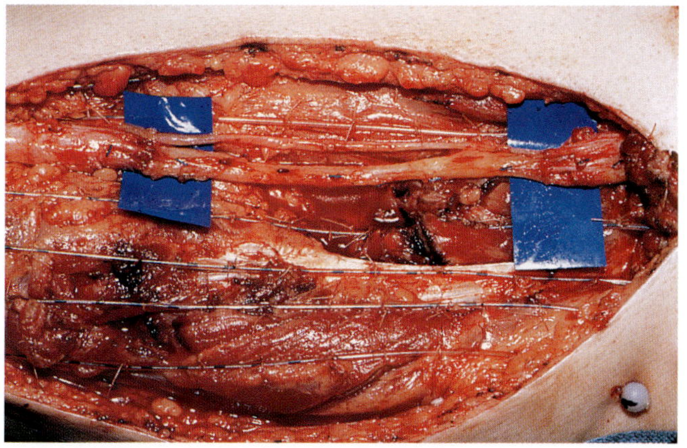

FIG. 1F. The defect after microsurgical placement of multiple sural nerve cable grafts.

3. Nerve repair must be tension free. Nerve gaps occur by nerve retraction. If this gap is too large or if there is a nerve deficit (loss of nerve), nerve grafting may be necessary. The sural nerve is the most frequently used nerve for grafting in our practice, allowing the reconstructive surgeon to harvest the nerve grafts as tumor extirpation continues. If nerve grafting or primary repair is required, postural positioning of the extremity to facilitate repair is discouraged. The extremity should be in the neutral position without tension. Alterations from this neutral position for nerve repair may alter the tension on the repair once the patient is awake and motion to the extremity is begun.

4. Primary nerve repair is preferred over nerve grafting. This nerve repair is best done at the time of tumor resection. Delayed repair is complicated by the addition of tissue scarring and postirradiation fibrosis.

5. Motor and sensory reeducation will maximize the results of nerve grafting. Rehabilitation is critical in the functional restoration of an extremity and should be started before surgical extirpation is contemplated. Adjuvant postoperative therapy may complicate the timing of this rehabilitation; however, it should not serve a passive role.

Technical Considerations

With the current state of technology, preoperative nerve involvement should be identified by physical and radiographic examination (Fig. 1A–F). If nerve involvement is suspected, intraoperative direct nerve stimulation should be arranged. The tumor is identified by the oncologic surgeon, and nerve involvement is assessed intraoperatively by determining whether deficits are caused by compression of an adjacent nerve or by direct neural invasion (Fig. 1C). If the tumor directly involves the nerve, nerve stimulation proceeds (Fig. 1D). The nerve is isolated both proximal and distal to the tumor invasion, and, using loupe magnification and microsurgical instruments, groups of fascicles can be identified and dissected. Vessels loops are placed around each group of fascicles for easy identification and to prevent the electric current from jumping to an adjacent fascicular group. Proximally, a group of fascicles is isolated and placed into the bipolar direct stimulator probe. These probes are connected to an electromyograph (EMG) system that can deliver controlled stimuli (Neuropack 4 [Nihon Kohden, Tokyo, Japan]). A neurophysiologist or technician should interpret the results. Distal to the tumor, each fascicular group is individually isolated with vessel loops, and the receiving bipolar electrode is placed on a selected fascicular group. Direct electrical nerve stimulation is performed on the proximal fascicular group, while the receiving electrode waits for the electrical current. It is important to make sure that the positive and negative currents are appropriately connected. If no electrical current is received by the distal electrode, the fascicle is noted and the distal electrode is place on another fascicular group. The procedure is repeated. If a current is received by the distal electrode, both the proximal and distal group of fascicles are marked. Nerve reconstruction that would proceed after tumor extirpation should include grafts placed between these two marked fascicular groups. If no current is received from any of the distal fascicular groups isolated while stimulating a proximal group, tumor involvement within that fascicular group has probably occurred and the nerve fascicles are nonfunctional. The same procedure is then repeated with another proximal fascicular group until all of the proximal fascicular groups have been tested.

Once tumor extirpation has proceeded, microsurgical repair of the nerve ends should be performed (Fig. 1F). The operative microscope is brought into the field, although loupe magnification can be employed, and if previous nerve fascicular groups have been identified as above, direct neurorrhaphy should be performed between these fascicular groups. A variety of donor nerve graft sites are available. If the tumor defect is small, cutaneous sensory nerves (lateral antebrachial and the anterior division of the medial antebrachial cutaneous nerve) from the extremity can be

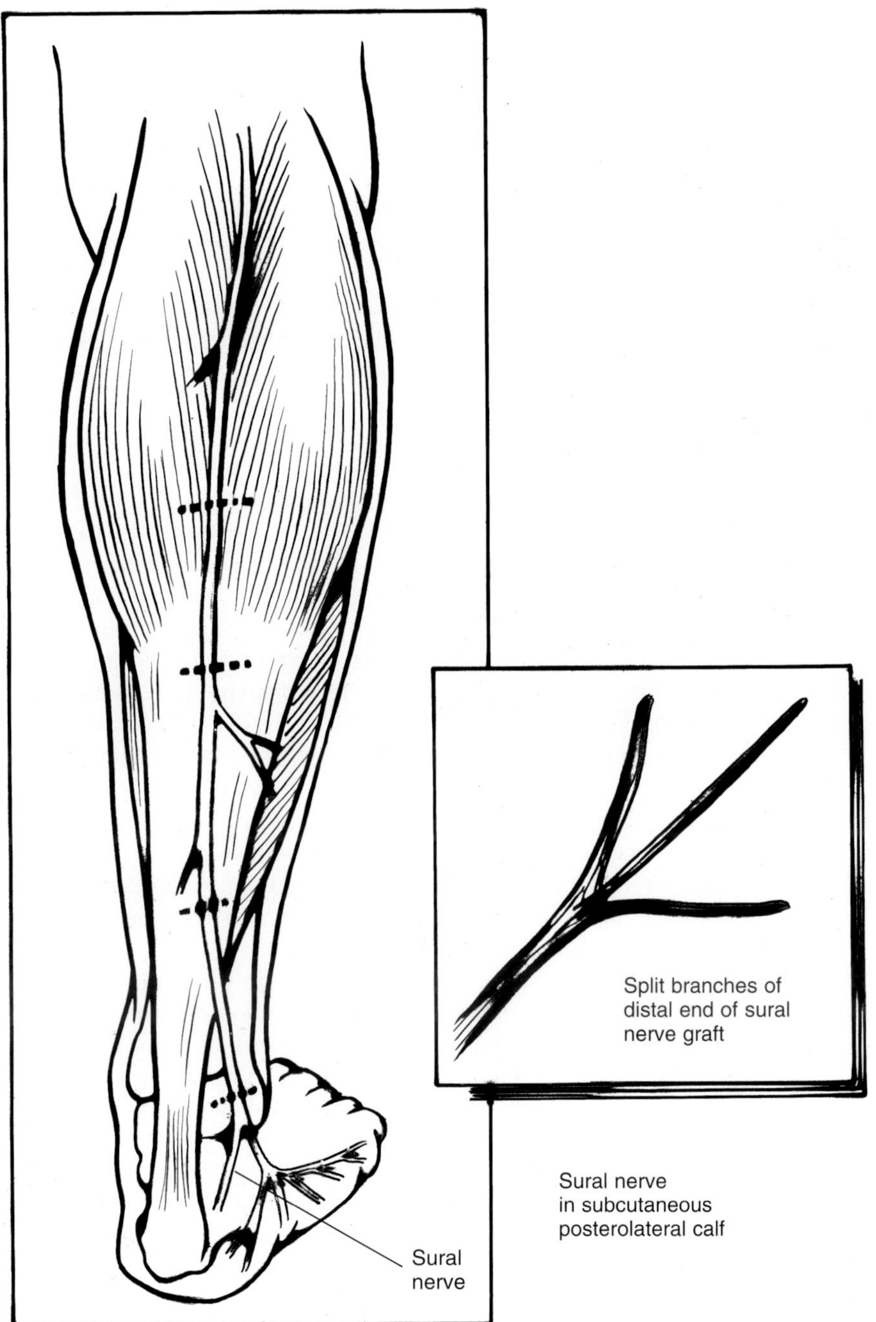

FIG. 2. Harvest of the sural nerve for grafting.

used. The lateral antebrachial cutaneous nerve lies adjacent to the cephalic vein. The forearm can be marked into thirds and the nerve lies in between the lateral and medial third. Alternatively, the cephalic vein is identified and dissected. The nerve lies on either side of the cephalic vein. Approximately 5 to 8 cm of nerve can be harvested. The medial antebrachial cutaneous nerve lies adjacent to the basilic vein.

The sural nerve is the most frequently used nerve for grafting in our practice, allowing the reconstructive surgeon to harvest the nerve grafts as tumor extirpation continues (Fig. 2). The sural nerve may provide up to 30 to 40 cm of nerve length. Dissection begins just below the lateral malleolus. A long incision or several small incisions may be used to isolate the nerve. A long incision may be more appropriate, as this allows the surgeon to identify the two branches of the nerve (medial sural cutaneous and peroneal communicating branch). Dissection continues to the popliteal fossa, the point at which the nerve exits the muscle. If nerve grafting or primary repair is required, postural positioning of the extremity to facilitate repair is discouraged. The extremity should be in the neutral position without tension. Alterations from this neutral position for nerve repair may alter the tension on the repair once the patient is awake and the extremity is moved. The clinical role of vascularized nerve grafts is yet to be determined; however, it may offer some advantage in a hostile environment. Once the nerve graft has been isolated, it is reversed and placed between our previously identified fascicular groups. If no groups of fascicles could be identified by nerve stimulation, the surgeon should attempt to line up fascicular groups that appear to have the same volume of fascicles. This should be done under microscopic vision. If no fascicle can be identified due to previous fibrosis from irradiation or damage from the tumor resection, the nerve ends must be cut back until groups of fascicles can be found. Our common method of nerve repair includes the use of 10-0 nylon suture. Epineural repair is advocated between the groups of fascicles. Nerve ends should be approximated and not tied so tight that axonal material is extruded on the contralateral side. Two to four sutures are usually required. Again, care must be taken not to tightened the suture too much, for the nerve repair or nerve graft must lie comfortably within the defect.

Once nerve repair is completed, closure of the soft tissue proceeds. Well-vascularized tissue is required over nerve repair. Closure of the skin over the brachial plexus or nerve repair must be performed with caution. Postoperative splinting is mandatory for 7 to 10 days. Once healing has begun, aggressive motor/sensory reeducation will maximize the results of nerve grafting. Muscle stimulation with external electrical stimuli to continue muscular motor end plate functioning should be contemplated if nerve reinnervation is suspected to take longer than 12 to 18 months. Unfortunately, this is frequently painful and not tolerated well by the patient. Postoperative physical examination for Tinel's sign and electrical nerve conduction will provide the reconstructive surgeon with information on the progress of the nerve repair.

Secondary Reconstruction After Nerve Repair

Despite the advances in nerve reconstruction, our best efforts do not always yield a functional extremity. Complicating factors such as the patient's age, medical condition, excess scarring, nutrition, and motivation can cloud a technically perfect nerve repair. In addition, proximal nerve injury and repair generally yield poorer functional restoration results than more distal reconstruction. Reconstruction of bone and nerve are the first two steps in the reestablishment of a functional extremity. The final common step is to provide adequate stable soft tissue coverage.

FLAP SELECTION

A variety of flaps are available for extremity reconstruction. Selection is based on the correct marriage between the defect and the donor flap. Muscle flaps or musculo-

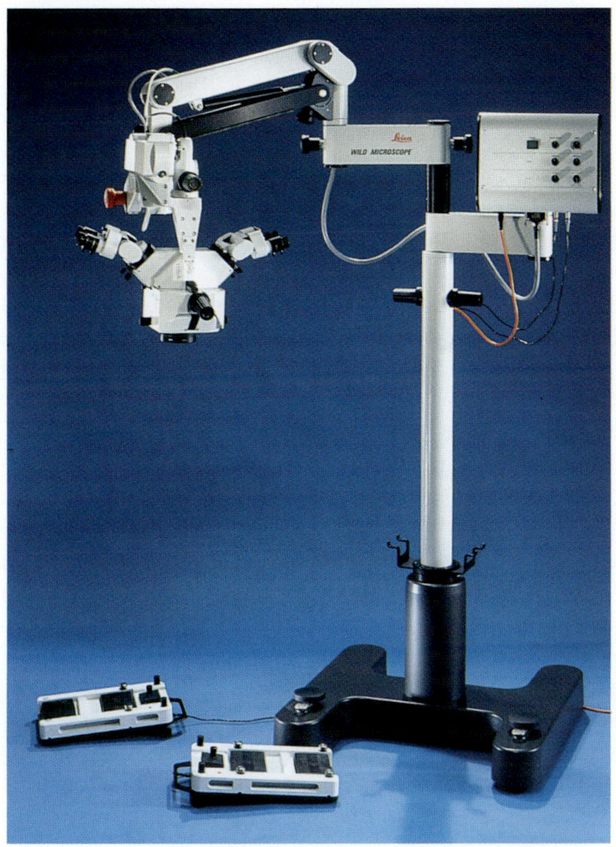

FIG. 3. The Wild Leitz 680 operating microscope.

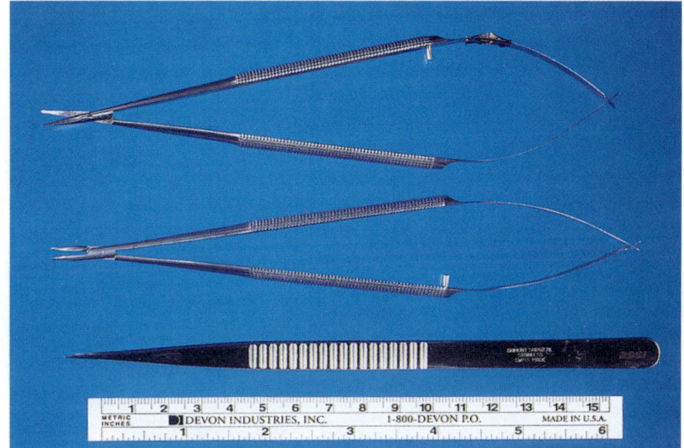

FIG. 4. Long microsurgical instruments (15 cm) are useful for dissection and anastomosis in difficult to reach places.

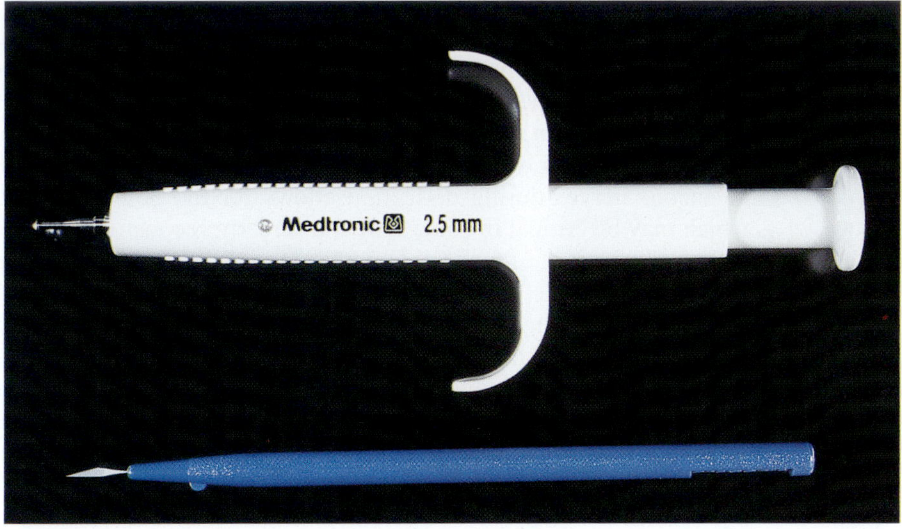

FIG. 5. The microknife and 2.5-mm aortic punch used to make the arteriotomy.

cutaneous flaps are used preferentially, especially for larger defects. Muscle provides highly vascularized tissue that promotes healing, especially in hostile wound environments. It also conforms well to deep complex wounds and is helpful in obliterating dead space. Fasciocutaneous flaps are used for smaller more superficial defects, especially if cosmesis is a primary concern.

The latissimus dorsi muscle offers a wide area for coverage and is one of the more versatile flaps used in microsurgery. This muscle can be rolled, turned, and tailored to conform to the defect. The latissimus dorsi muscle offers the microvascular surgeon the ability to fill large cavitary defects, obliterating the dead space. When the serratus anterior muscle is included within the dissection, a greater area can be covered, such as in defects comprising both the anterior and posterior extremity. When not used as a free tissue transfer, the pedicled latissimus may offer functional restoration to the shoulder, arm, or forearm. The muscle may be used with or without a skin paddle. If the muscle is used alone, it is readily covered with a skin graft. The skin paddle, if used, may be extended over the thoracodorsal fascia allowing more area for defect coverage. The donor site can be closed primarily in the absence of or small design of a skin paddle.

Another popular and reliable large muscle flap is the rectus abdominis flap. Like the latissimus dorsi flap, it can be harvested with or without a cutaneous skin paddle and it can serve to fill dead space as well as cover exposed structures after surgical extirpation. If required, both a transverse and vertical oriented skin paddle may be designed with the rectus abdominis muscle. This skin paddle is based on perforating vessels from the muscle and may include the medial and/or lateral row of perforators. Thus, larger defects can be covered with the addition of a cutaneous paddle. In multicavitary defects, the use of the muscle with a skin graft may be more appropriate to allow muscle conformity to the defect's variability. The chief advantage of the rectus abdominis flap is that it can be harvested with the patient in the supine position, thus making it the flap of choice in patients with large anterior defects. If the patient is positioned laterally or prone, the latissimus dorsi flap is the preferred large muscle flap.

Unlike the latissimus dorsi and rectus abdominis muscles, the gracilis muscle in long and thin. This muscle is ideal for smaller defects of the lower one-third of the extremity, ankle, foot, or elbow. Its lack of bulk is more suited to defects with a more aesthetic quality. The gracilis muscle also has the capability of a functional transplant, particularly in the forearm. The distal one-third of a cutaneous skin paddle must be used with caution, as the vascular supply is frequently unreliable.

Several fasciocutaneous flaps are also readily available. The radial forearm flap can provide a thin layer of skin and/or fascia. Inclusion of the lateral or medial antebrachial cutaneous nerves during dissection allows for the potential of sensory innervation, which may be critical in some foot and forearm reconstruction. The thin nature of the flap allows gliding of tendons and muscles and is ideal for coverage over functionally sensitive areas. The flap may also be elevated on a pedicle, which would allow coverage of more proximal defects around the elbow. A distally based radial forearm for reverse coverage to the hand and digits can be employed; however, with tumor resection, one must be cautious of the vascular supply. Up to 10 cm of bone may be harvested with the flap, but donor site morbidity in the form of fracture of the remaining radius is a significant problem. This bone is ideal for metacarpal and metatarsal reconstruction, because of the additional supply of well-vascularized soft tissue.

The scapular flap has a large and consistent vascular pedicle, which is one reason for its popularity. Although occasionally bulky, the scapular flap offers durable skin and soft tissue for moderate defects. The skin can be removed, which offers fascia and soft tissue for more functionally sensitive areas such as the dorsal hand and foot. The scapular flap is ideal for the patient placed in the prone position. The parascapular flap can also be designed and included within the dissection allowing for coverage of two defects. Up to 12 cm of bone can be harvested with the flap; furthermore, the flap offers ideal vascularized bony tissue for small defects of the hand, enabling the bone to be sandwiched between soft tissue.

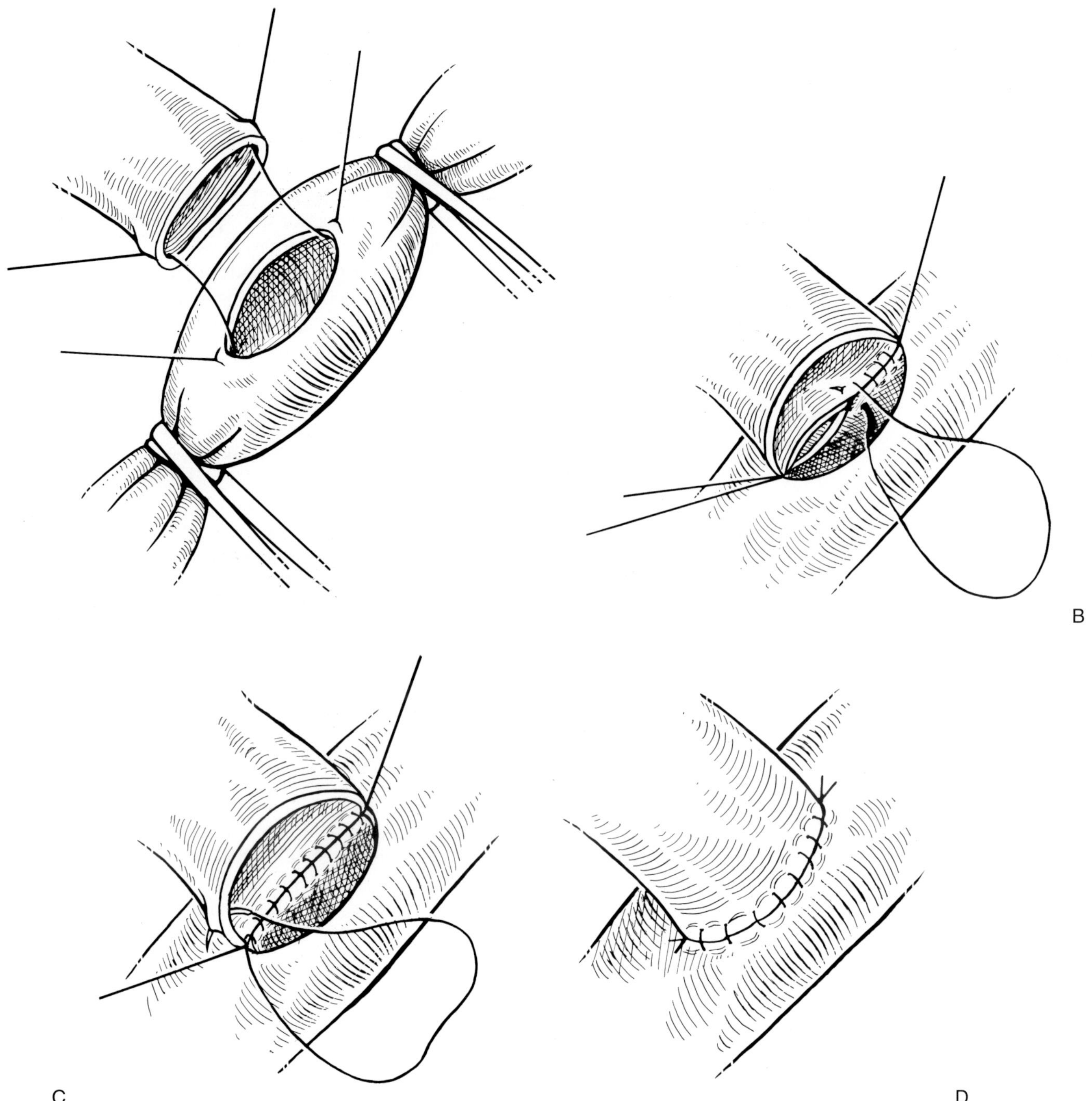

FIG. 6A–D. The running end-to-side anastomosis.

The dorsalis pedis flap can provide thin skin, which may include tendons, bone, and joints. Sensory innervation is also possible with inclusion of the superficial peroneal nerve. This makes the dorsalis pedis flap an attractive flap option for hand reconstruction. The major disadvantage of this flap is the donor site morbidity as the skin graft required for the dorsal foot may inhibit ambulation due to frequent breakdown. The radial forearm flap has much less donor site morbidity in our hands and therefore has been used preferentially to the dorsalis pedis flap.

The temporoparietal fascia flap offers a large sheet of thin pliable tissue available from the temporal, parietal, and occipital areas of the scalp. Its advantage is in the reconstruction of tissue defects where large, bulky tissue would diminish the desired results. The temporoparietal flap is ideal for the hand and foot reconstruction covering exposed tendons, nerves, and bone for salvage. This flap is used commonly for trauma defects, but because of the nature of the tumors encountered, this type of defect is seldom seen in the oncology setting, and therefore this flap is mentioned only for completeness sake.

If vascularized bone is needed, several donor sites are available as mentioned above, but we have preferentially used the free fibula transfer. The fibula can fill defects up to 25 cm and is appropriate for hostile environments. The straight, tubular, and compact characteristics of the fibula make it an ideal candidate for early weight bearing. Evaluation of the donor lower extremity vascular supply is necessary prior to bony harvest. A large skin paddle and some muscular bulk can be designed with the flap to provide soft tissue requirements. Donor site morbidity is minimal and the flap is ideal for long segmental defects.

TECHNICAL CONSIDERATIONS

Unlike other operative procedures, reconstruction of the extremities requires several additional measures in the preparation of the operating room. The upper extremities can be placed on hand tables or double arm boards if forearm and hand reconstruction is required. Care must be taken not to hyperextend the upper extremity during positioning. More proximal lesions may be more suitable for resection and reconstruction in the lateral decubitus position. In this situation, the use of the back as a donor site for reconstruction would be ideal. The patient should be placed on a beanbag and adequate foam padding provided, allowing both protection and stabilization during surgery. Axillary rolls are necessary to protect the brachial plexus while in the lateral decubitus position. Frequently, taping the iliac crest to the operating room table allows for further patient stabilization.

Reconstruction of the lower extremities may entail placing the patient prone or placing the legs in a frog-leg position. Hyperabduction of the legs should be avoided. If the patient is placed prone, chest rolls are required to relieve pressure and allow adequate ventilatory excursion. Attention should be paid to the endotracheal tube. Adequate padding to the face will lower the incidence of endotracheal tube kinking and facial trauma. While prone, the upper extremities should not be hyperextended and the arms should be placed volar with the elbows flexed. The full extremity is prepped into the field to allow for mobility and ease of access. If skin grafting or vein harvest is required, the opposite leg should also be prepped. If oncologically sound, the same extremity may satisfy the donor requirements. Providing there is no oncologic contraindications, tourniquets can be placed on the proximal extremity to assist with the dissection or if excessive blood loss is anticipated. Tourniquet inflation is generally kept under 250 mm Hg for a maximum of 2 hours.

The operative microscope with a 200- to 250-mm lens is optimal for performing the reconstructive procedures (Fig. 3). Long microvascular instruments are necessary, especially for those areas where cavitary defects may required coverage (Fig. 4). A direct nerve-to-nerve stimulator using an EMG system with bipolar direct electrodes should be available for tumor involvement. A technician or neurophysiologist should

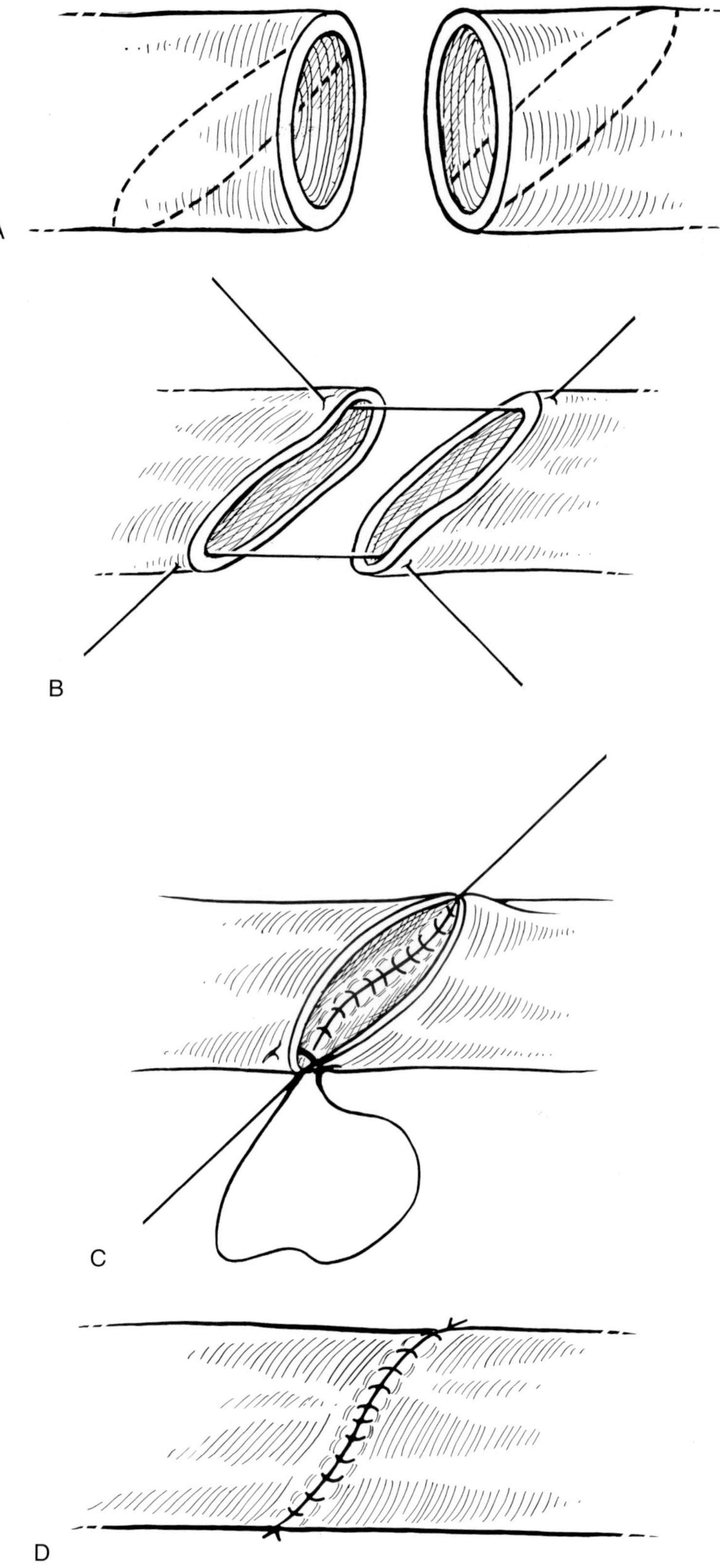

FIG. 7A–D. The running end-to-end anastomosis.

be present to interpret and monitor nerve stimulation. This allows for determination of fascicular involvement and the opportunity for selective group fascicular grafting if nerve resection is required.

Large-caliber vessels are used for the anastomosis. The femoral, axillary, brachial, and popliteal vessels are all appropriate for recipient vessels. An end-to-side anastomosis is preferred. With distal wounds, the posterior or anterior tibial vessels, as well as the radial and ulnar artery, may be used. An end-to-end anastomosis can be performed into these vessels providing the blood flow to the distal extremity is adequate. More commonly, an end-to-side anastomosis is done, allowing for flap and distal extremity perfusion. Vessels are isolated with vessels loops. This allows the vessels to be elevated out of the defect. Vessel loops also avoid crush injuries that may occur with the use of a peripheral vascular clamp. This is especially important for those vessels subjected to previous irradiation. For the end-to-side anastomoses, an arteriotomy can be performed with the microvascular scissors; however, more commonly used is a microknife and a 2.5 mm diameter aortic punch (Fig. 5). Depending on the size of the donor vessels, the vessels may require spatulation. Two running sutures of 9-0 nylon are placed on either end and the posterior and anterior wall of the anastomosis is done (Fig. 6A–D). If an end-to-end anastomosis is used, sutures are placed 180° apart and the posterior and anterior wall sutured in a running fashion (Fig. 7A–D). Care must be taken not to narrow the anastomosis with this end-to-end technique and spatulating the vessels may be necessary. Alternatively, an interrupted anastomosis may be more appropriate. Although loupe magnification can be used, the operative microscope allows two surgeons to perform the anastomosis. A variety of veins for the venous anastomosis is available in the upper and lower extremity, so an end-to-end anastomosis is usually performed. Occasionally, the superficial system is more accessible than the deep venous system. The use of the superficial venous system, however, requires caution, as previous surgical and adjuvant therapy may lead to venous occlusion. The cephalic and saphenous vein can be used as an in situ vein loop for deep-seated defects or for those areas in the site of injury or resection. In addition, these vessels may be reversed and used as traditional vein grafts. Thought should be given to performing the anastomosis outside the field of injury depending on the flow and size of the recipient vessel. The use of vein grafts in areas where the recipient vessels have been previously damaged or are small is encouraged. Although previous adjuvant therapy does not preclude the use of these vessels, care must be taken in performing an anastomosis to previously irradiated structures. The use of systemic anticoagulants is controversial; local heparin irrigation appears to offer some protective antithrombotic role, and concentrations between 10,000 and 50,000 units have been employed.

The extremity should be mobilized following the microvascular transfer. If possible, the foot should be placed in 90° of dorsiflexion. The hand should be placed in the neutral position or position of function. The joint above and below the flap should be immobilized. Whatever splinting technique is employed, the flap must be visible and easily monitored. Flap monitoring is most commonly performed by hand-held Doppler examination or with the use of the laser Doppler if a skin paddle is present. Despite all of these techniques, clinical observation is the most important. Immobilization should be continued until the wound appears stable. Because of this immobilization, it is important to use prophylactic measures to prevent deep venous thrombosis. This can be performed by low-dose heparin infusion or subcutaneous injections. The upper extremity should be elevated most commonly on an intravenous pole. For the lower extremity, bed rest with elevation of the extremity above the pelvis is required for approximately 5 days. After allowing for healing and neointimilization during this period, the patient begins dangling the extremity for 15-minute periods. Standing proceeds with the assistance of physical therapy. The lower extremity should be wrapped with an elastic bandage to assist with venous pooling secondary to ambulation. Extreme venous congestion demands a reappraisal of the therapy. After a period of crutch training, weight is gradually increased over the following several weeks. Specialized shoes need to be considered for those flaps required for foot reconstruction.

Diligence and frequent examinations for lesions and flap breakdown needs to be performed as ambulation proceeds.

ADJUVANT THERAPY

The use of adjuvant therapy has allowed a great number of leg salvage surgeries. External beam radiotherapy and brachytherapy are common in the postoperative course in the cancer patient with extremity malignancy. With the use of free tissue transfers and the ability to bring well-vascularized tissue into the wound, we have not found an increased complication rate with the use of adjuvant therapy. In fact, microvascular surgery has allowed the use of higher radiation doses and more frequent limb salvage by the prevention of some secondary wound complications.

CONCLUSION

This chapter provides the reconstructive microsurgeon with background for, and an approach to, the patient with extremity malignancy. The reconstruction is as important as the ablative procedure. The primary goal of the surgical plan is to adequately ablate the cancer; the reconstruction is secondary only in chronology, not in importance. The reconstructive techniques chosen should have the following characteristics: reliability, expediency, and maintenance of function and aesthetics. The advocacy of microvascular reconstruction of the patient undergoing limb-sparing surgery cannot be overemphasized, and fulfills all of these characteristics.

Oncologic surgery is a multidisciplinary approach with a variety of specialists involved in the care of the patient. It is vital that communication is established in the preparation and execution of the surgery and in the postoperative planning for the patient. Microvascular surgery has facilitated the multidisciplinary approach to extremity neoplasms. With careful patient selection and forethought, improved quality of life can be achieved through functional and aesthetic restoration.

SELECTED READINGS

Aldea PA, Shaw WW. Lower extremity nerve injuries. *Clin Plast Surg* 1986;13(4):691–699.

Aldea PA, Shaw WW. Management of acute lower extremity nerve injuries. *Foot Ankle* 1986;7(2):82–94.

Breidenbach WC. Emergency free tissue transfer for reconstruction of acute upper extremity wounds. *Clin Plast Surg* 1989;16(3):505–514.

Brennan MF. Management of extremity soft-tissue sarcoma. *Am J Surg* 1989;158:71.

Cordeiro PG, Neves RI, Hidalgo DA. The role of free tissue transfer following oncologic resection in the lower extremity. *Ann Plast Surg* 1994;33(1):9–16.

Dellon AL. Think nerve in upper extremity reconstruction. *Clin Plast Surg* 1989;16(3):617–662.

Doi K, Sakai K, Ihara K, Abe Y, Kawai S, Kurafuji Y. Reinnervated free muscle transplantation for extremity reconstruction. *Plast Reconstr Surg* 1993;91(5):872–883.

Hidalgo DA, Carrasquillo IM. The treatment of lower extremity sarcomas with wide excision, radiotherapy, and free-flap reconstruction. *Plast Reconstr Surg* 1992;89(1):96–101.

Lee GW, Mackinnon SE, Brandt K, Bell RS. A technique for nerve reconstruction following resection of soft-tissue sarcoma. *J Reconstr Microsurg* 1993;9(2):139–144.

Mackinnon SE. Surgical management of the peripheral nerve gap. *Clin Plast Surg* 1989;16(3):587–603.

Reece GP, Kroll SS, Miller MJ, Baldwin BJ, Pollock RE, Romsdahl MM, Ross MI, Janjan NA, Schusterman MA. Lower extremity salvage in cancer patients with free tissue transfer. *Riv Ital Chir Plastica* 1992;25:441–446.

Shiu MH, Castro EB, Hajdu SI, Fortner JG. Surgical treatment of 297 soft tissue sarcomas of the lower extremity. *Ann Surg* 1975;182:597–602.

Skibber JM, Lotze MT, Seipp CA, Salcedo R, Rosenberg SA. Limb-sparing surgery for soft tissue sarcomas: wound related morbidity in patients undergoing wide local excision. *Surgery* 1987;102(3):447–452.

Stinson SF, DeLaney TF, Greenberg J, Yang JC, Lampert MH, Hicks JE, Venzon D, White DE, Rosenberg SA, Glatstein EJ. Acute and long-term effects on limb function of combined modality limb sparing therapy for extremity soft tissue sarcoma. *Int J Radiat Oncol Biol Phys* 1991;21(6):1493–1499.

Stotter A, McLean NR, Fallowfield ME, Breach NM, Westbury G. Reconstruction after excision of soft tissue sarcomas of the limbs and trunk. *Br J Surg* 1988;75:774–778.

Terzis JK, Maragh H. Strategies in the microsurgical management of brachial plexus injuries. *Clin Plast Surg* 1989;16(3):605–616.

Usui M, Ishii S, Naito T, Yamashita M, Yamamura M. Microsurgical reconstruction in limb salvage procedures: comparison between primary and secondary reconstruction. *J Reconstr Microsurg* 1993;9(2):91–101.

Microsurgical Reconstruction of the Cancer Patient, edited by M.A. Schusterman.
Lippincott-Raven Publishers, Philadelphia © 1997.

13

Upper Extremity Reconstruction

Gregory R.D. Evans and Michael J. Miller

Despite the success of limb preservation with extremity malignancies, the approach to the patient with an upper extremity mesodermal tumor is challenging, and presents the reconstructive microsurgeon with a variety of complexities in the restoration of function. Several factors are responsible for this increased reconstructive complexity in the upper as compared with the lower extremity: (a) the muscle mass is less, (b) major nerves and vessels are more superficial, and (c) there are more nerves responsible for both sensory and motor function.

This chapter describes our approach for microvascular reconstruction of the upper extremity. Fortunately, most defects of the upper extremity can be reconstructed by use of pedicled flaps from the shoulder girdle or forearm. Despite the rare need for microvascular free tissue reconstruction of the upper extremity, we will explain our approach to this difficult problem.

SHOULDER AND UPPER ARM RECONSTRUCTION

In our experience the most common location for presentation of tumors in the upper extremity is the shoulder and upper arm. Patients that require free tissue transfer for lesions in this area are those that require large tumor resection, which would necessitate use of large flaps such as the latissimus dorsi or rectus abdominis myocutaneous flaps (Fig. 1A–E). The brachial plexus and any exposed vascular and bony structures require coverage. Large fasciocutaneous flaps such as the scapular flap can also be used with good success (Fig. 2A–E). The brachial, axillary, and subclavian vessels are

G.R.D. Evans and M.J. Miller: Department of Plastic Surgery, The University of Texas, M.D. Anderson Cancer Center, Houston, Texas 77030.

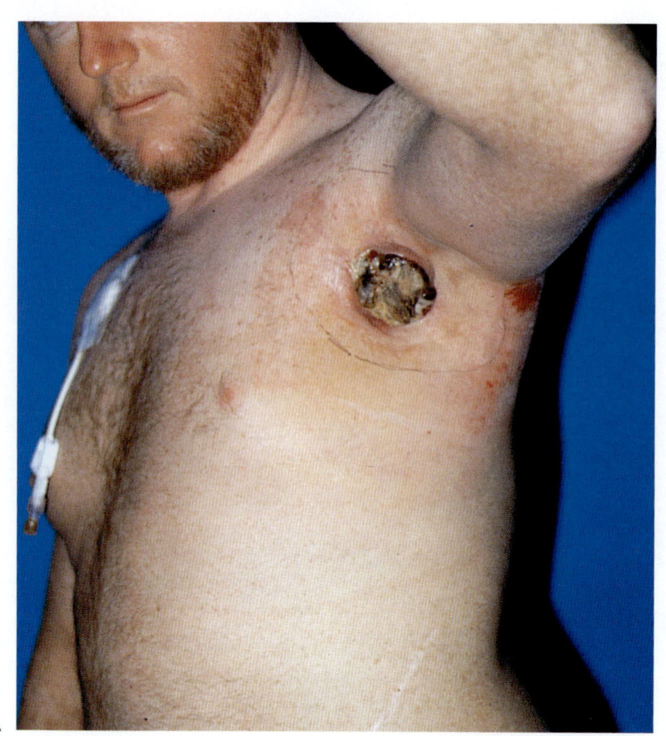

FIG. 1A. Melanoma of left axilla.

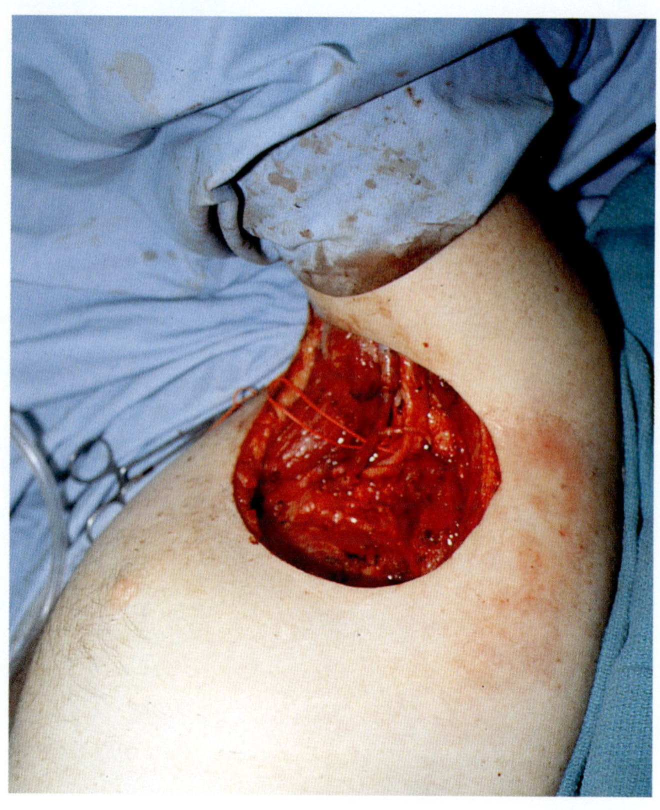

FIG. 1B. Defect after resection.

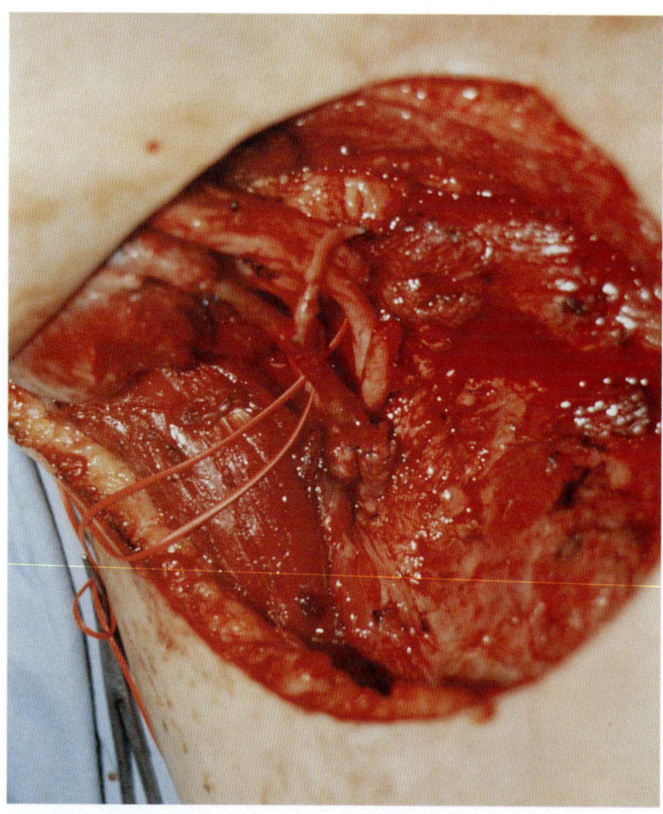

FIG. 1C. Closeup view of defect showing axillary vessels to be used as recipient vessels.

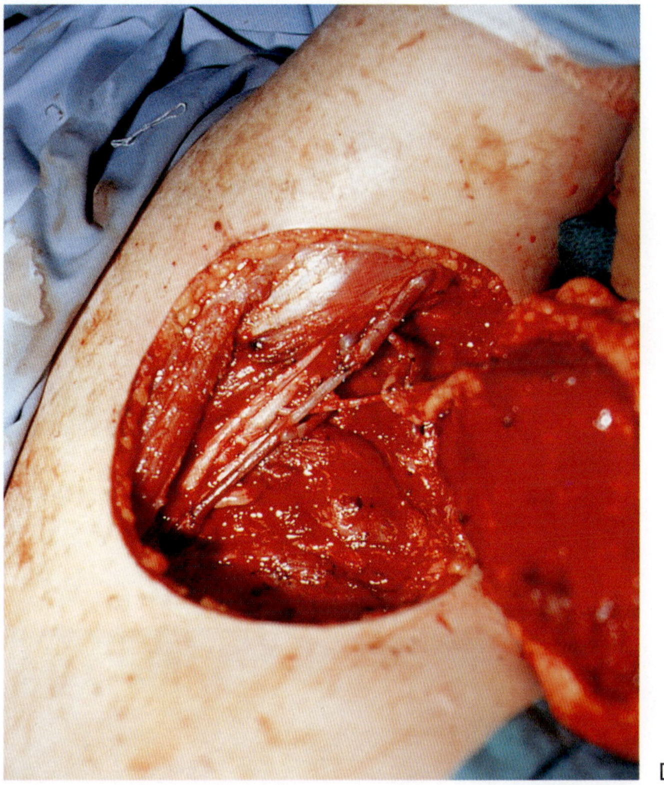

FIG. 1D. View of defect site after completion of anastomosis of free rectus abdominis myocutaneous flap.

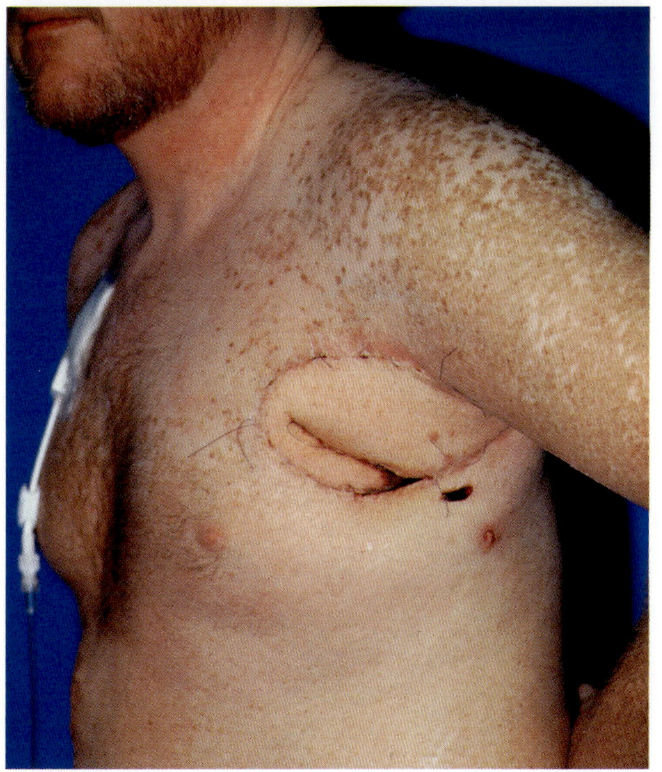

FIG. 1E. Postoperative view of reconstructed axilla.

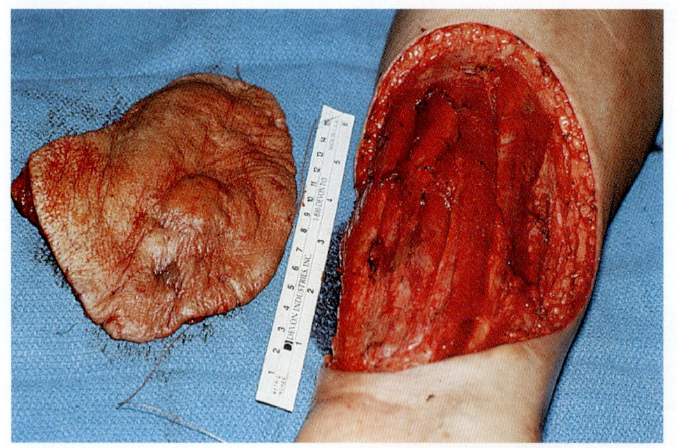

FIG. 2A. Recurrent leiomyosarcoma of right anterior arm. Defect after resection of tumor.

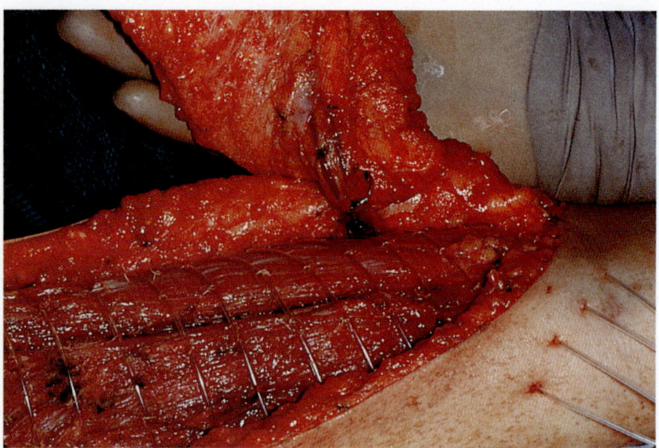

FIG. 2C. Recipient site after completion of anastomosis. Note the use of brachytherapy catheters, which are placed prior to flap inset.

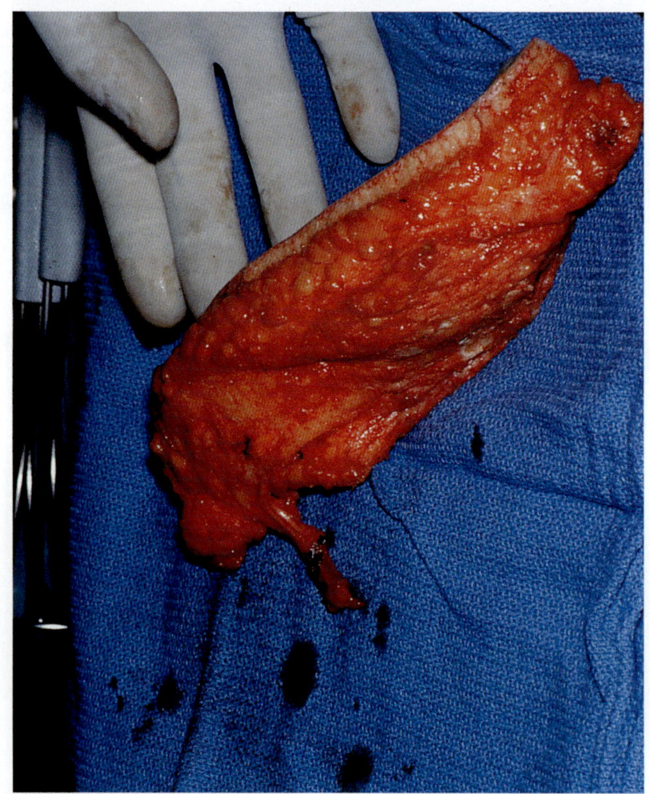

FIG. 2B. Scapular flap to be used for reconstruction.

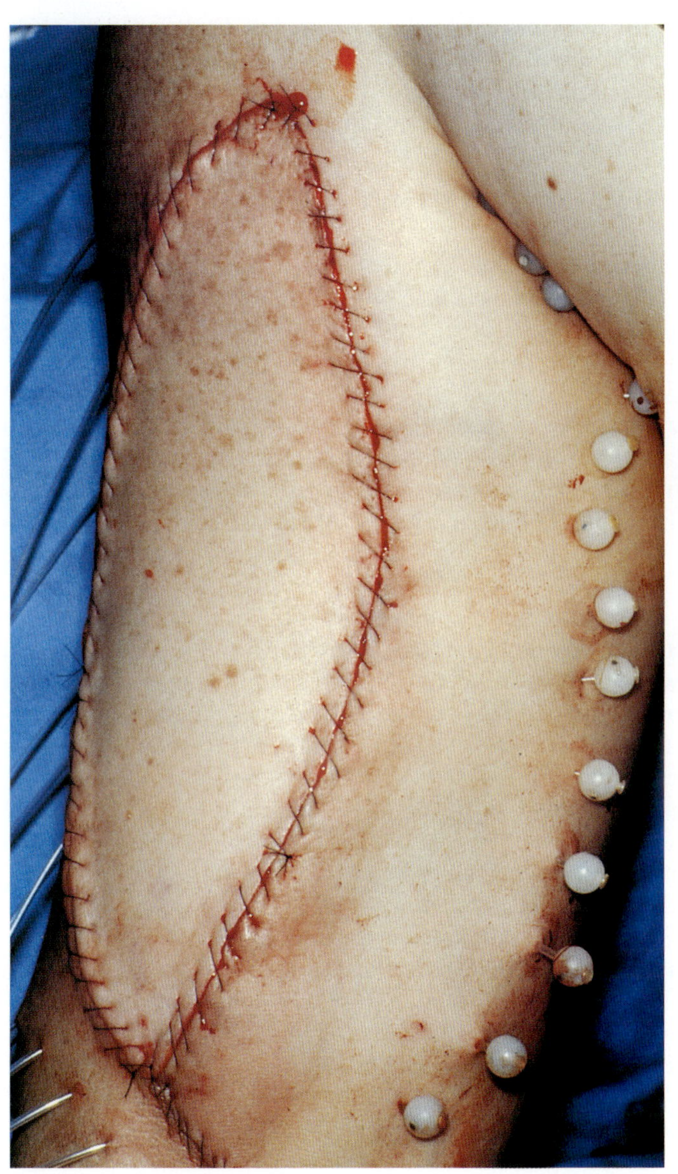

FIG. 2D. Flap inset completed, brachytherapy catheters in place.

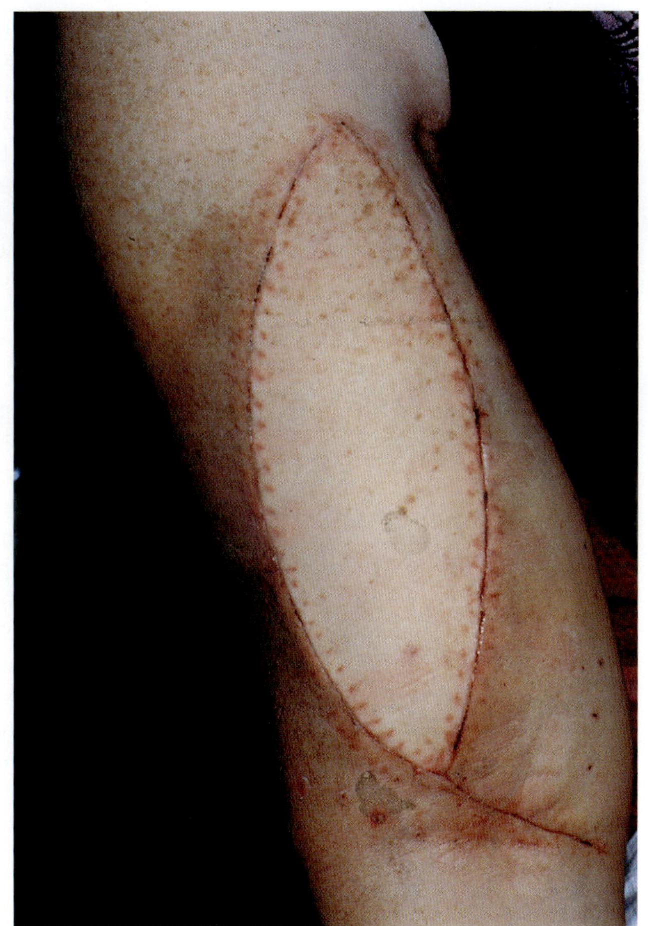

FIG. 2E. Long-term postoperative result.

ideal for recipient vessels for free tissue transfer. An end-to-side anastomosis is most commonly performed. Consideration should be given, however, to primary amputation with coverage if the tumor is extensive and restoration of functional structures is impossible. The use of the skin and muscle of the amputated forearm can be transferred as a free tissue transfer for coverage of the shoulder.

Postoperative care requires shoulder immobilization. This can be performed with gauze rolls or elastic bandage wraps securing the elbow to the chest wall. If a free tissue transfer has been performed, the immobilization must not exert excess pressure on the flap. Early mobility of the area may cause flap dehiscence, leading to complications with wound healing. Mobility is usually begun 1 to 2 weeks after surgery and sutures are routinely left within this area for 2 weeks. Aggressive occupational therapy is vital after surgery to assist with the restoration of function.

ELBOW AND FOREARM RECONSTRUCTION

Reconstruction involving the elbow is more challenging, as functional preservation is more difficult. Incisions should avoid the antecubital fossa, where scarring may preclude full extension and flexion. Free tissue transfer provides well-vascularized tissue in elbow reconstruction (Fig. 3A–D). In the forearm free tissue transfer may be appropriate for defects that have been compromised with adjuvant therapy. The branchial artery or one of its many branches can be employed in an end-to-side or end-to-end anastomosis (Figs. 4A–F and 5A–C). The well-vascularized tissue allows for minimal tension on the surrounding skin and provides an opportunity to simply remove any skin at the wound edges that appears ischemic. If a prosthesis is used, free tissue transfer provides appropriate coverage decreasing the chance of exposure and possible infection.

The resection of flexor or extensor muscles may hamper the postoperative function of the patient. Suture approximation of the muscle groups between the superficial and deep structures may allow restoration of function. Alternatively, tendon transfers and functional free tissue transfers (gracilis) may allow for functional restoration in addition to the soft tissue coverage. If the median or ulnar nerves are resected, these must be reconstructed with nerve grafts (Fig. 4).

Postoperative immobilization with the extremity elevated is critical. This can be accomplished with splinting or casting of the extremity. The elbow should be splinted to allow for a decrease in tension on the suture line and to protect the reconstructed structures. Splinting should be preformed such that the flap is accessible to the microsurgeon. This will allow caring for the skin graft and flap monitoring while the extremity is immobilized. Immobilization should continue for 1 to 2 weeks and sutures should remain for approximately 2 weeks. Hand or digit motion may be possible during this immobilization to prevent joint stiffness. Once immobilization is removed, occupational therapy is critical for the establishment of future function.

HAND RECONSTRUCTION

Tumors of the hand that are extensive enough to require free tissue transfer are usually too advanced for limb salvage and thus necessitate amputation. If free tissue transfer is required, thin small flaps such as the radial forearm or gracilis may provide appropriate soft tissue coverage in this area. Larger flaps with bulk such as the rectus should be avoided unless the defect requires the excess tissue. Frequently the free tissue transfer may encompass bone in addition to the soft tissue, allowing for simultaneous reconstruction of the bony and cutaneous defect (e.g., radial forearm and scapular flap). The radial and ulnar artery provide excellent recipient vessels in an end-to-end or end-to-side fashion. Debulking of the free tissue transfer is occasionally required; however, the correct choice of tissue transfer may prevent this. Functional muscle transfer (gracilis) as well as tendon transfers may be appropriate in this area.

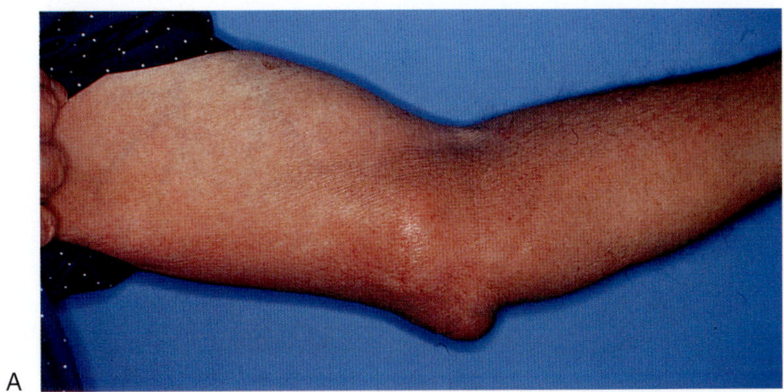

FIG. 3A. Recurrent squamous cell cancer involving the epitrochlear lymph nodes.

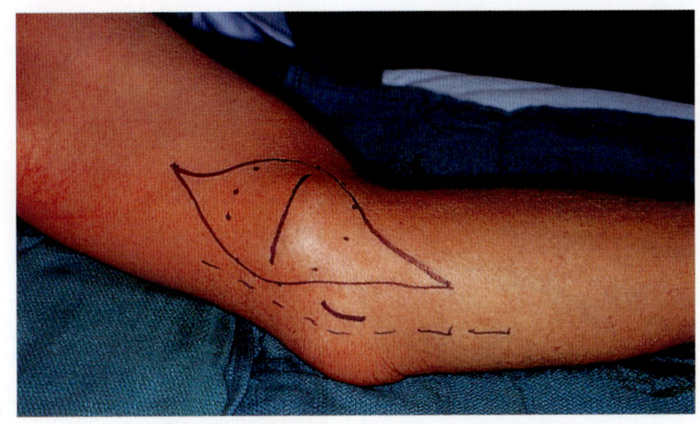

FIG. 3B. Planned area of resection.

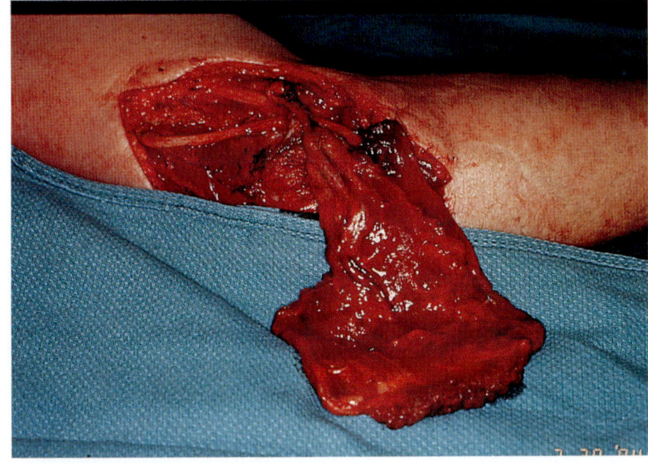

FIG. 3C. Free rectus abdominis muscle flap after completion of anastomosis.

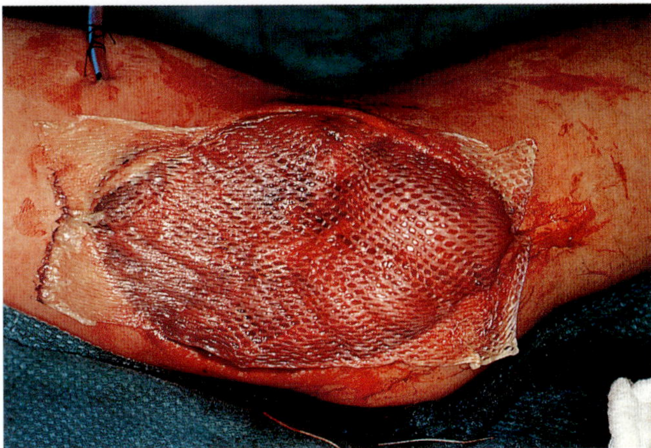

FIG. 3D. Free rectus abdominis muscle flap after inset and placement of skin graft.

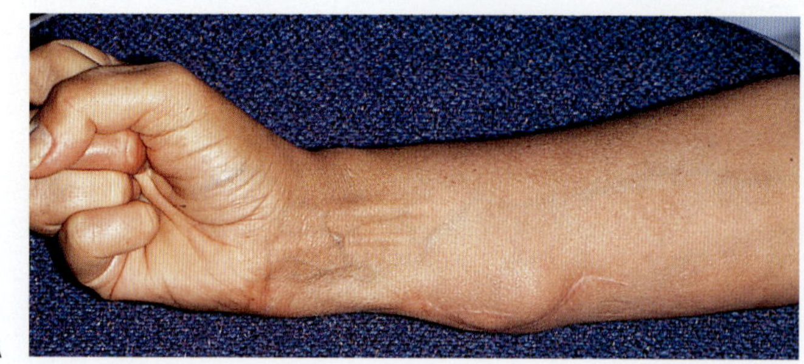

FIG. 4A. Recurrent liposarcoma right forearm.

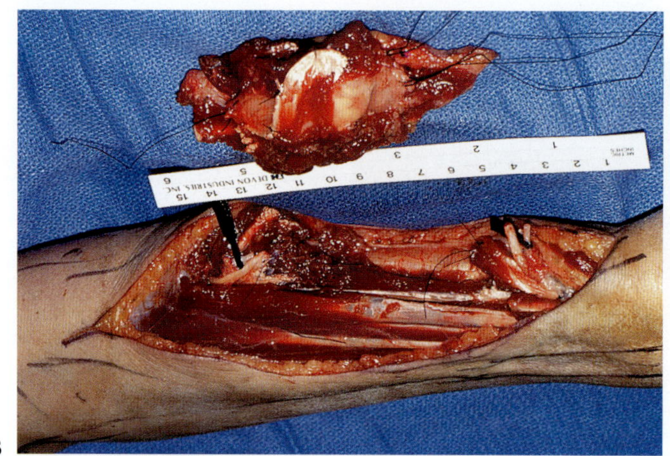

FIG. 4B. Defect after resection.

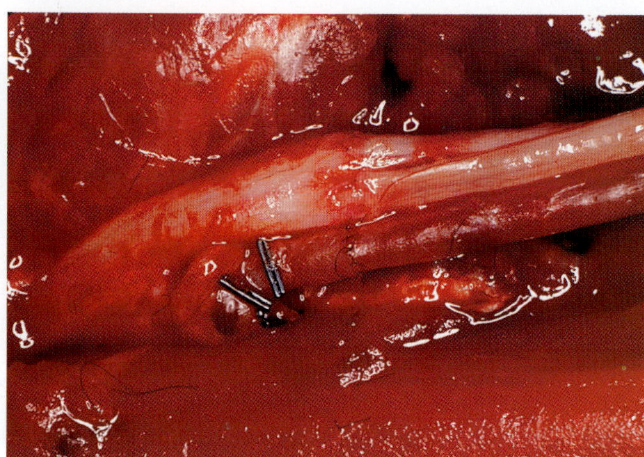

FIG. 4C. Reconstruction of ulnar nerve with sural nerve grafts.

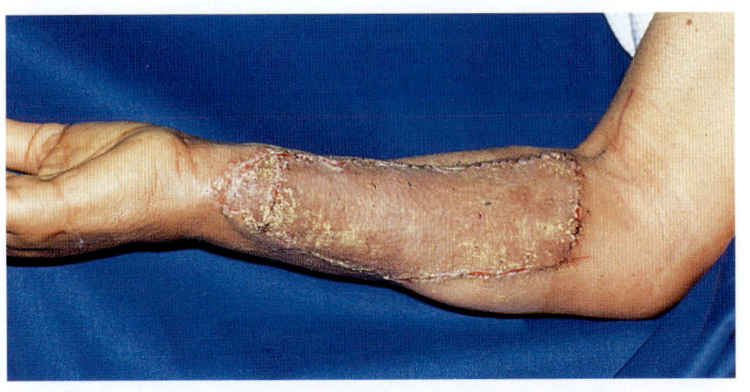

FIG. 4D. Free gracilis muscle and skin graft coverage.

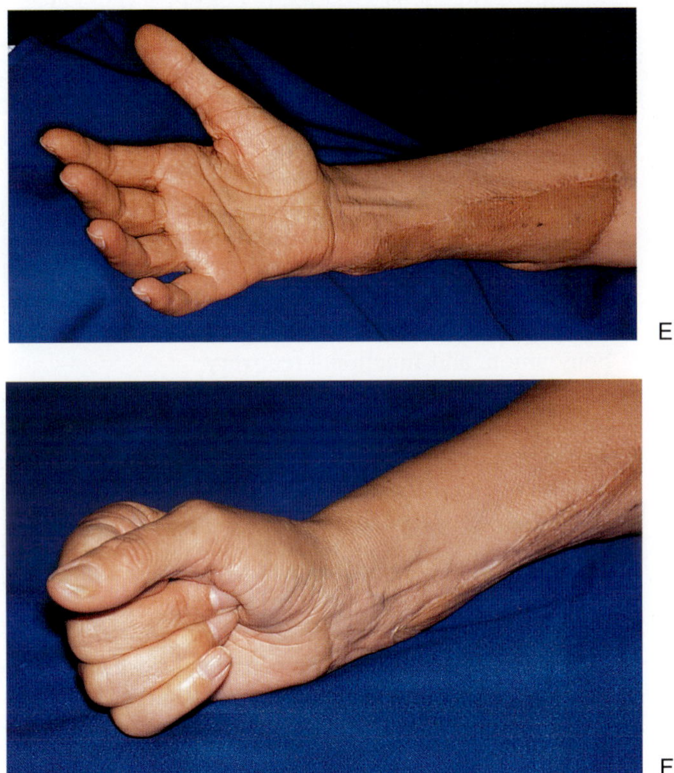

FIG. 4E,F. Long-term functional result.

Immobilization is required in the position of function for 1 to 3 weeks. Occasionally, passive mobility of certain digits may be desired to prevent possible stiffness. If tendon repair or transfer is performed, passive motion is begun at 2 to 3 weeks after surgery, unless an initial postoperative regimen of motion was begun. Active motion soon follows and extensive occupational therapy is required.

SKELETAL STABILITY

Satisfactory reconstruction of osseous defects in the upper extremity requires restoration of stability and length while maintaining mobility. Several methods are available to accomplish these goals. Bone shortening may be considered if the defect is limited to the humerus and is shorter than 3.5 cm; however, it is rarely an option in upper extremity tumors. Conventional bone grafting is also an option for segmental defects of limited length (< 8 cm), but it requires stable soft tissue coverage and a well-vascularized bed. This method should be avoided in irradiated tissues. Cadaver allografts may be used for large defects that may involve joint surfaces, and they heal like conventional bone grafts (creeping substitution). Because of their large volume and possible low-grade immune activity, cadaveric allografts may require up to 1 year for healing and are more prone to complications. Resection and arthroplasty may yield a functional extremity in cases of tumors in proximity to the ends of long bones. An example of this is the Tinkoff/Linberg proximal humeral interscapulothoracic resection and shoulder arthroplasty. Vascularized bone transfer provides a useful alternative to some of these techniques or may be used in conjunction with them to enhance successful bone healing. Vascularized bone provides healing even in compromised tissue beds and reduces the volume of bone to heal by creeping substitution, speeding stable bony union, and functional recovery.

Several donor sites have been described for vascularized bone transfer. Generally, the most useful one for the upper extremity is the fibula (Fig. 6A–F). The diameter approximates that of the radius and ulna. Up to 25 cm of bone may be easily obtained, and the thick cortex allows reliable fixation with plates and screws. In cases requiring soft tissue, a skin paddle may be harvested with the bone as a reliable composite.

Fibula Flap

The fibula is based on the peroneal artery and venae comitantes (Fig. 7A,B). There are rare anatomic abnormalities that a surgeon must be aware of. Difficulties with the vascular supply of the fibula should be anticipated on clinical examination. In cases of severe atherosclerosis, the patient will have altered distal pulsations, and an angiogram may be indicated. However, we do not obtain routine angiograms on patients prior to mobilization of the flap.

The fibula is mobilized by placing a hip roll underneath the patient on the side of the anticipated harvest. The extremity is flexed and bent at the knee. The head of the fibula and the lateral malleolus are identified. One should plan harvest of the bone in such a way that approximately 8 to 10 cm of bone is preserved proximally and distally to avoid impairing function at the ankle and knee joint (Fig. 8A–G). The bone is palpable on the lateral aspect of the leg. An incision is designed overlying the fibula. The plane of dissection proceeds between the soleus muscle posteriorly and the muscles of the lateral compartment anteriorly. Working from the proximal aspect, the bone is identified in this groove. If a skin paddle is to be harvested with the flap, then care is taken to identify perforating vessels and the pattern of their anatomy as the skin flap is mobilized. For most patients, the skin paddle is supplied primarily through pedicle branches in the septum. If, however, the pedicle goes through the soleus muscle, a cuff of muscle is harvested with the flap.

After complete identification of the bone along the entire length of the area to be harvested, the muscles in the lateral compartment are divided sharply from the fibula.

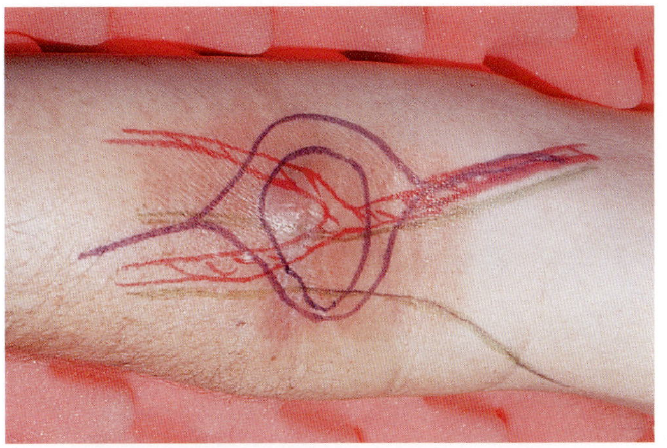

FIG. 5A. Recurrent leiomyosarcoma of forearm.

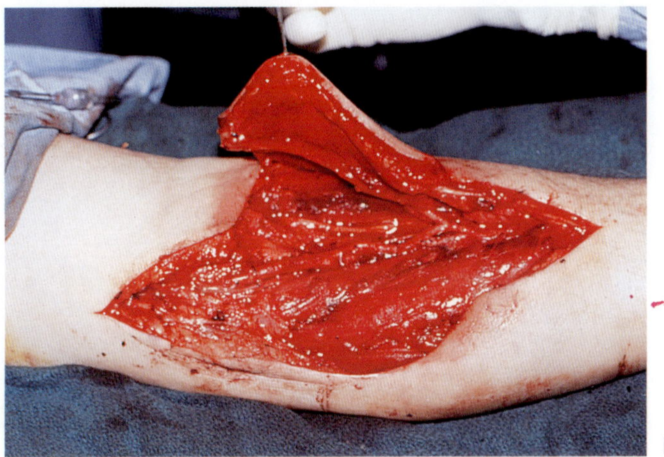

FIG.5B. After resection and transfer of contralateral radial forearm flap. The contralateral side was used due to the tumor involvement of the ipsilateral flap vessels.

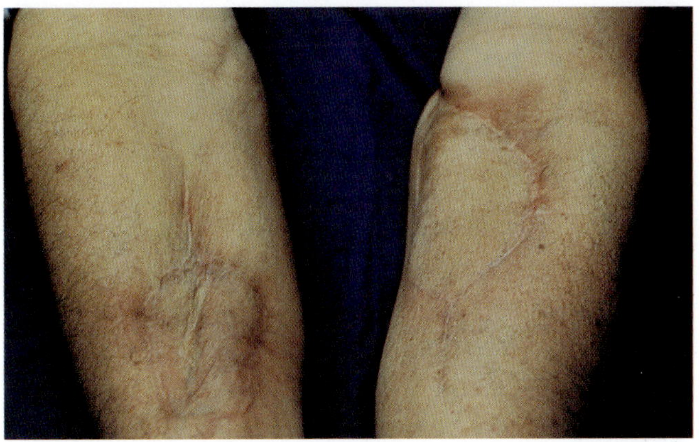

FIG. 5C. Postoperative result of recipient and donor sites.

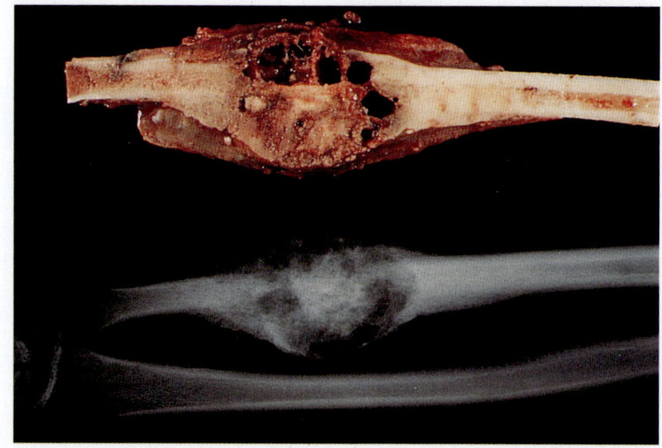

FIG. 6A. Osteosarcoma of right ulna, radiograph of forearm and photograph of resected specimen.

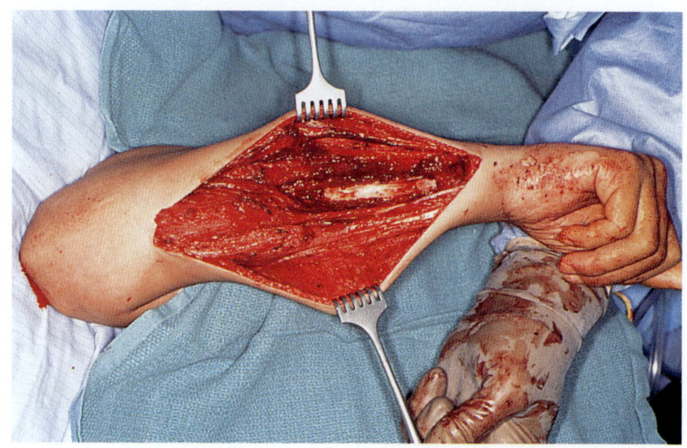

FIG. 6B. Defect after resection.

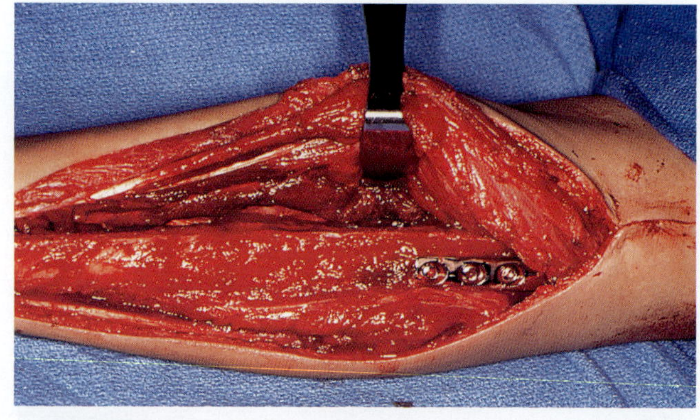

FIG. 6C. Free fibula transfer performed to reconstruct ulna, with use of internal plate fixation.

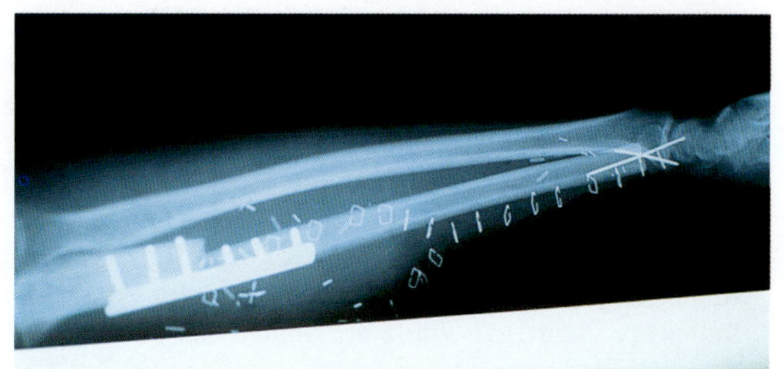

FIG. 6D. Radiograph of reconstructed forearm.

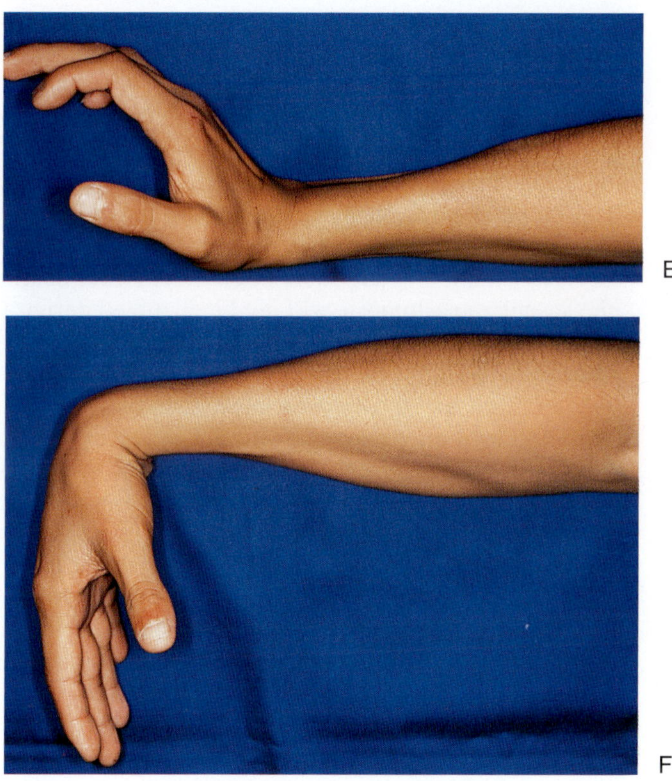

FIG. 6E,F. Functional result.

Care is taken to preserve the periosteum. The muscles are divided sharply, leaving a small cuff of muscle attached to the periosteum. Once the septum between the lateral compartment and the anterior compartment is encountered, it is then divided along the length of the muscle. Care must be taken at this point to avoid injury to the anterior tibial neurovascular structures running in the base of the anterior compartment. The anterior compartment muscles are divided from the fibula, and the interosseous membrane is encountered. The membrane is divided along the entire length of the fibula to be harvested. The dissection may be carried posteriorly at this point to expose the area proximally and distally where the bone will be divided. The peroneal artery and vein are identified proximally and a site on the fibula above the entry point of the vascular pedicle is identified. Using a power or a Gigli saw, the bone is divided proximally and distally. With retraction of the bone laterally, the distal peroneal artery and vena comitantes are identified. These are ligated and divided and then the medial musculature is divided. The anatomic landmark to guide this division is the median raphe of the tibialis posterior muscle. If the dissection is carried along this chevron-shaped area in the muscle, it is unlikely that the vascular pedicle will be injured. After complete division of all the muscles medially, the flap is fully mobilized, and if a tourniquet has been used, it is released at this point. It usually takes between $1\frac{1}{2}$ and 2 hours to mobilize the bone. The peroneal artery and venae comitantes are then traced proximally up to the level of the bifurcation from the posterior tibial vessels, where the pedicle may be ligated and divided.

It is possible to tailor the bone to fit the defect appropriately by preserving the periosteum and the connections with the vasculature proximally. The periosteum may be stripped from the bone and the bone cut to the appropriate size. This procedure also lengthens the vascular pedicle, allowing for easier inset. The bone is transferred into the anatomic defect in the upper extremity and stabilized with internal fixation devices. Fixation is advisable prior to revascularization if possible. This ensures that the vascular anastomosis will not be disrupted during fixation of the flap.

After the flap is inset and revascularized, care is taken with the skin closure. If skin closure is too tight, the vascular pedicle may be compromised. It is better to place a skin graft on an exposed area rather than compromise the vascular pedicle. The skin graft will contract postoperatively and can be excised later, if necessary. If a skin paddle has been employed, it provides a suitable means for flap monitoring. However, if no skin paddle is available, a percutaneous point for Doppler examination is identified. Alternatively, an implantable 20-MHz Doppler may be used. The extremity is kept in an elevated position postoperatively. The patient must avoid use of the extremity for up to 7 days postoperatively. This allows optimal healing after the microvascular anastomosis to ensure a good blood supply. The patient is then treated as if he/she had sustained a fracture of the upper extremity, and may be maintained in a splint for a period of 8 weeks to ensure adequate osseous healing. At that point, physical therapy may commence to ensure full range of motion. If physical therapy can be performed on noninvolved joints after fixation of the fracture, it is advisable to proceed throughout the period of the healing.

For problems related to osseous reconstruction of the upper extremity proximal to the hand, we work closely with our colleagues in orthopedic oncology planning the resection and reconstruction. For segmental humeral defects, the fibula may be set into the medullary cavity of the retained portions of humerus and fixed with plates and screws. For proximal humeral defects for which a shoulder prosthesis is not selected, scapulohumeral arthrodesis in approximately 35° abduction, 25° forward flexion, and rotation to allow hand-to-mouth excursion is usually preferred. Revascularization may be accomplished by an anastomosis into a side branch of the brachial artery or directly end to side. A flow-through reconstruction of the brachial artery is also possible using the peroneal artery.

The fibula is ideally suited for forearm reconstruction. Stable fixation is provided by plates and screws. If, however, the proximal or distal remnants are too short, crossed Kirschner wires and casting may be employed to protect the osteosynthesis

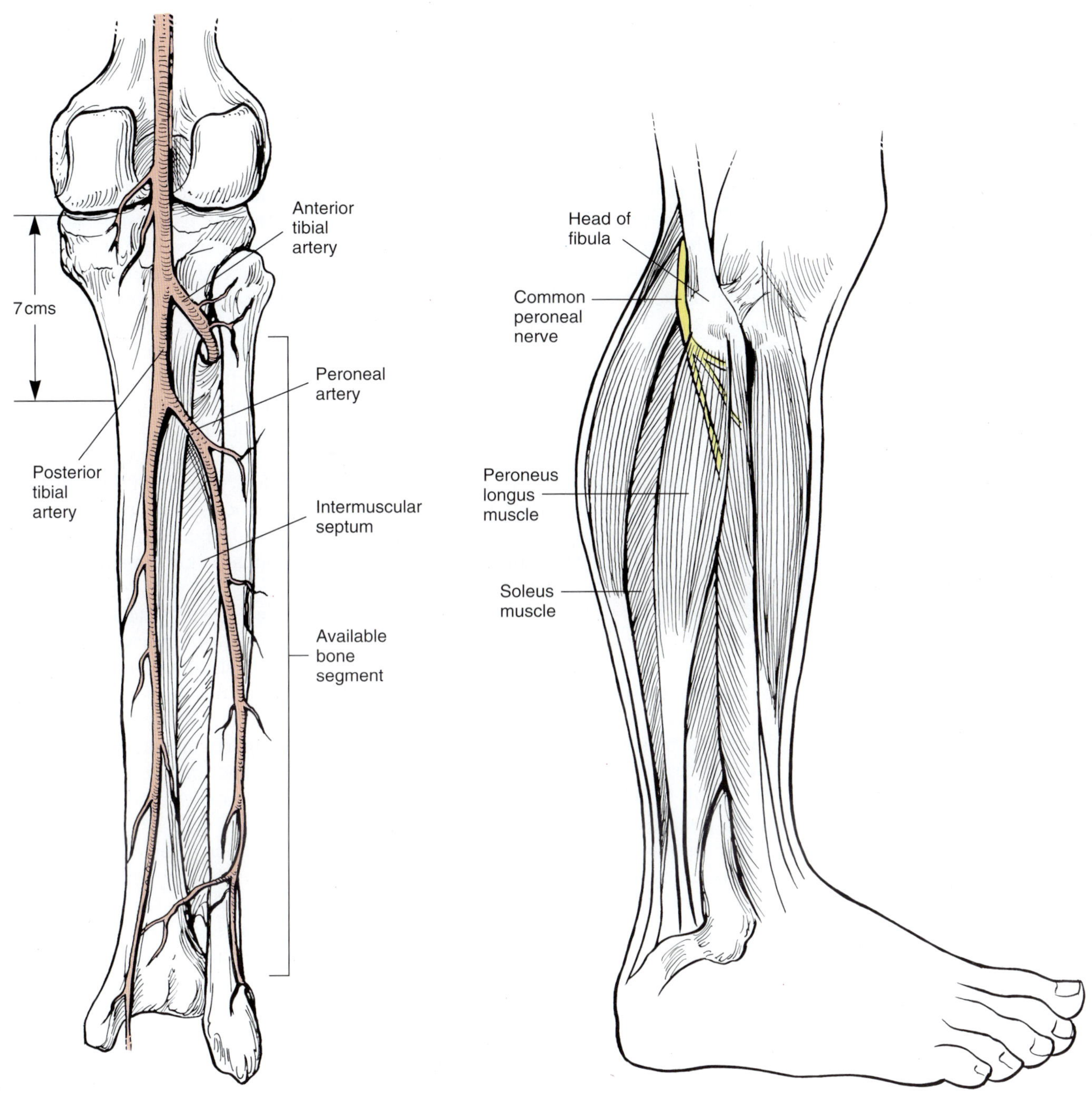

FIG. 7A. The anatomy of the leg vasculature. The peroneal artery branches off the popliteal trunk 7 cm from the knee joint.

FIG. 7B. The common peroneal nerve courses around the fibula head and must be avoided during the dissection.

and allow bony union. A single plate should not be used to span the entire length of the fibula, as stress shielding will prevent the fibula from hypertrophy and remodeling, which provides more natural support in its new location.

Latissimus Dorsi Muscle Flap

The latissimus dorsi muscle flap is based on the thoracodorsal artery and vein (Fig. 9A–C). This vessel is the terminal branch of the subscapular artery after the bifurcation of the serratus branch to the serratus anterior. The vascular pedicle enters the muscle approximately 8 cm distal to the humerus. Flap harvest is facilitated with the patient in the lateral position. The arm is prepped into the field to allow ease of access to the axilla. The landmarks to identify for flap design are the spinous processes posteriorly and the inferior tip of the scapula. The superior medial border of the muscle can then be sketched on the skin using a curvilinear line from the proximal humerus extending toward the scapula tip and transversely to the midline. The lateral border of the latissimus can often be palpated through the skin and is marked extending toward the iliac crest. A skin paddle is designed over the more lateral aspect of the latissimus muscle. Medial and inferior skin paddle designs are less reliable and blood flow is dependent on lumbar perforators rather than the musculocutaneous perforators from the latissimus. A skin paddle of almost any shape can be designed if it is located over the muscle. Often, depending on the mobility of the patient's skin, a paddle of 8 to 10 cm is possible.

The perimeter of the skin paddle is incised and carried down to the superficial surface of the latissimus muscle. The skin and subcutaneous tissues are mobilized to identify the superior medial and the lateral borders of the latissimus. The deep surface of the latissimus is developed by extending underneath the muscle, beginning laterally. This ensures that a proper plane is developed between the serratus anterior and the latissimus muscle. After complete mobilization of the superficial and deep surfaces of the muscle, the perimeter is divided with electrocautery and the muscle is now mobilized with its humeral attachment and its vascular pedicle intact. The dissection continues toward the axilla, where the vascular pedicle and the deep surface of the latissimus muscle are identified. The muscle above the vascular pedicle can be divided, thus isolating the latissimus completely on its thoracodorsal artery and vein. The serratus branches are also identified and carefully ligated. The vascular pedicle can be dissected toward the axillary vessels, ensuring a long pedicle of large caliber vessels. The pedicle is then ligated and the muscle transferred to a suitable location. Often the muscle can be rotated to cover the upper arm; however, if it is needed for coverage of the forearm or hand, then the free tissue technique is mandatory. Pedicle rotation of the latissimus dorsi to the proximal arm may provide some functional restoration. Donor site closure simply involves reapproximation of the skin. Closed suction drains are placed exiting the tissues laterally to ensure that the patient does not lie upon them. The major morbidity associated with this flap is marginal skin necrosis from the donor site if too wide a skin paddle is taken. Seromas may also be problematic, with an incidence of 10% to 15% in our patient population.

Scapular Flap

The scapular flap is one of the most reliable fasciocutaneous donor sites. If osseous reconstruction is desired, the lateral border of the scapula may be harvested to provide vascularized bone. The scapular flap system is highly versatile, providing various combinations of skin, fascia, muscle, and bone. Up to 14 cm of corticocancellous bone is available from the lateral border of the scapula, and a thin bicortical bone can also be harvested from the body of the scapula to reconstruct specific areas, such as the orbital floor and the maxilla (Fig. 10A–C).

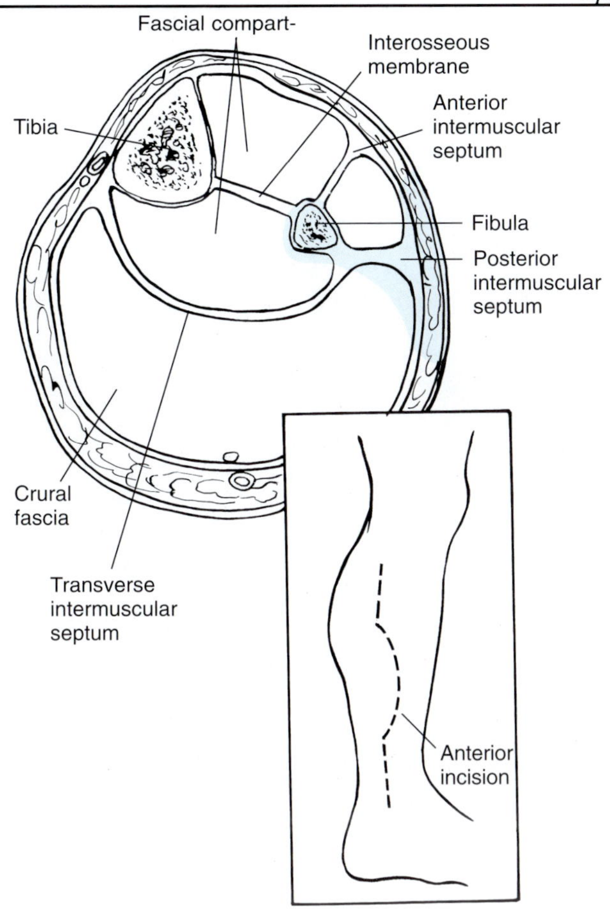

FIG. 8A. The flap harvest is approached from the lateral aspect of the leg. This schematic demonstrates harvest of the flap with a skin paddle. Harvest of bone alone is straightforward and described in the text.

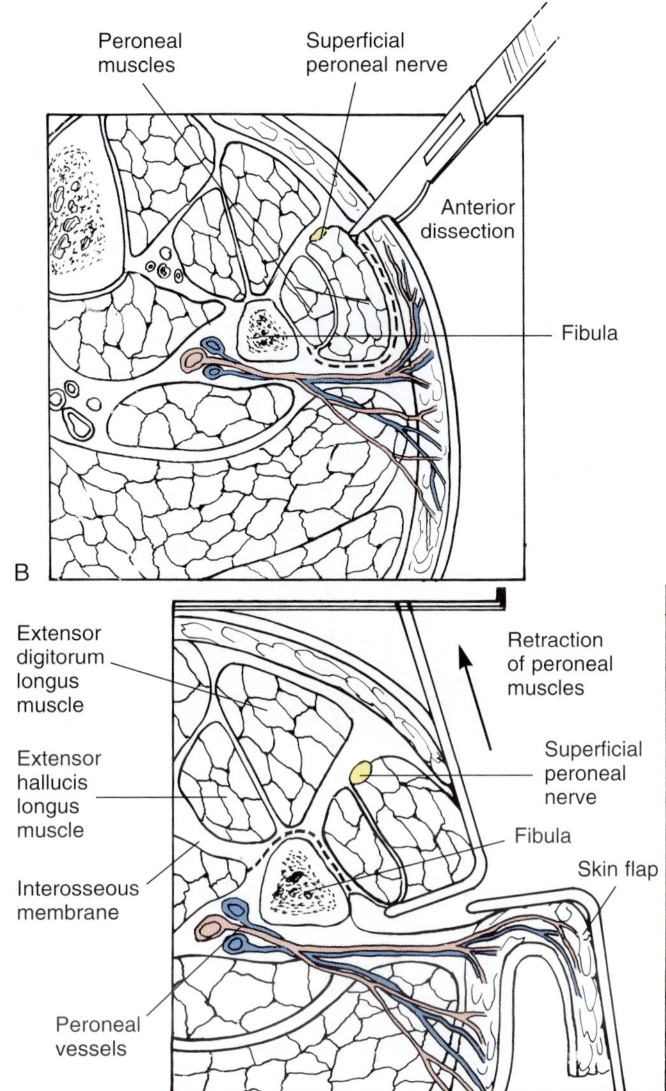

FIG. 8B,C. B: The anterior incision is made over the peroneal musculature, with care taken to avoid injury to the superficial branch of the peroneal nerve. **C:** The incision is made down through the deep muscle fascia and the flap is then elevated toward the posterolateral intermuscular septum, which is preserved because the skin perforators travel in this fascia.

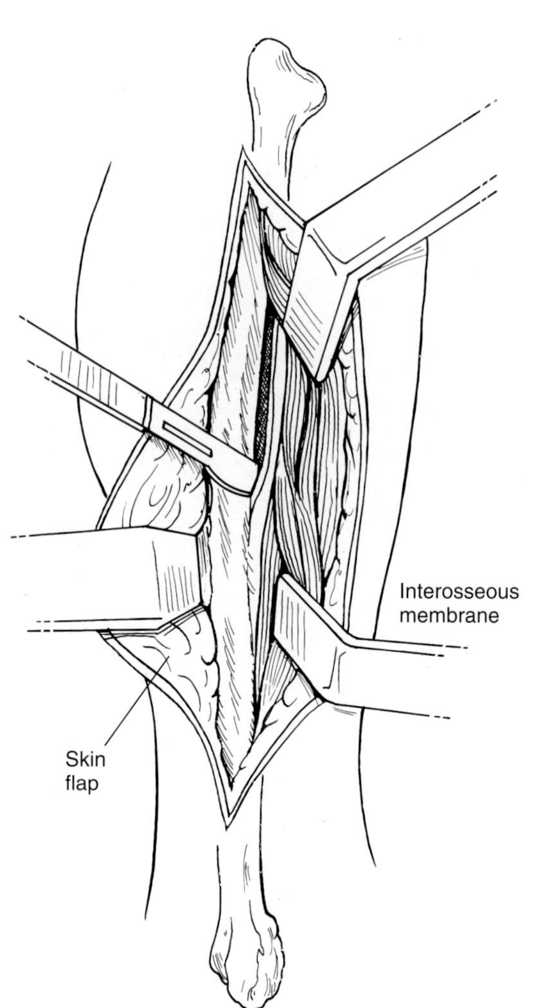

FIG. 8D. The muscles are elevated from the septum up over the top of the fibula, dividing the anterolateral intermuscular septum and the interosseous membrane.

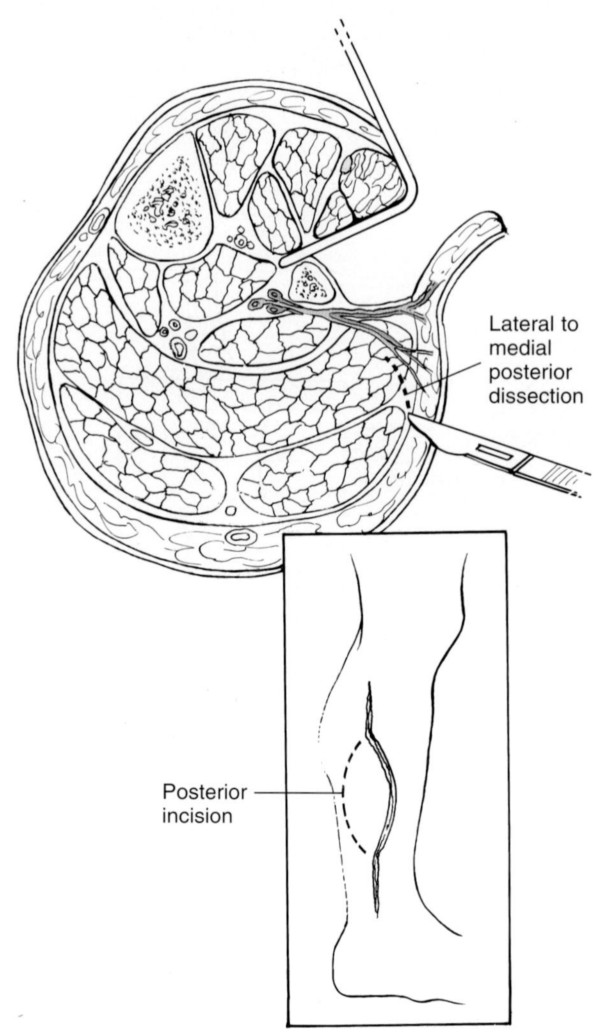

FIG. 8E. After the interosseous membrane has been divided, the posterior skin incision is made again including the deep muscle fascia, but the elevation is stopped 1 cm from the edge of the soleus. At that point the soleus muscle is incised for a depth of about 1 cm, then the bone cuts are made.

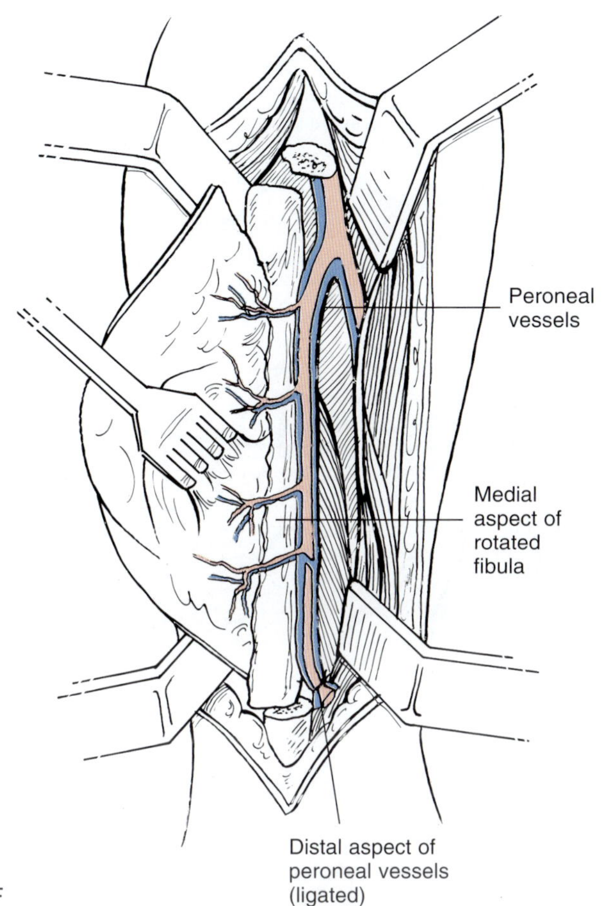

FIG. 8F. The osteotomies are done allowing for traction on the flap, which exposes the deep musculature and helps with the medial dissection. The peroneal vessels are ligated distally, and the musculature is then divided from distal to proximal, taking care to avoid injury to the flap vessels.

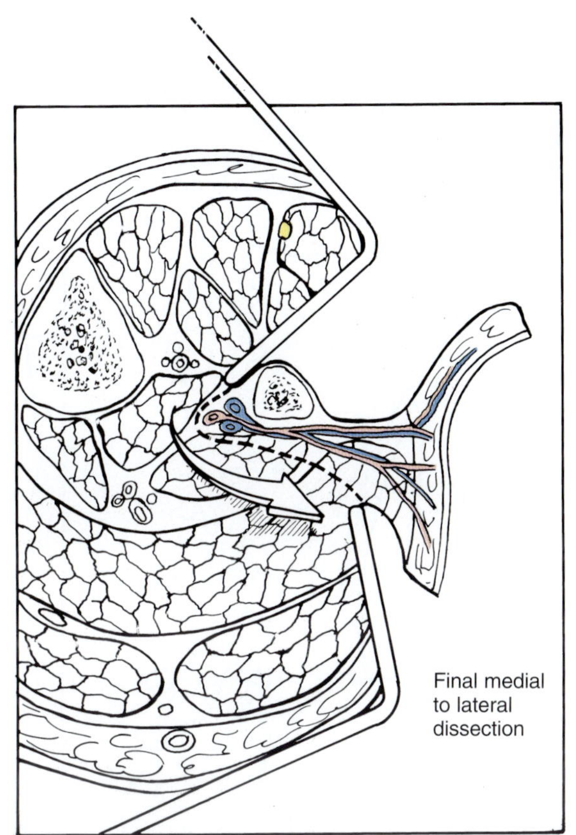

FIG. 8G. The remainder of the posterior dissection can then be done from medial to lateral, which helps prevent injury to the skin perforators.

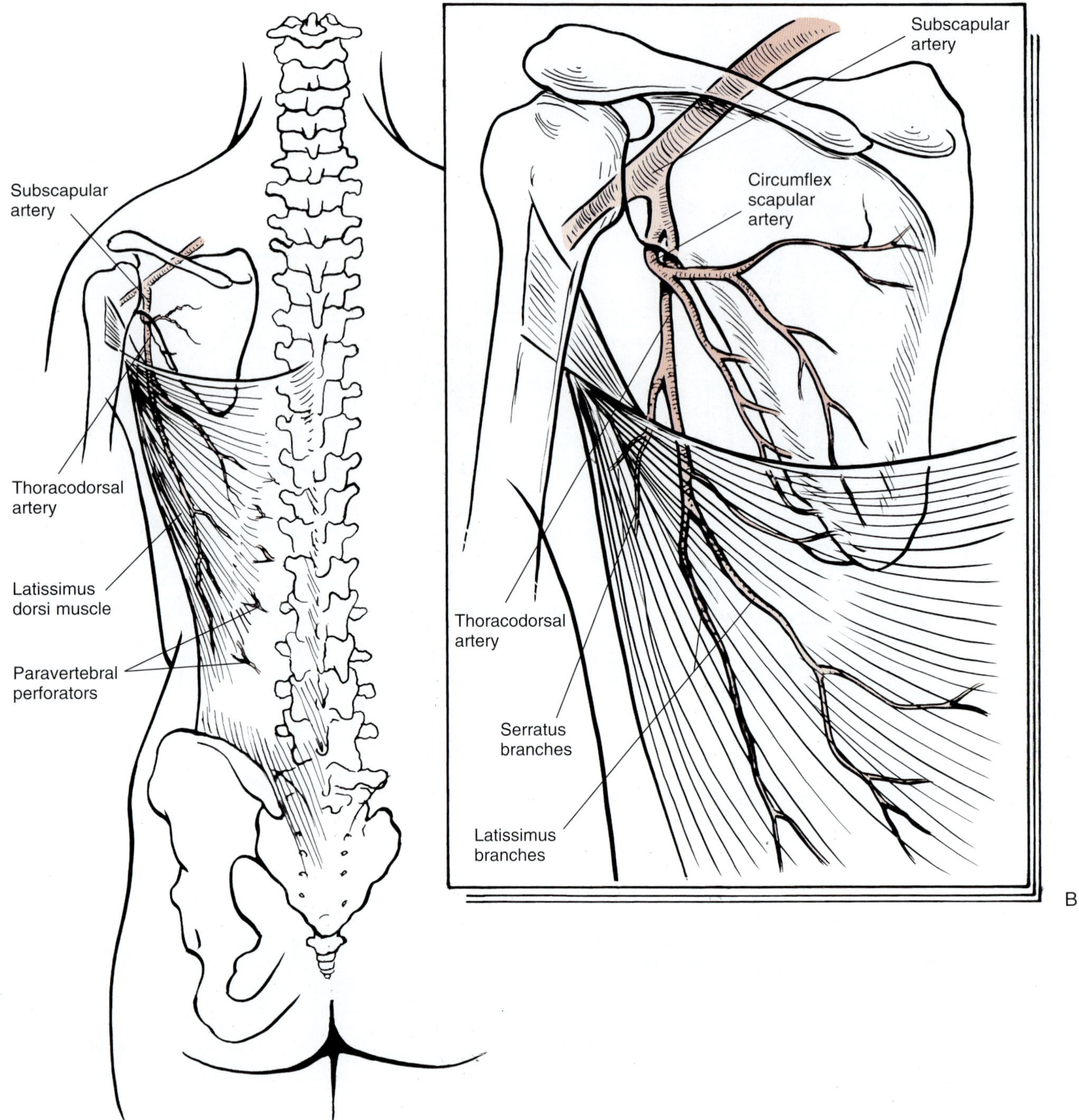

FIG. 9A–C The latissimus dorsi muscle flap is based on the thoracodorsal vessels. It can be transferred as a myocutaneous flap, or a muscle flap that requires skin graft coverage.

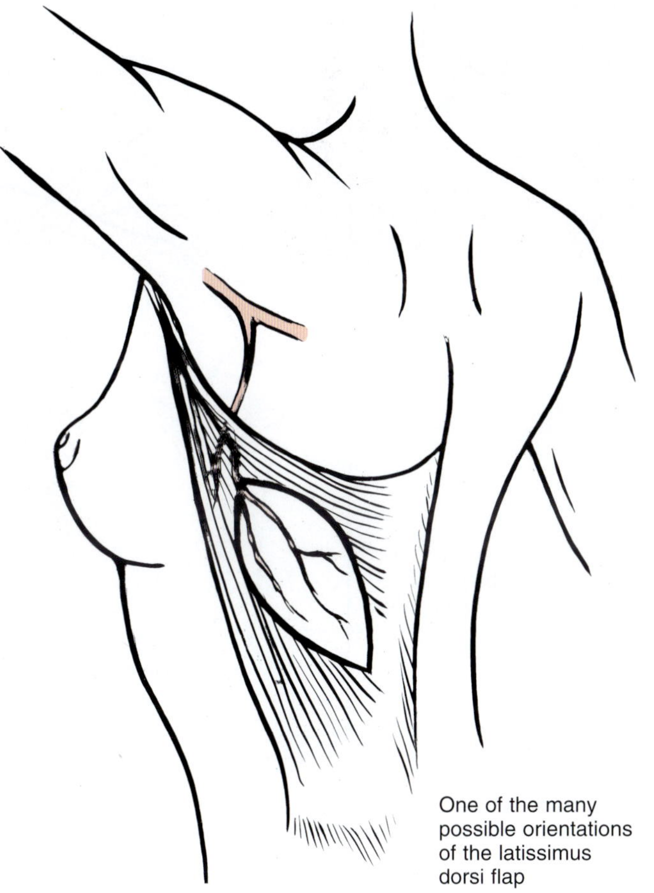

FIG. 9 *(Continued).*

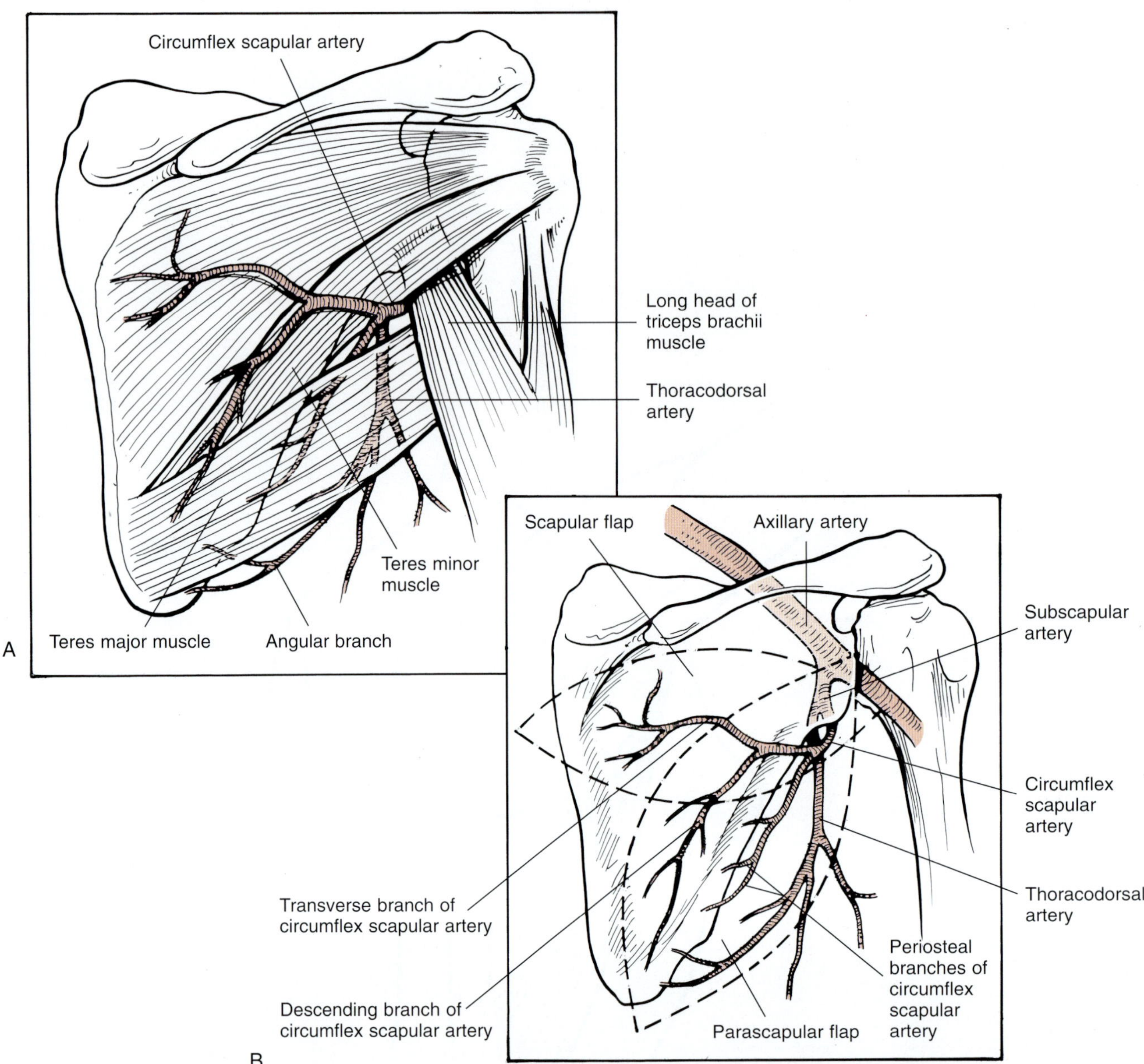

FIG. 10A,B. A: The circumflex scapular artery comes through the triangular space and gives off two skin branches and one bone branch. **B:** The anatomic arrangement allows for design of one bone paddle and two skin paddles.

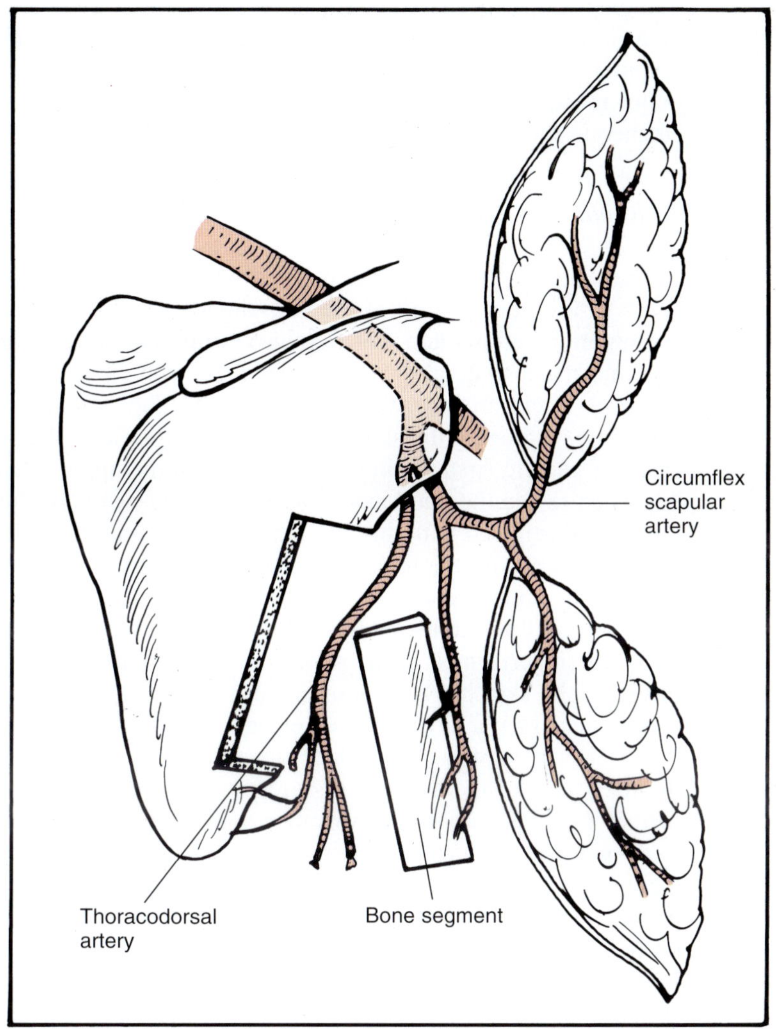

FIG. 10C. Each one of these vascularized units has its own pedicle, thus allowing for greater independent inset of each individual unit.

Pertinent Anatomy

The cutaneous territory of the flap extends from the triangular space laterally to the midline of the back. A flap of approximately 20 cm in length and 10 cm in width can be harvested. The vascular anatomy of the scapular flap is dependent on circumflex scapular artery. It arises from the subscapular artery and passes posteriorly through the triangular space, bordered by the teres minor above and the teres major below, and the long head of the triceps. The artery arborizes in several major branches: the infrascapular artery supplying the subscapular muscle, the branches for the teres major and minor muscles, the descending branch that gives off the cutaneous scapular, and the cutaneous parascapular branches.

Technique of Dissection

The scapular landmarks are marked with the patient in the sitting position. Medial and lateral border and tip of the scapula are noted. The triangular space is identified by palpation and marked. For flap harvesting, the patient is placed in the lateral position and the ipsilateral arm is prepped into the field. The torso is stabilized with a beanbag. There are two ways to elevate the flap, starting from the vascular pedicle (prograde) or raising the skin paddle first (retrograde). We prefer the dissection of the vascular pedicle first. An incision is made on the upper lateral skin marking, and it is deepened to the thoracodorsal fascia, which is just superficial to the deep muscular fascia, and is raised with the flap. The posterior margin of the deltoid is identified and retracted, exposing the teres minor. The dissection proceeds along the surface of the teres minor, and the cutaneous branches of the circumflex scapular artery are exposed. At this point the skin incision is prolonged superomedially and inferiorly and the flap elevation is performed in the space between the thoracodorsal fascia and the muscle fascia. If the skin marking is oriented horizontally, the parascapular artery is ligated and divided, or if a larger skin extension is needed, this branch is conserved to supply the inferior part of the flap. Once the entire flap has been freed from the chest wall, the long head of the triceps, the teres major, and the minor are retracted to facilitate further the exposure of the vascular pedicle. The vascular branches directed to the teres major and minor and the infrascapular branch are ligated and divided, allowing 6 cm of pedicle. At this point the recipient vessel is inspected, the circumflex scapular pedicle is ligated and divided, and the flap is transferred to the surgical defect and partially inset. A microvascular anastomosis of the vein is performed first, using standard microsurgical techniques. The occluding clamps are released after the vein anastomosis and the presence of a back flow is noted. The anastomosis of the artery is performed next. The blood flow in the vessels is then assessed using an ultrasonic Doppler. Often a pulsation is felt on palpating the artery. The inset of the flap is then completed and one or two drains are left in place. The donor site is closed primarily with interrupted absorbable sutures and with staples.

Flap Inset

The flap is oriented to fill the defect and allow perfect approximation of the vascular pedicle and the recipient vessels. If bone is included in the flap, it is fit into the defect first. The surfaces are shaped with a powered saw or bur, and the bone is fixed using microplates and/or screws. Next, the soft tissue of the flap is partially inset using absorbable sutures. The flap is revascularized, and then attention is turned to completing the inset. Again, it is usually advisable to place closed suction drainage catheters beneath the flap. Care is taken to avoid excessive tension on the skin margins of the flap as it is secured over the elbow or shoulder. The blood flow of the flap is then again assessed using capillary refill and perhaps a percutaneous ultrasonic Doppler. A reliable point for obtaining a Doppler signal on the skin of the flap may be marked using

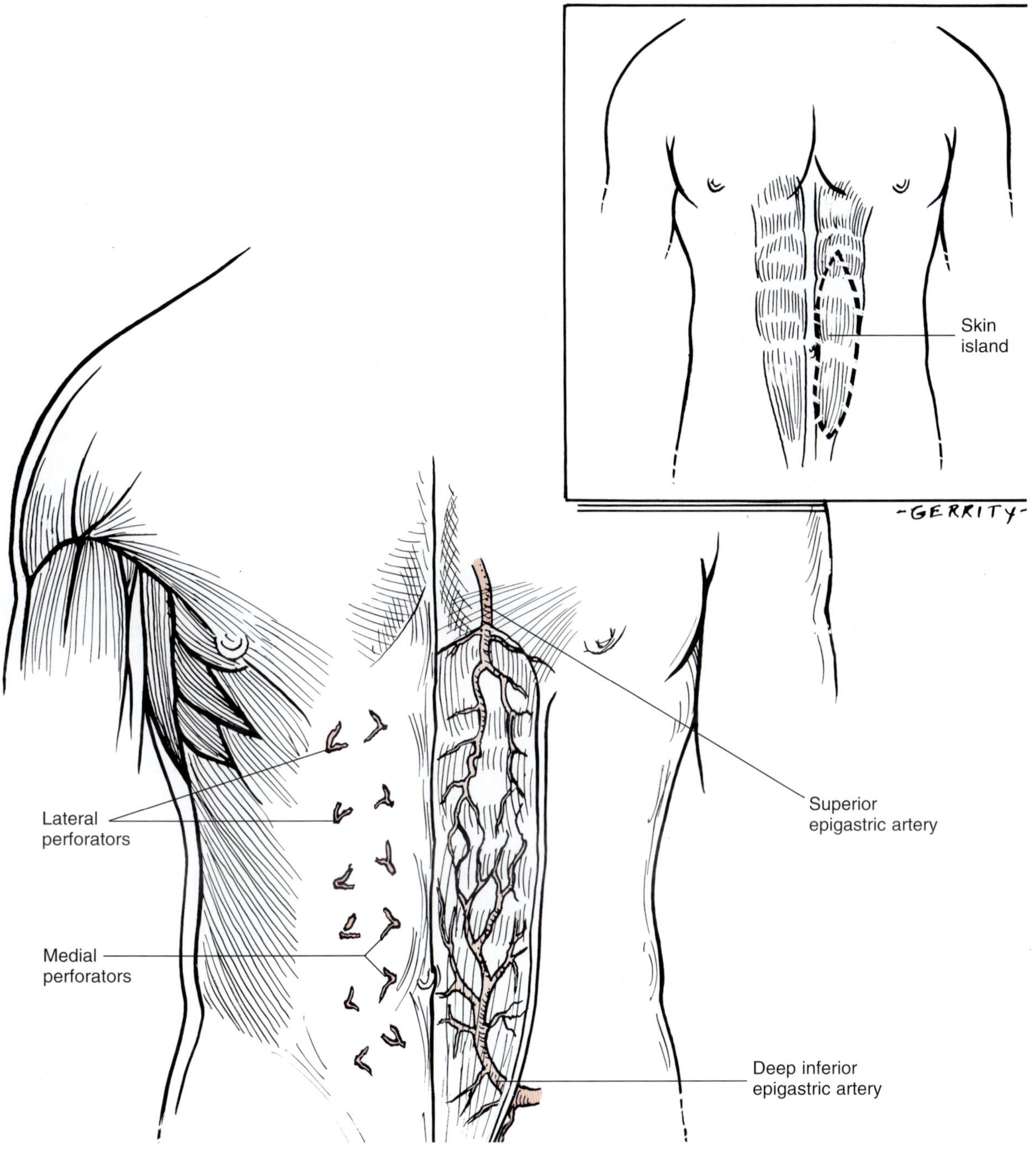

FIG. 11. The anatomy of the rectus abdominis muscle flap.

a absorbable suture. A dressing is usually not applied, so that flap monitoring may be facilitated, but the extremity should be immobilized with a plaster splint.

Rectus Abdominis Free Tissue Transfer

The rectus abdominis free tissue transfer is one of the most versatile flaps in the armamentarium of the microvascular surgeon. It can be raised with a large skin paddle that can be outlined in a transverse, vertical, or oblique direction. The origins of the rectus abdominis muscle are the pubic symphysis and iliac crest, and it inserts into the fifth through seventh costal cartilages, interdigitating with the pectoralis muscle (Fig. 11). It is enclosed by a rectus sheath, except below the arcuate line where a posterior fascial cover is not present. The number of tendinous insertions vary, but usually three are present. The average muscle is 30 cm long, 6 cm wide, and 0.5 cm thick, but varies depending on the physical status of the patient. Arterial supply is from two sources: the superior and deep inferior epigastric arteries. The superior epigastric artery pierces the rectus abdominis muscle on the posterior surface near the muscle's origin, and is accompanied by two venae comitantes. The inferior epigastric artery arises from the external iliac artery immediately above the inguinal ligament. It ascends obliquely and penetrates the transversalis fascia from the arcuate line. The inferior epigastric vessel usually divides into a lateral and medial branch; consequently, the rectus abdominis free flap can be raised on either of these branches, leaving the remaining muscle in situ. The average arterial diameter is 2.7 mm, with a pedicle length of up to 15 cm. The artery has two vena comitantes that occasionally join prior to their origin off the external iliac vein. The cutaneous paddle above the rectus abdominis muscle is classically supplied by a lateral and medial row of perforators. These perforators tend to be concentrated around the umbilicus and, despite their constancy in anatomical dissections, variations can occur that alter the reliability of the cutaneous paddle. The innervation of the rectus abdominis muscle is supplied by the ventral rami of the lower six or seven segmental thoracic spinal nerves. Consequently, the ability to transfer the rectus abdominis muscle for functional recovery is limited due to this segmental innervation.

The flap is elevated with or without a skin paddle. If a skin paddle is taken, the skin can be elevated on both the lateral or medial perforators, which are identified as they course through the anterior fascia. The anterior muscular fascia is identified, incised, and elevated off the medial and lateral muscle, with care taken not to injure the perforating vessels (Fig. 12A–C). The intercostal vessels are divided along with the flap innervation. The flap is divided superiorly and elevated in a superior to inferior direction. The fascia is split down towards the inguinal ligament and the inferior epigastric vessels are identified within some properitoneal fat. The vessels are dissected and the inferior portion of the muscle is divided from the pubic tubercle. If skin is the primary reconstructive tissue, only a small portion of muscle needs to be included on the inferior epigastric pedicle and perforator.

Frequently, inclusion of the skin creates a flap that is too bulky, and skin grafting the muscle usually conforms well to the defect. During abdominal fascial closure using nonabsorbable sutures, the internal oblique layer must be included within the closure, or an abdominal bulge may develop postoperatively. Plication of the anterior rectus fascia on the opposite side of the muscle harvest may be required if umbilical asymmetry is noted, or if a transverse skin paddle is used and the umbilicus is included within the closure, the umbilicus can be re-created in the abdominal tissue using absorbable dermal and skin sutures. The use of onlay Marlex mesh may also be necessary in some patients with abdominal wall weakness. Closed suction drainage is indicated after harvest of the rectus abdominis muscle until the drainage output is less than 30 cc in a 24-hour period.

The muscle tolerates irradiation well and enhances wound healing in areas preoperatively treated with adjuvant therapy. The rectus abdominis muscle is a true workhorse

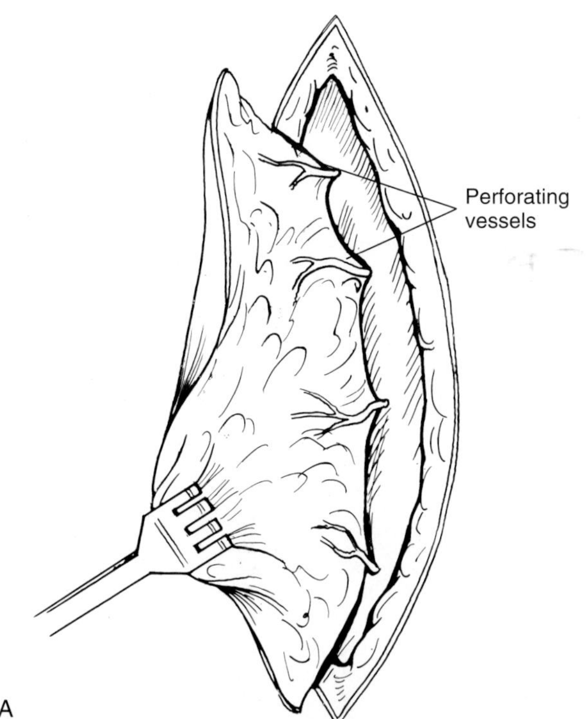

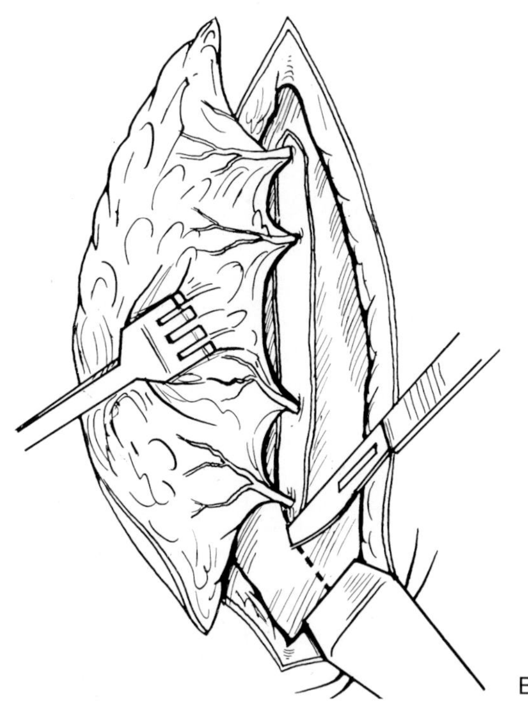

FIG. 12A. Elevation of the rectus abdominis flap using the vertical rectus abdominis muscle (VRAM) skin paddle design. The perforators are exposed laterally and medially.

FIG. 12B. The fascia is incised circumferentially.

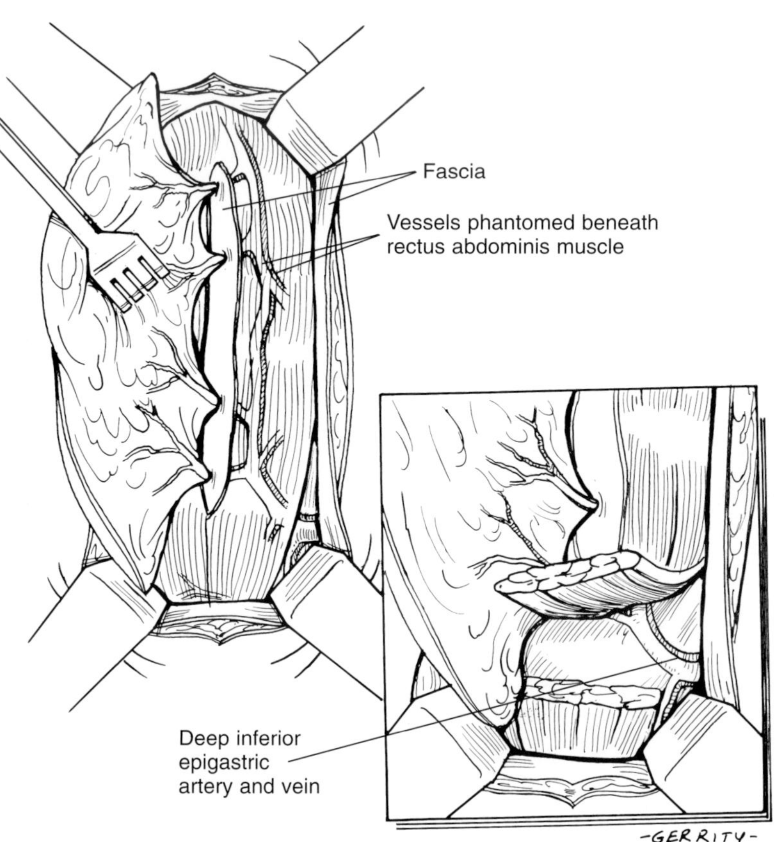

C

FIG. 12C. The deep inferior epigastric vessels are identified in the lower lateral aspect of the muscle. **Inset:** Once the lower aspect of the muscle is divided, the vessels are traced to their origin.

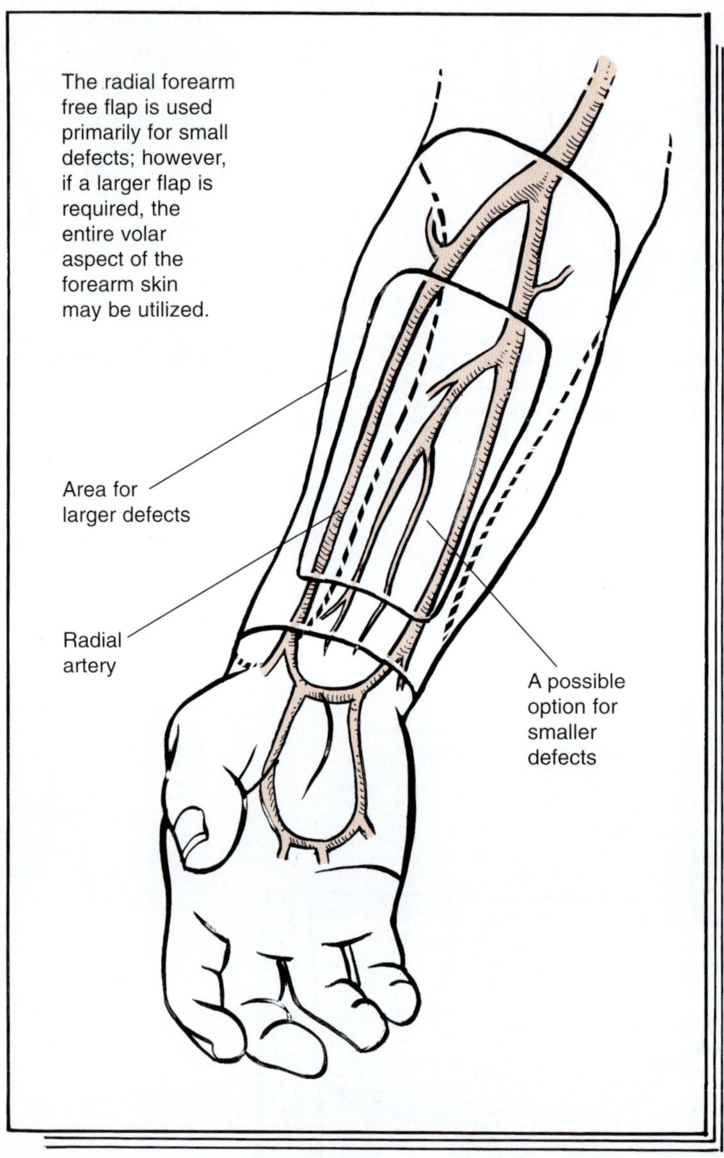

FIG. 13A. Anatomy of the radial forearm flap. Flap design is located over radial vessels.

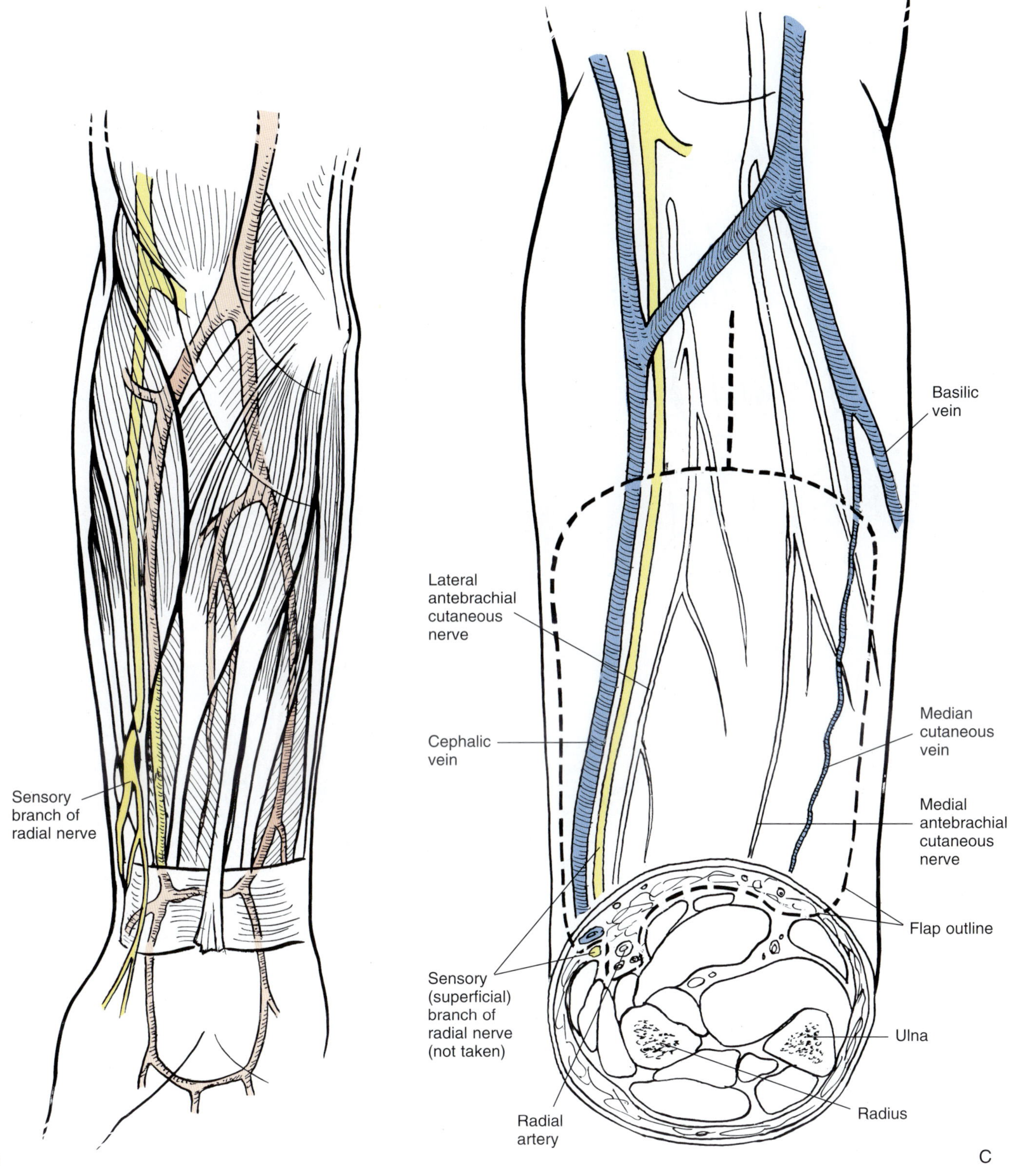

FIG. 13B. Vascular anatomy of the radial forearm flap. Note location of superficial radial nerve.

FIG. 13C. Cross-sectional anatomy of proposed flap elevation.

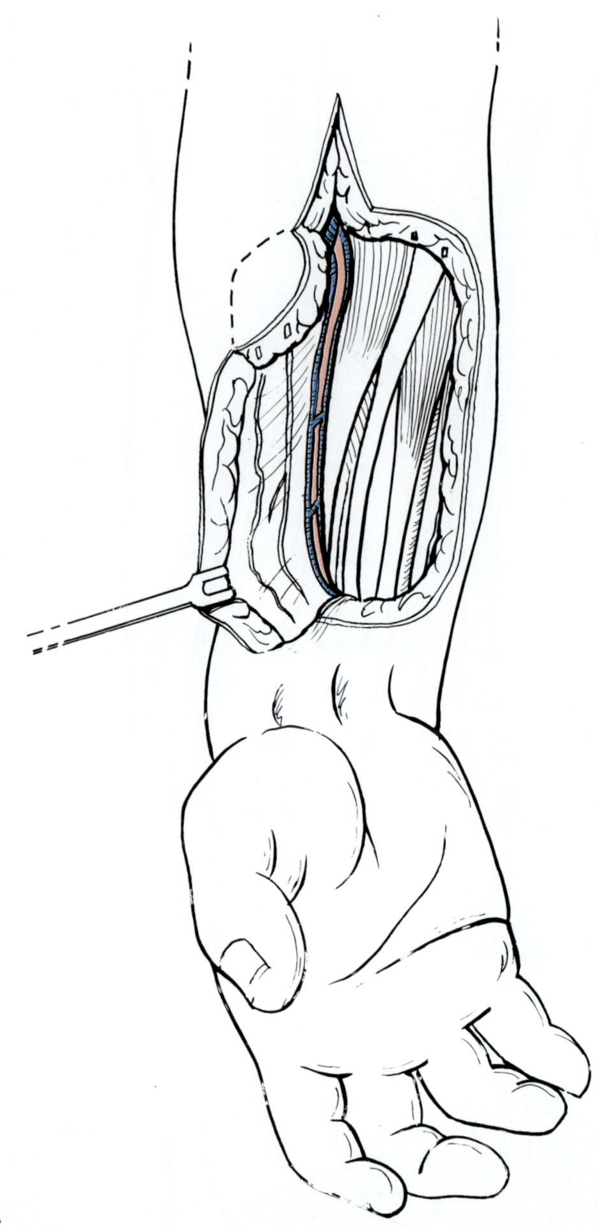

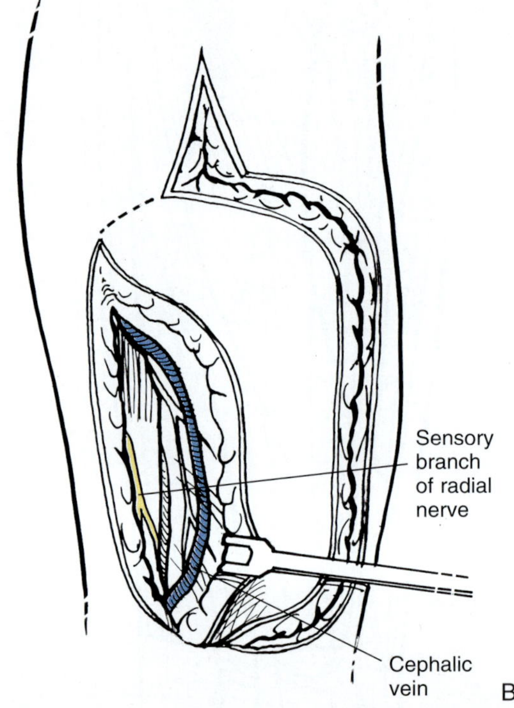

A

FIG. 14A. Radial forearm flap elevation. Medial incision and flap elevation with exposure of radial vessels.

B

FIG. 14B. Lateral incision with exposure of cephalic vein and identification and preservation of radial nerve.

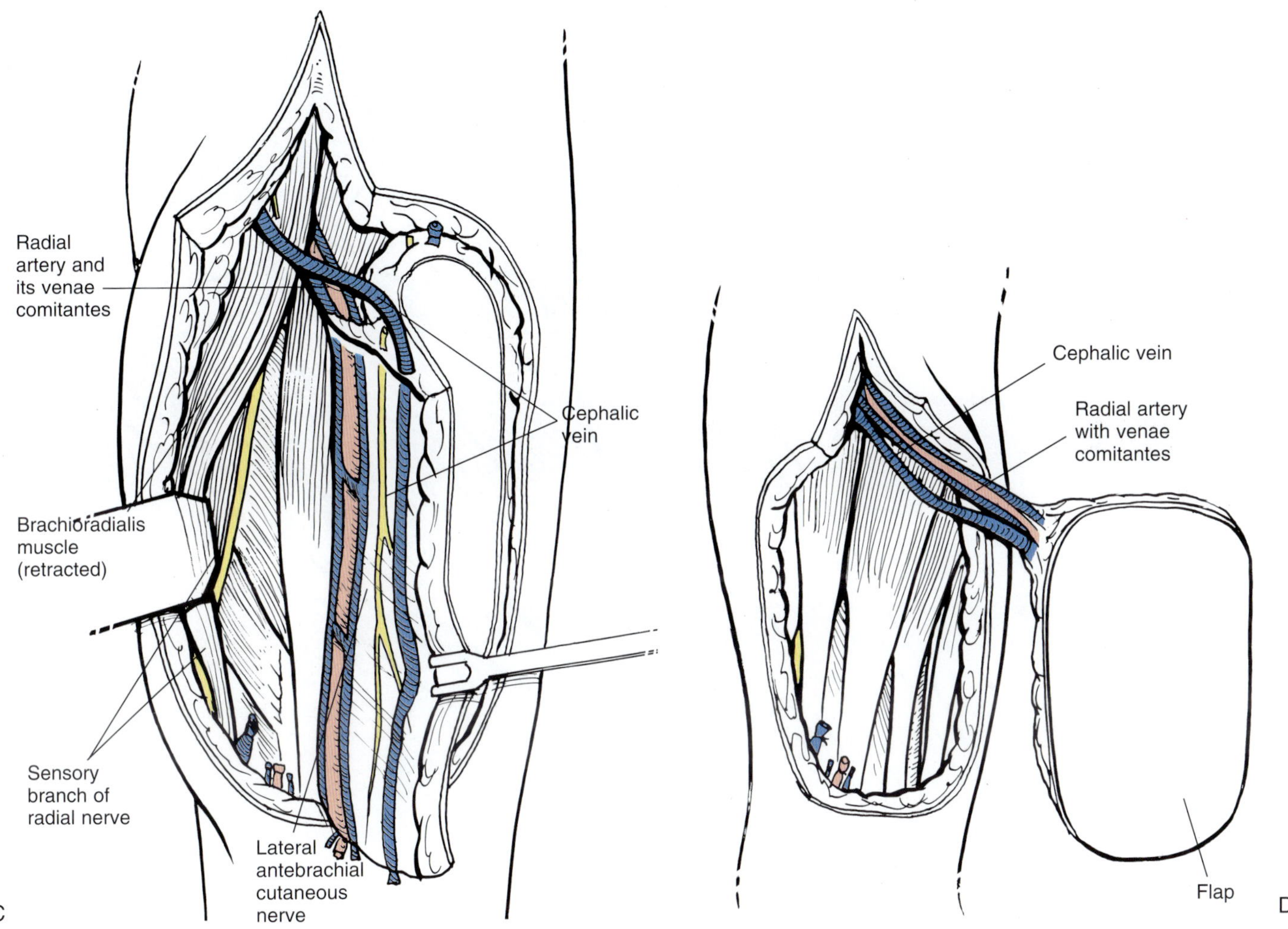

FIG. 14C. Ligation of vessels distally, with elevation of remainder of flap.

FIG. 14D. Donor vessels are then traced to their origin.

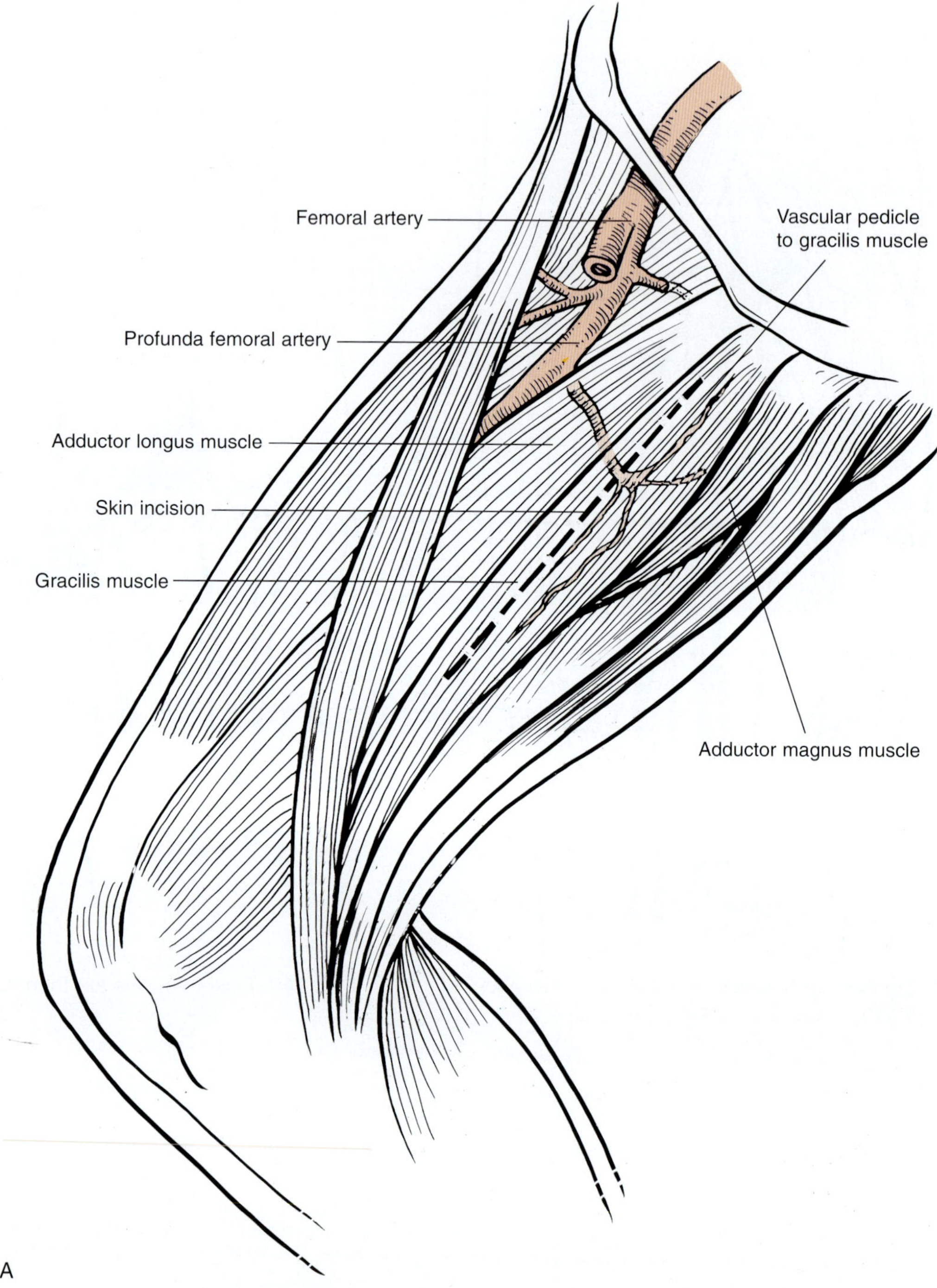

FIG. 15A,B. Anatomy of the gracilis muscle transfer.

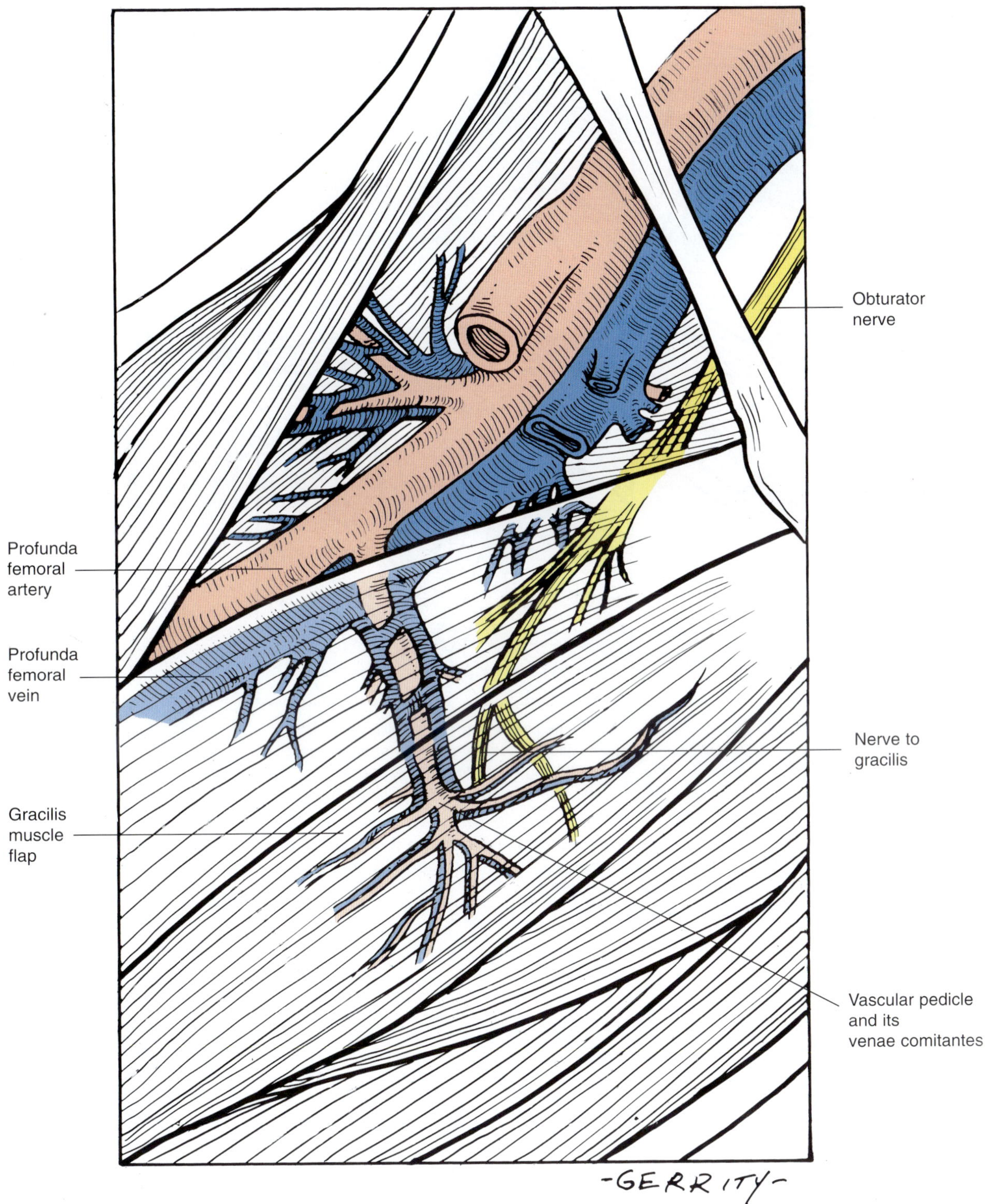

FIG. 15. *Continued.*

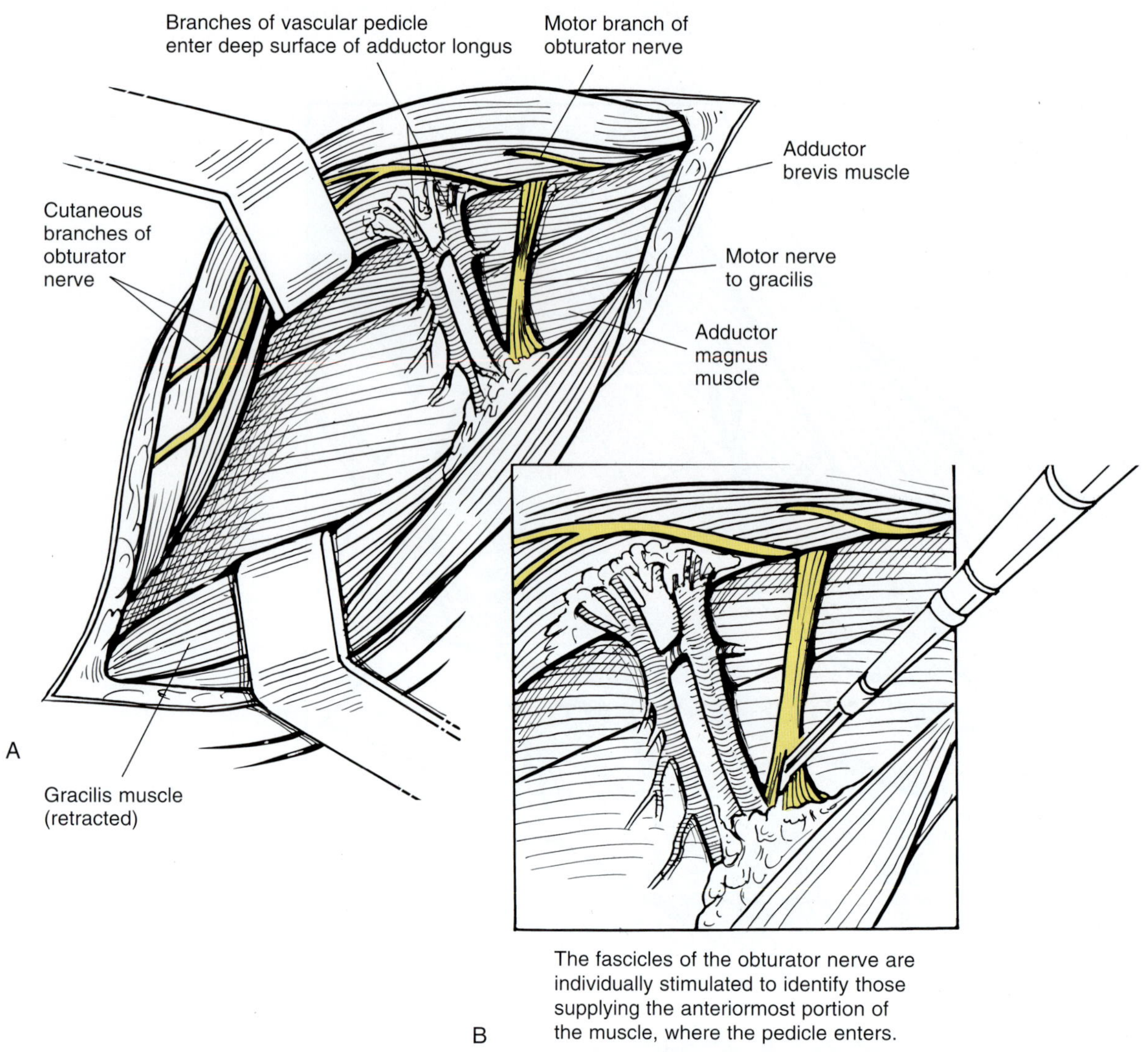

FIG. 16A,B. A: Relationship of the adductor longus and magnus muscles to the gracilis muscle neurovascular pedicle. **B:** The branches of the obturator nerve are individually stimulated to identify those innervating the anterior most portion of the muscle where the neurovascular pedicle enters.

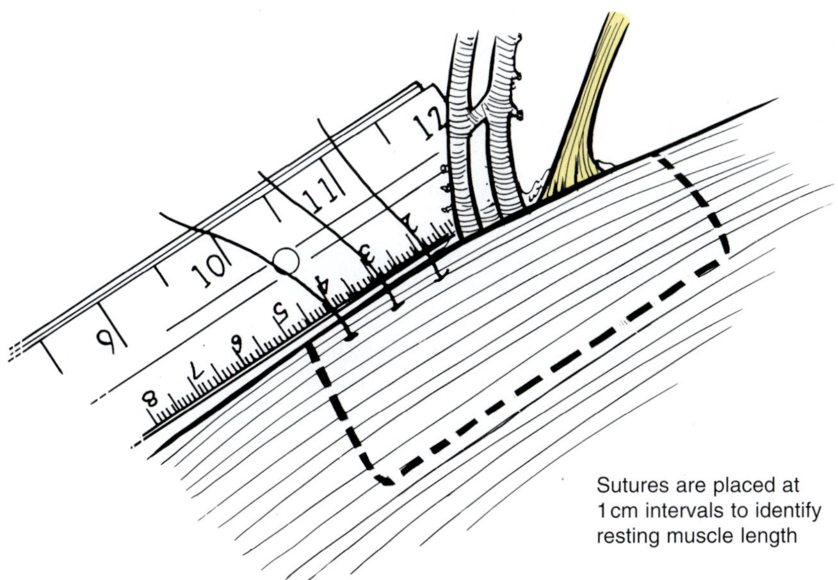

FIG. 16C. Sutures placed at 1-cm intervals to identify the resting muscle length.

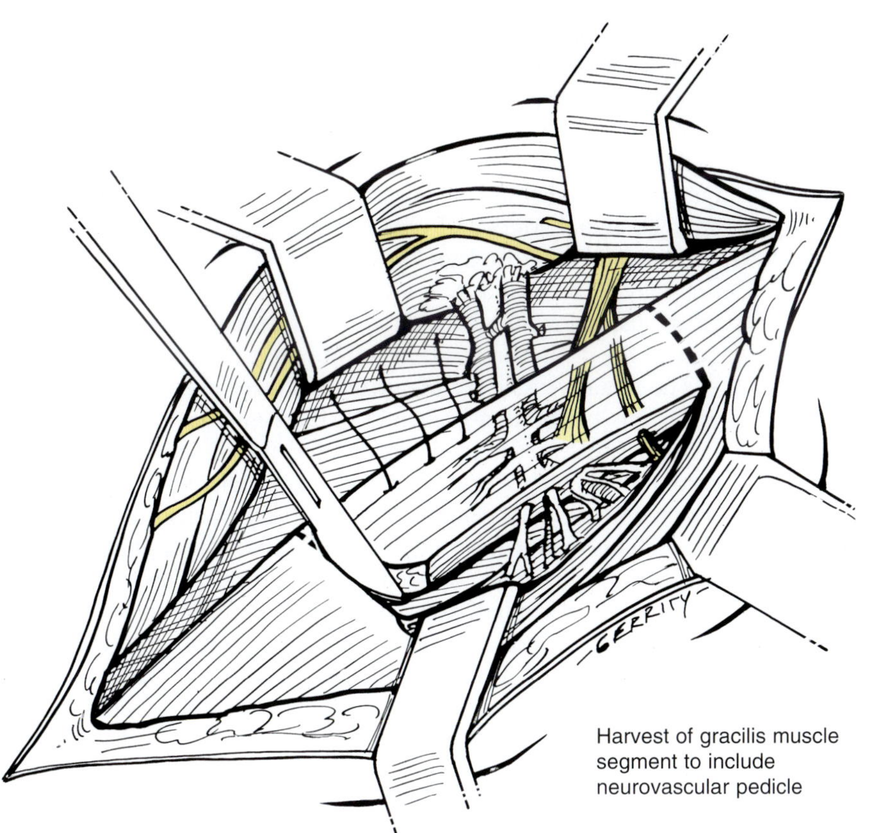

FIG. 16D. Harvest of the gracilis muscle segment to include the neurovascular pedicle.

for extremity reconstruction. Its versatility, ease of dissection, tolerance, and well-vascularized fibers are enticing and consistent for the reconstructive microsurgeon.

Radial Forearm Free Flap

Technical Considerations

The radial forearm flap is supported by a fascial plexus that is supplied by multiple small perforators that stretch along its length and reach it from the radial artery passing along the fascial septum. The radial artery has 9 to 17 branches in the forearm with an average diameter of 0.5 mm that form a rich vascular plexus. The venous drainage of the radial forearm flap is based on both deep and superficial systems (Fig. 13A–C). The superficial system is composed of the cephalic and basilic veins. The cephalic vein arises from the radial border of the forearm and receives tributaries from the entire forearm. Medially it communicates with the basilic vein and below the elbow it communicates with the deep system through the median cubital vein. The deep system is usually composed of two venae comitantes accompanying the radial artery. Frequently, these veins are small (average diameter 1.3 mm), necessitating the elevation of one of the superficial veins with the flap.

Preoperative Allen's test is necessary to ensure the patency of collateral circulation, as absence of flow through the collateral system precludes the use of the flap or, at least, requires arterial reconstruction. The territory of the flap may be extended from the lower third of the anterior aspect of the proximal forearm to the proximal wrist flexion crease distally. The width of the flap can be taken from the lateral to medial humeral epicondyle. Proximal placement of the flap on the forearm allows for increased thickness of the flap and decreased pedicle length. Dissection is performed under tourniquet control, which is inflated to 250 mm Hg for a maximum of 2 hours. Our preferred method of elevation begins at the distal border (Fig. 14A–D). The flexor tendons, radial artery and vena comitantes, cephalic vein, brachioradialis, and median nerve are all identified, and initial ulnar elevation is performed, although radial elevation may be preferred by some. The antebrachial fascia is incised, and dissection proceeds just below the fascia along the flexor tendons. Preservation of the peritenon is critical for the adherence of a full- or split-thickness skin graft.

The radial vessels are identified and care must be taken not to damage the fasciocutaneous perforating branches as they emerge from the intermuscular septum. The radial vessels are divided distally and the dissection continues toward the extensor carpi radialis longus muscle. Care must be taken not to injure the radial sensory nerve, which emerges between the tendons of the extensor carpi radialis longus and the brachioradialis tendon near the juncture of the distal and middle third of the forearm. The superficial vein is also divided distally, and the flap is elevated in a distal to proximal direction on its radial artery pedicle with venae comitantes and the superficial vein intact. The incision along the forearm may extend to the antecubital fossa if a long pedicle is desired. The increased vessel diameter around the antecubital fossa (2 to 4 mm) facilitates microvascular anastomoses.

After dissection, the tourniquet is released and the hand evaluated for collateral circulation. The radial forearm free flap is transferred to the defect site by standard microvascular techniques. An end-to-end or end-to-side anastomosis is used. Full- or split-thickness skin grafting can be used for the donor site on those areas that cannot be closed primarily. A volar splint is maintained for 5 days with the hand in position of function, and active and passive motion may then begin, if the graft appears to be viable.

The radial forearm free flap is ideal for three-dimensional defects; the thin and pliable skin is used for coverage of vital structures over the dorsum of the hand. The flap is inset with 3-0 Vicryl suture along the dermis and 4-0 or 5-0 nylon sutures for skin approximation. The skin may also be taken off the flap and the fascia alone used for coverage. Split- or full-thickness grafts can be placed on the fascia if bulk is not required. An anterolateral segment of the radial bone that lies between the insertions of the pronator teres and the brachioradialis muscle can be included in the radial forearm free flap (up to 10 cm). This flap allows nourishment of the radius by two fascioperiosteal branches through the intermuscular septum and musculoperiosteal branches through the flexor pollicis longus, and pronator quadratus from the radial artery. The flap is raised in a similar fashion while leaving the intermuscular septum intact. Medially, the muscle bellies of the flexor pollicis longus and pronator quadratus are divided and elevated to reach the periosteum. The periosteum is incised longitudinally beyond the attachment of the septum to the radius. Bony cuts are made in a beveled fashion and bony excision must not exceed one-third of the diameter of the radius to preserve radial bone stability. The osteocutaneous flap is elevated with attention paid to preserving the intermuscular septum with the flap and intact radius. Inclusion of the bone may allow for simultaneous repair of bone and skin coverage especially in the digits and hand. While not always possible in the extirpative extremity, the flap can be elevated on a proximal pedicle to cover large defects or exposed structures around the elbow. The lateral and medial antebrachial cutaneous nerves provide sensation to the forearm and provides the radial forearm flap with the potential for sensation as well. Primary neurorrhaphy is performed with 10-0 nylon suture under microsurgical technique to the sensory nerves in the upper extremity.

The versatility of the radial forearm flap has encouraged its use as potential coverage for upper extremity defects. Although the degree of resection frequently precludes the use of the radial forearm flap and necessitates the use of larger muscle for coverage, it remains a strong candidate for options in reconstruction.

Gracilis

Technical Considerations

Although the gracilis muscle does not provide bulk like the rectus abdominis muscle, the gracilis free tissue transfer does have the ability to provide function. The muscle originates from the pubis and the ischium, and inserts into the medial upper surface of the tibia, below the condyle. The muscle is thin and strap shaped, measuring approximately 42 cm in length. The gracilis tendon adds an additional 10 cm (Fig. 15A,B). The muscle is not wide, with an average width of 4 cm. There are two blood supplies to the gracilis muscle; the dominant vessel arises off the profunda femoris vessels, passing inferomedially between the adductor longus and the brevis and entering the upper third of the muscle consistently at 9 cm below the pubic tubercle. Several additional minor branches from the femoral vessels supply the distal muscle belly; however, only the dominant proximal vascular supply reliably nourishes the entire muscle. The anterior branch of the obturator nerve runs between the adductor longus and the brevis and splits into the motor and sensory nerves near the dominant vascular pedicle. The motor nerve enters the muscle with the dominant vascular pedicle and divides into two branches. The sensory branch crosses the gracilis muscle to innervate the overlying skin.

A cutaneous paddle can also be raised with the gracilis muscle; however, the distal third of the skin paddle does not receive sufficient blood supply from the muscle to be consistently reliable. The muscle is harvested with the patient in the frog-leg position; however, the patient should be premarked in the standing position. This is critical, as difficulty delineating the boundaries of the gracilis can occur when the patient is supine. The anterior border of the gracilis corresponds to a line between the posterior border of the tendon of the adductor longus at the pubic tubercle. The muscle lies approximately 3 cm below the adductor longus. The distal end lies between the sartorius anteriorly and the semimembranosus posteriorly. The greater saphenous vein traverses the medial thigh and can be a source of vein grafts for this muscle. The muscle is identified and the adductor longus is retracted superiorly. The dominant vascular pedicle is identified and lies between 10 and 12 cm below the inferior border of the pubic tubercle. The anterior branch of the obturator nerve is identified on the adductor brevis. Approximately 10 cm can be dissected. The muscle is elevated and small perforating branches from the pedicle to the adductor muscle are ligated. The muscle is dissected from its origin and insertion until it is isolated on its neurovascular pedicle.

The gracilis is ideal for smaller defects around the elbow and forearm. Since it does not have the bulk the rectus abdominis does, it can fill small defects and provide a good aesthetic result. The versatility of the gracilis muscle lies in its functional transfer. The sine qua non of functional muscle transfer is the availability of an undamaged motor nerve. It should be remembered that patients who undergo free muscle transfer for functional reestablishment will require up to 2 years to develop maximal power in the transplanted muscle. Oncologic criteria must meet these reconstructive requirements. A pure motor nerve must be chosen for the recipient site. This includes the musculocutaneous and axillary nerve in the upper arm and the anterior and posterior interosseous nerve or equivalent branch in the forearm. Good active and passive movement of joints is required. Motor nerve repair should be near the muscle to decrease the time of innervation. The donor muscle tension is premarked with sutures placed at 5- or 10-cm intervals prior to severance of the origin and insertion (Fig. 16A–D). A suitable recipient artery and nerve are identified. Microvascular transfer is performed with 9 to 0 nylon suture with an end-to-side or end-to-end anastomosis. Primary neurorraphy is performed using 10-0 nylon suture between the muscle and the recipient nerve. This same tension is set once the muscle has been transferred to the recipient site, and can be measured by the premarked sutures. The wrist is placed in flexion or extension depending on volar or dorsal placement and the fingers in the position of function. This allows the relief of undue tension. If the skin cannot be closed over the muscle belly, skin grafting is required. Postoperative monitoring is performed, and at approximately 3 weeks active and passive finger and wrist motions are initiated. A program of extensive rehabilitation to improve grip strength is initiated once a good range of motion is established.

In conclusion, the gracilis provides a long, thin, and functional muscle for free tissue transfer. Although most frequently used for traumatic injury to the brachial plexus, the possibility exists for partial functional restoration after tumor extirpation.

ADDITIONAL FLAPS

Although ideal for forearm and hand reconstruction, the following flaps are infrequently utilized at our institution. Consequently, they are only brief reviewed here.

Dorsalis Pedis Flap

Another useful source of thin skin coverage for the upper extremity is the dorsum of the foot. The dorsum of the foot is supplied primarily by the dorsalis pedis artery. The flap should be considered only if it is certain that the posterior tibial artery provides the dominant blood supply to the foot. The donor site on the dorsum of the foot is the primary source of morbidity with this flap. Meticulous care in securing and preparing the bed is necessary. A skin graft with 100% take is the best insurance to avoid delayed wound healing and morbidity in this area.

Temporoparietal Fascial Flap

The temporoparietal fascia provides an excellent, well-vascularized, and thin piece of tissue for coverage of the upper extremity. An area of coverage approximately 8 × 8 cm may be anticipated. This is most useful for areas on the hand, particularly on the dorsum. It is possible to harvest both the deep fascia (fascia of the temporalis muscle) and the temporoparietal fascia as a double fascial flap. This is possible if the vascular connection is preserved just as the superficial artery proceeds over the zygomatic arch. After flap transfer, the fascia may be skin grafted to provide satisfactory thin coverage over the dorsum of the hand.

SUMMARY

Reconstruction of the upper extremity involves a complex set of functional and anatomic structures that require attention during tumor resection. It is our duty as microsurgeons to address each of these potential defects in the restoration of function and improvement in the quality of life.

SELECTED READINGS

Bennett JB, Crouch CC. Compression syndrome of the recurrent branch of the median nerve. *J Hand Surg* 1982; 7:407–409.

Breidenbach WC. Emergency free tissue transfer for reconstruction of acute upper extremity wounds. *Clin Plast Surg* 1989;16(3):505–514.

Buncke HJ. *Microsurgery: transplantation-replantation. An atlas text.* Philadelphia: Lea and Febiger, 1991; 276–294.

Cormack GC, Lamberty BGH. A classification of fasciocutaneous flaps according to their patterns of vascularization. *Br J Plastic Surg* 1984;37:80–87.

Dellon AL. Think nerve in upper extremity reconstruction. *Clin Plast Surg* 1989;16(3):617–662.

Doi K, Sakai K, Ihara K, Abe Y, Kawai S, Kurafuji Y. Reinnervated free muscle transplantation for extremity reconstruction. *Plast Reconstr Surg* 1993;91(5):872–883.

Evans GRD, Brandt K, Ang KK, Cromeens DM, et al. Peripheral nerve regeneration: the effects of postoperative irradiation *Plast Reconstr Surg (in press).*

Heiner J, Rao V, Mott W. Immediate free tissue transfer for distal musculoskeletal neoplasms. *Ann Plast Surg* 1993;30(2):140–146.

Hentz VR, Pearl RM, Grossman JAI, Wood MB, Cooney WP. The radial forearm flap: a versatile tissue source of composite tissue. *Ann Plast Surg* 1987;19(6):485–498.

Jabaley ME, Wallace WH, Heckler FR. Internal topography of major nerves of the forearm and hand. A current view. *J Hand Surg (Br)* 1980;51:1.

Jones NF. Ischemia of the hand in systemic disease: the potential role of microsurgical revascularization and digital sympathectomy. *Clin Plast Surg* 1989;16(3):547– 556.

Kutz JE, Shealy G, Lubbers I. Interfascicular nerve repair of peripheral nerve injuries in the upper extremity. *Orthop Clin North Am* 1981;12:277–286.

Lanz V. Anatomic variations of the median nerve in the carpal tunnel. *J Hand Surg* 1977;2:44– 53.

Lilla JA, Phelps DB, Boswick JA. Microsurgical repair of peripheral nerve injuries in the upper extremity. *Ann Plast Surg* 1979;2:24–31.

MacKinnon SE. New directions in peripheral nerve surgery—a collective review. *Ann Plast Surg* 1989;22:257.

MacKinnon SE. Surgical management of the peripheral nerve gap. *Clin Plast Surg* 1989;16(3):587–603.

MacKinnon SE, Dellon AL. Medians nerve entrapment in the proximal forearm and brachium. In: MacKinnon SE, Dellon AL, eds. *Surgery of the peripheral nerve.* New York: Thieme, 1988.

Manktelow RT. Functioning microsurgical muscle transfer. *Hand Clin* 1988;4:289.

Rose EH. Small flap coverage of hand and digit defects. *Clin Plast Surg* 1989;16(3):427– 442.

Stotter A, McLean NR, Fallowfield ME, Breach NM, Westbury G. Reconstruction after excision of soft tissue sarcomas of the limbs and trunk. *Br J Surg* 1988;75:774–778.

Strauch B, Yu HL. *Atlas of microvascular surgery: anatomy and operative approaches.* New York: Thieme, 1993; 44–82.

Swartz WM. Restoration of sensibility in mutilating hand injuries. *Clin Plast Surg* 1989;16(3):515–529.

Swartz WM, Izquierdo R, Miller MJ. Implantable venous Doppler microvascular monitoring: laboratory investigation and clinical results. *Plast Reconstr Surg* 1994;93:152–163.

Tang CH. Reconstruction of the bones and joints of the upper extremity by vascularized free fibular graft: report of 46 cases. *J Reconstr Microsurg* 1992;8(4):285–292.

Terzis JK, Maragh H. Strategies in the microsurgical management of brachial plexus injuries. *Clin Plast Surg* 1989;16(3):605–616.

Wei FC, Colony LH. Microsurgical reconstruction of opposable digits in mutilating hand injuries. *Clin Plast Surg* 1989;16(3):491–504.

Wei FC, Colony LH. Microsurgical restoration of distal digital function. *Clin Plast Surg* 1989;16(3):443–455.

Woodall B, Beebe WG. *In peripheral nerve regeneration, a follow-up study of 3,656 World War II injuries.* VA Medical Monograph. Washington, DC: US Government Printing Office, 1956.

*Microsurgical Reconstruction of the Cancer
Patient,* edited by M.A. Schusterman.
Lippincott-Raven Publishers, Philadelphia © 1997.

14

Lower Extremity Reconstruction

Geoffrey L. Robb and Gregory P. Reece

Standard therapy for most patients presenting with sarcoma or other tumors of the lower extremity has become wide local excision with or without adjuvant therapy. This approach has markedly reduced the number of amputations performed at most medical centers. In most cases, eligibility for limb salvage surgery is determined by the ability to obtain tumor-free surgical margins, the capacity for reconstruction of the resulting defect, and the feasibility of reasonable limb function after resection. Many of these extremity sarcoma patients present with large but resectable tumors that require extensive soft tissue resection with possible exposure of structures that are vital to limb function. Limb salvage for these patients is possible only if the wound can be covered by nonirradiated, well-vascularized tissue.

Although closure of extensive wounds can sometimes be obtained by using local muscle flaps, the use of local tissues in these patients is frequently limited by previous radiation therapy and/or surgery, the volume of local tissue available for transfer, and the ligation of the blood supply of many of these local flaps during the tumor dissection. Moreover, if the patient requires postoperative radiation therapy, the use of local muscle for wound coverage increases the surgical wound area exposed to tumor cells and thus increases the volume of tissue that must be irradiated. Similarly, should an amputation be necessary at a later time, the use of local tissue for reconstruction potentially raises the level of amputation. Finally, the use of multiple local muscles for wound closure can interfere with the ultimate functional quality of ambulation after surgery. Under these circumstances, a free tissue transfer is the most reliable and expedient method to close the wound and rehabilitate the patient.

G.L. Robb and G.P. Reece: Department of Plastic Surgery, The University of Texas, M.D. Anderson Cancer Center, Houston, Texas 77030.

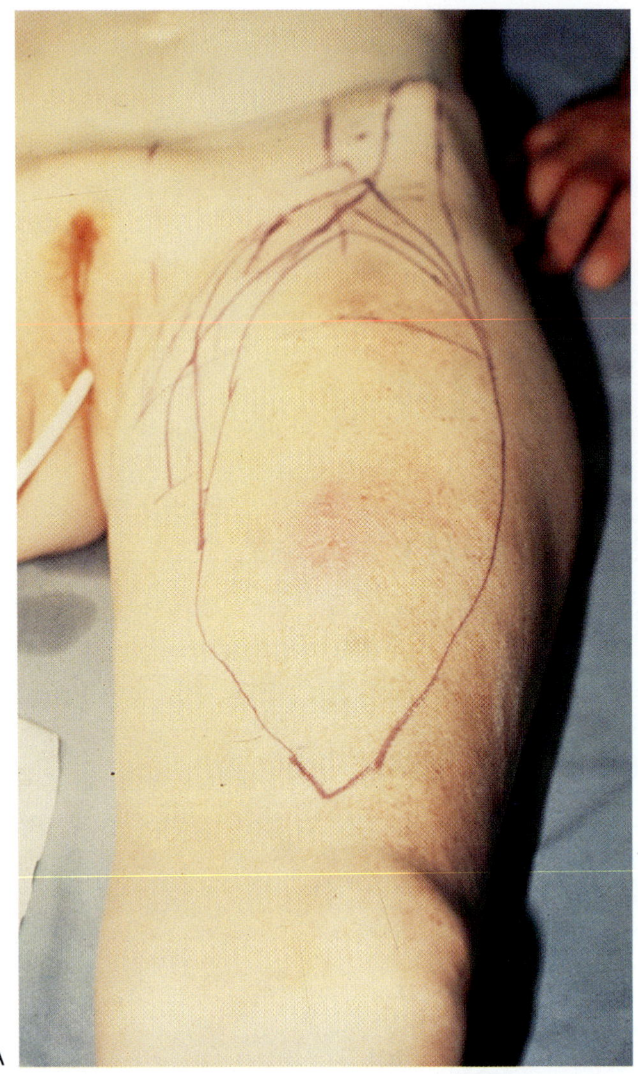

FIG. 1A. Large sarcoma on the left anterior thigh.

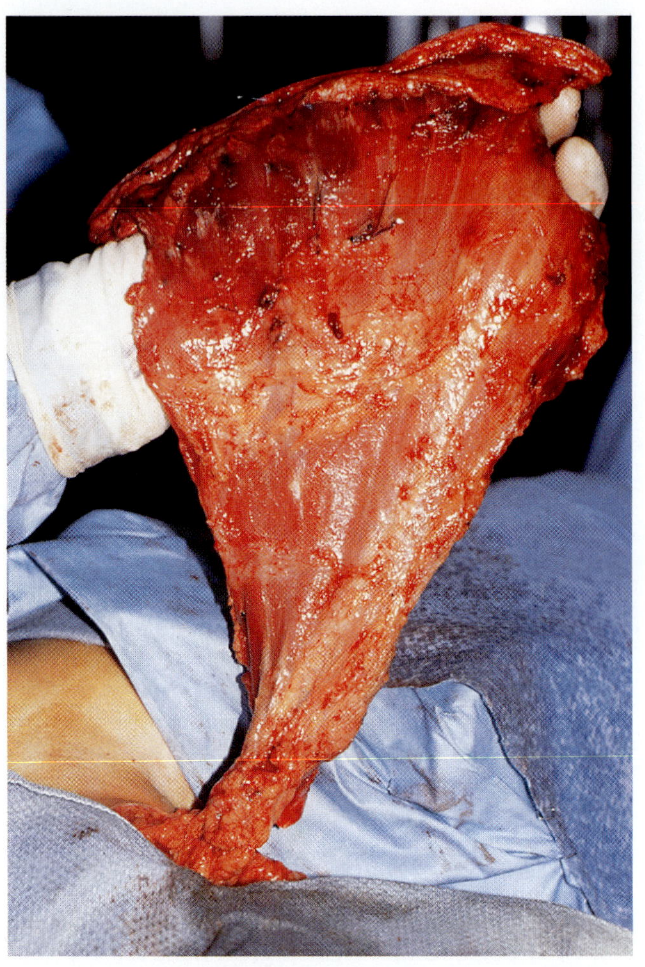

FIG. 1C. Latissimus dorsi myocutaneous donor flap.

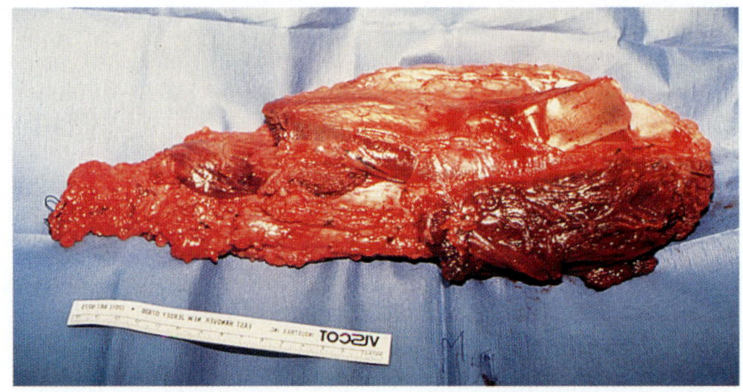

FIG. 1B. Extensive tumor specimen.

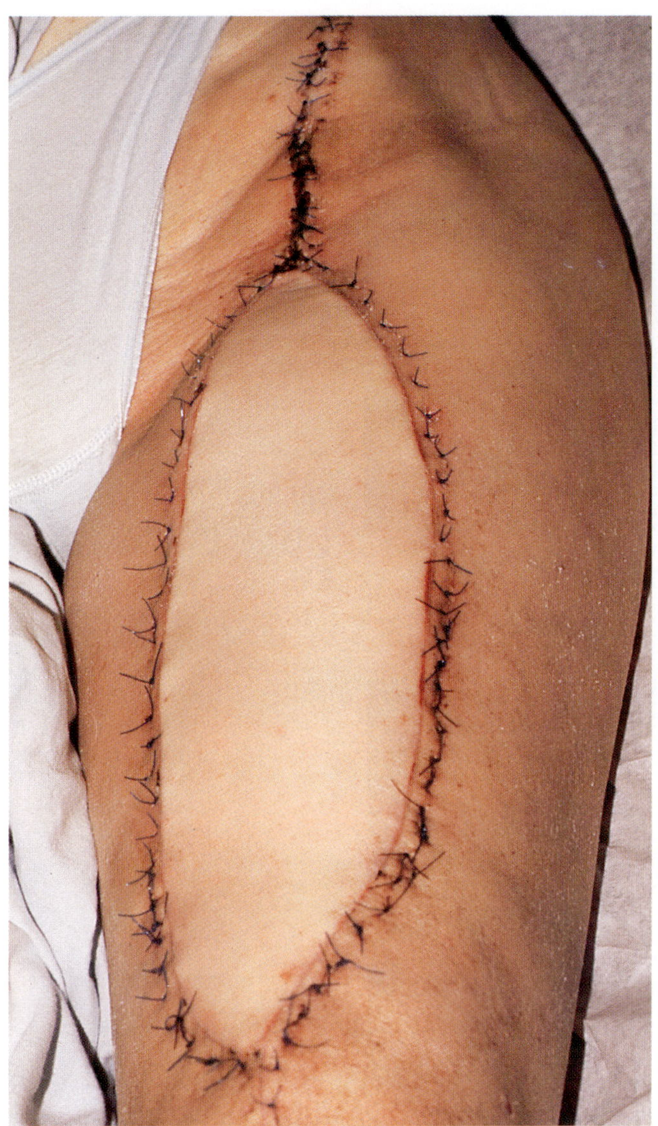

FIG. 1D. Free latissimus dorsi flap reconstruction of the thigh defect.

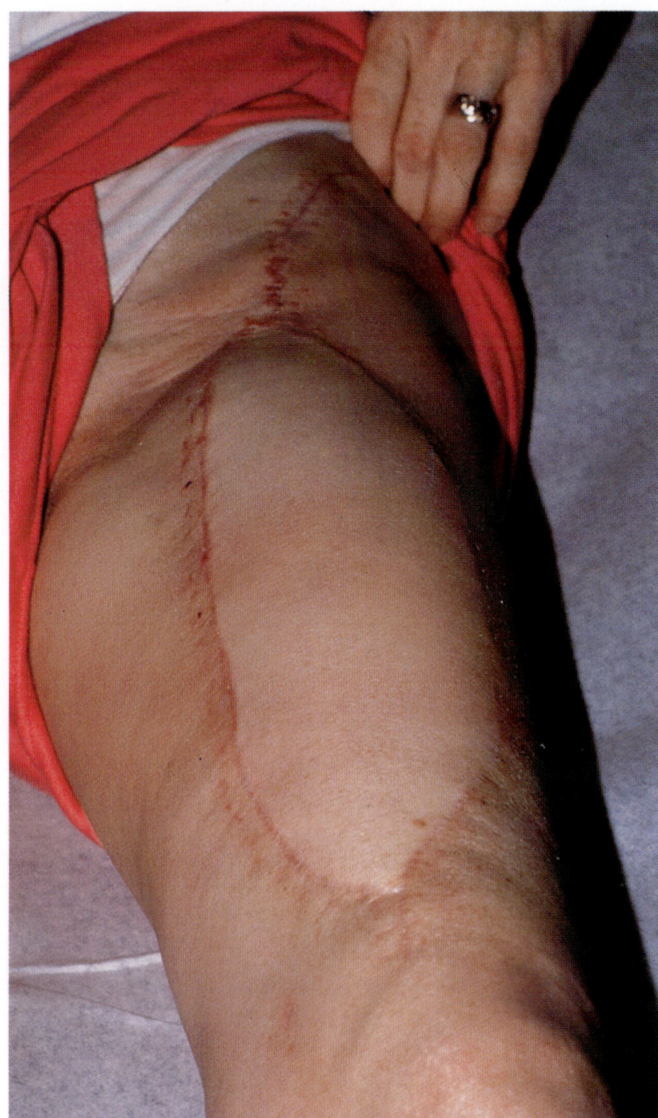

FIG. 1E. Well-healed myocutaneous flap at 1 month postoperative.

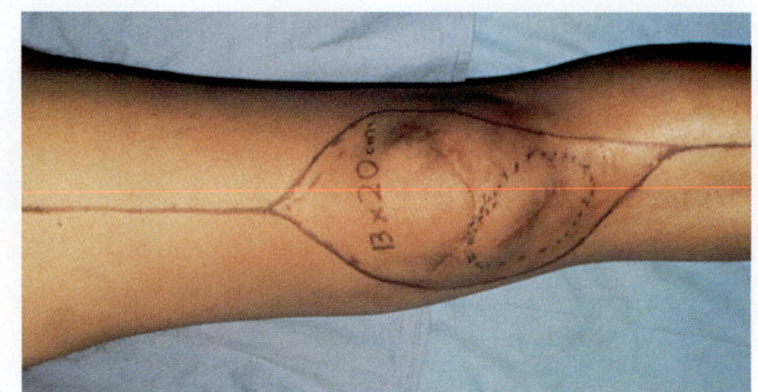

FIG. 2A. Malignant fibrous histiocytoma of left knee.

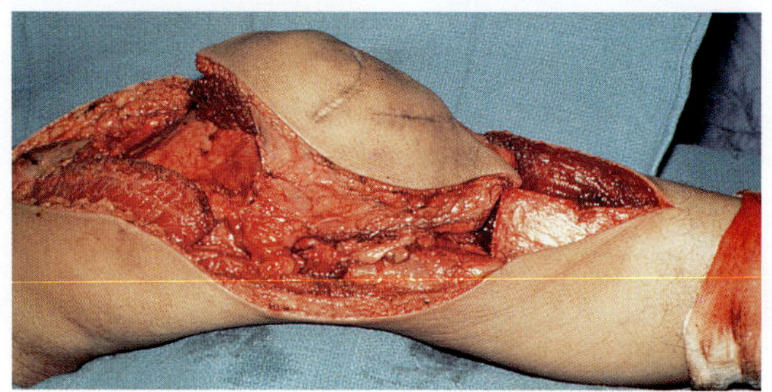

FIG. 2B. Extensive tumor resection.

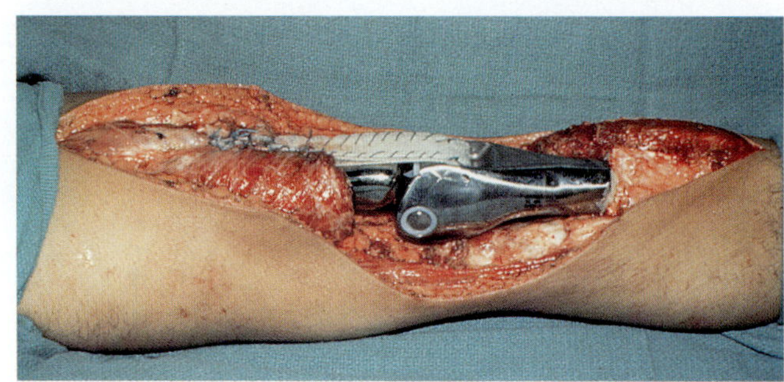

FIG. 2C. Defect with endoprosthesis in place.

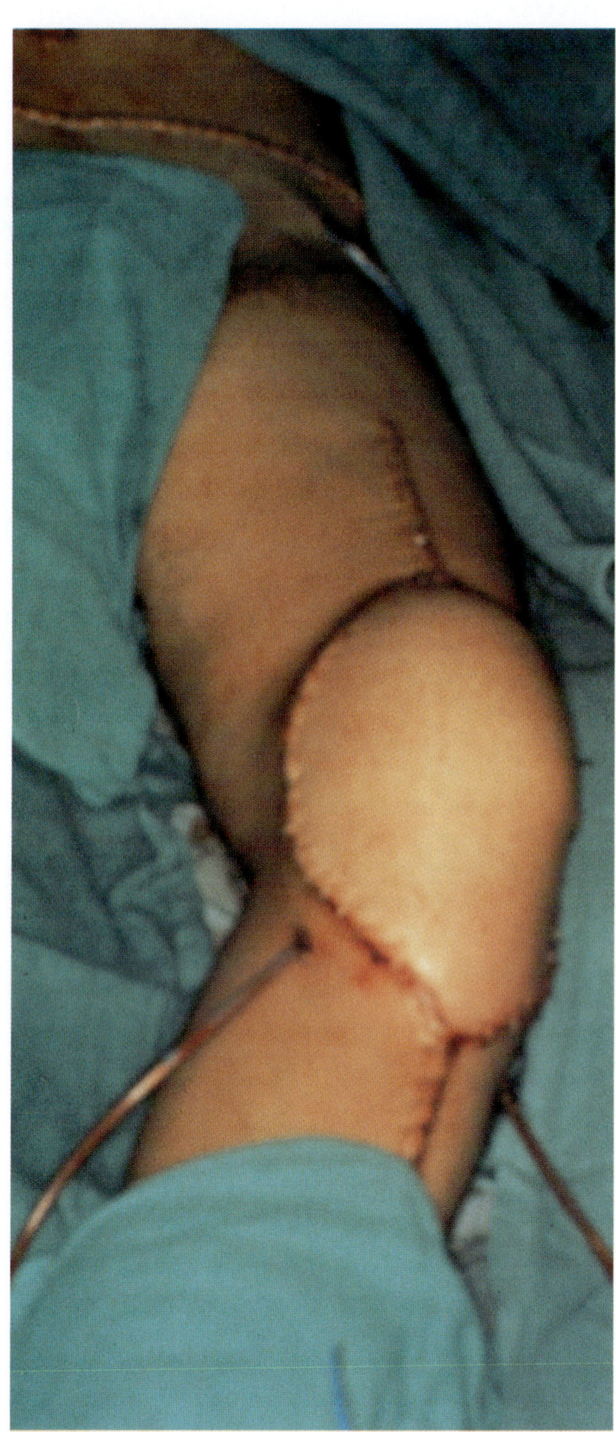

FIG. 2D. Free TRAM flap used for immediate reconstruction.

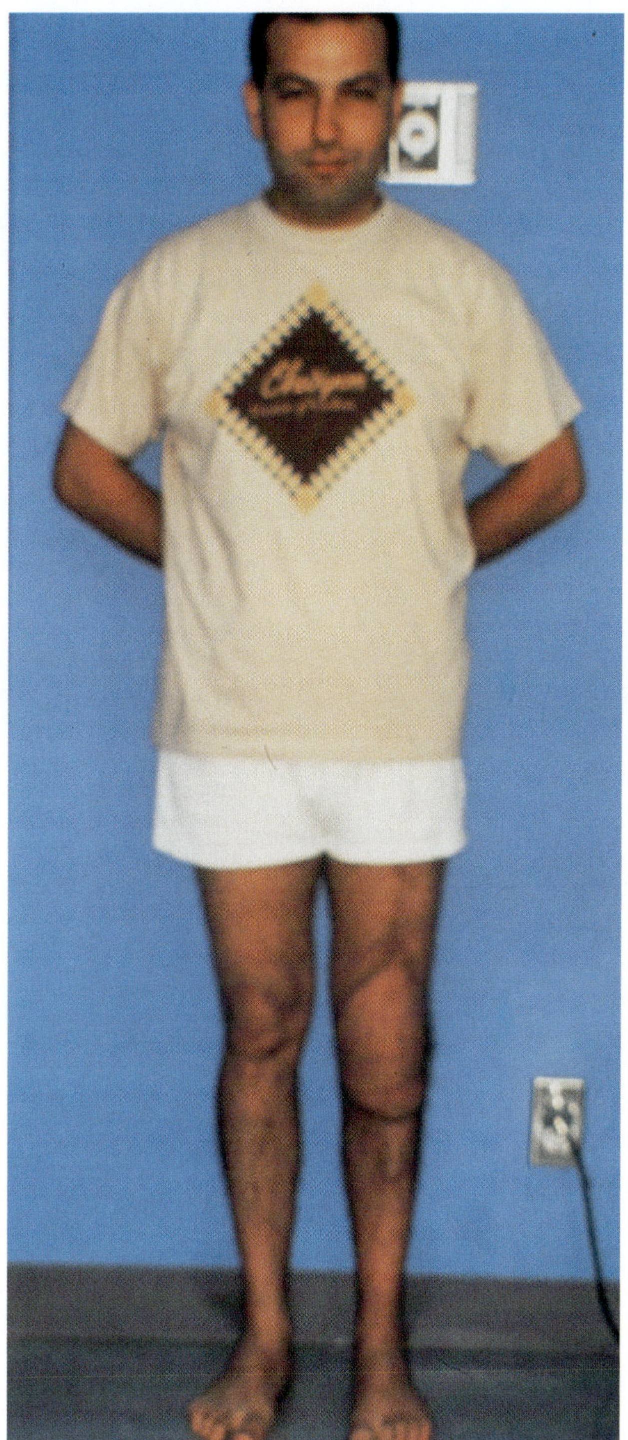

FIG. 2E. Well-healed flap and highly functional extremity at 9 months.

PREOPERATIVE CONSIDERATIONS

The success of the extremity reconstruction and the posttreatment quality of life for the patient strongly correlates with the functional level of the patient's ambulation after surgery. To this end, the anatomic complexity of the leg with its regional concentration of myoneurovascular structures crucial for function necessitates attention to several important preoperative considerations. Accurately estimating the anticipated size of the extremity defect following the tumor ablation allows more precise reconstructive planning in terms of the volume and type of microvascular tissue needed and the most likely location of the vascular anastomoses. This approach also allows the reconstructive surgeon to design a backup plan, should the first option become nonviable.

In assessing defect size, patients presenting with an extensive tumor clearly require a large free flap, such as the latissimus dorsi muscle flap, for wound closure. However, under some circumstances, a large free flap also may be required for patients with small tumors. Patients who were biopsied through an inappropriate incision placed transverse to the long axis of the extremity, who have had an incomplete tumor excision, or who develop a hematoma after biopsy often require extensive soft tissue resection to obtain surgical margins that are free of tumor. Similarly, patients who have a small tumor located in a bed of soft tissue that has been extensively damaged by radiation therapy may benefit from excision of most of the radiation-damaged tissue along with the tumor and placement of a larger flap into the defect to obtain better overall wound healing. In all of these situations, a much larger wound defect should be anticipated and the appropriate flap selected.

Other factors that must be considered when planning the reconstruction include the timing of the reconstruction, the total dose of radiation delivered to the tumor bed, the portals used for radiation therapy, the possible need for brachytherapy, the location and characteristics of the defect, the need to cover or repair any vital limb-function structures that may be exposed or removed during the tumor resection, the location and condition of the recipient vessels, the availability and characteristics of the donor tissue, the patient's position on the operating room table, the extent of extremity immobilization immediately after surgery, and the patient's potential for ambulation postoperatively. In most cases, careful examination of these details prior to surgery helps avoid many pitfalls in the reconstruction and results in a successful outcome.

THIGH RECONSTRUCTION

In our experience, the most common location for lower extremity tumors is the thigh. Patients who require a free flap for thigh reconstruction are usually those who present with large tumors that require wide local excision and result in extensive soft tissue defects or have a history of high-dose radiation therapy to a large area of the thigh, and are at high risk for wound healing problems. Clearly a local muscle flap or free flap is required for closure over any exposed vital limb-function structures. Defects resulting from tumor resection in the lower groin and for some lesions in the proximal medial or anterior thigh frequently can be repaired with an ipsilateral pedicled vertical or transverse rectus abdominis myocutaneous (VRAM or TRAM) flap, provided the pedicle to the flap has not been divided at the time of tumor dissection. However, large defects in other areas of the thigh require a large volume of well-vascularized tissue transferred from a distant site for satisfactory extremity reconstruction. At our institution, the two most commonly used free flap donor tissues for closure of thigh wounds are the latissimus dorsi and rectus abdominis muscles with or without a skin paddle (Fig. 1A–E). The femoral or profunda vessels are usually easily accessed as recipients either directly through the defect or by a superficial extension of the wound to the vessels that can also be covered by the flap. Small, low-flow recipient vessels are not generally considered as viable alternatives to the more dependable high-flow vessels in the thigh that can usually be reached without vein grafts.

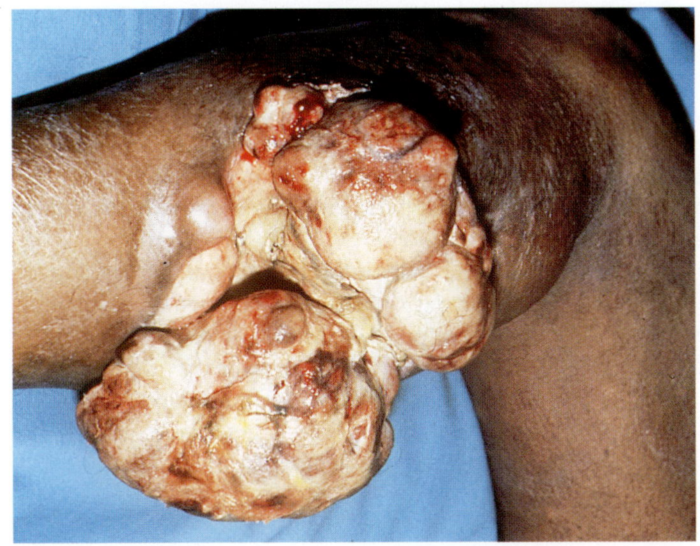

FIG. 3A. Neurofibrosarcoma of left calf.

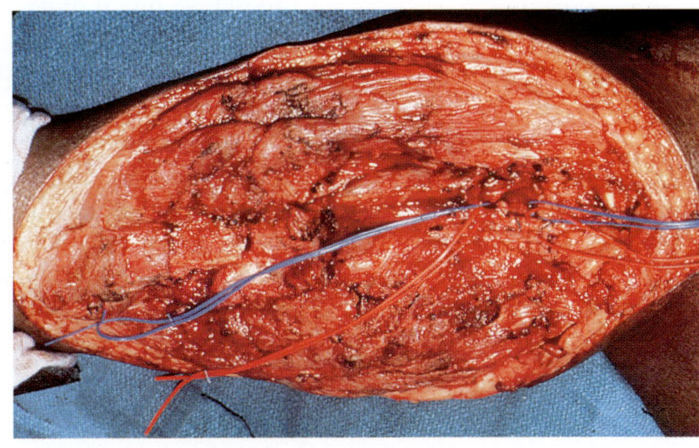

FIG. 3B. Extent of tumor resection with a viable extremity.

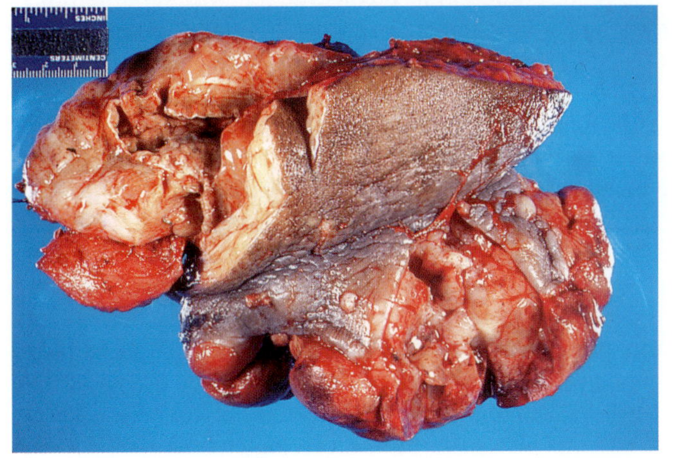

FIG. 3C. Tumor specimen.

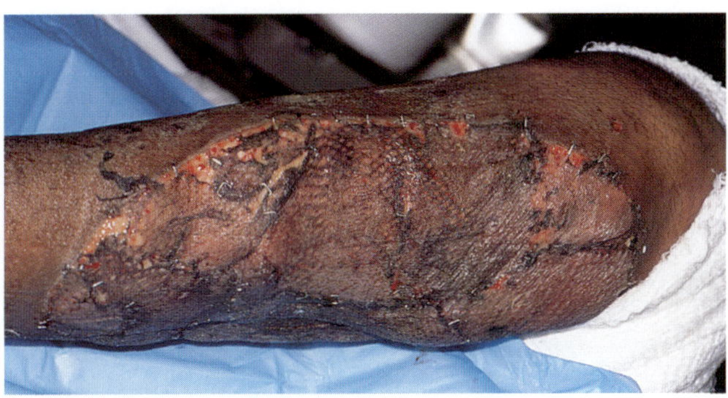

FIG. 3D. Healing skin-grafted latissimus dorsi/serratus muscle flap reconstruction at 1 week.

The insetting of the free flap into the wound relates to the geometry of the defect in the thigh. The muscle flaps should be ideally oriented so that the long axis of the muscle parallels that of the wound, which is usually longitudinal in the extremity. The muscle should be rolled up longitudinally and stretched tautly across the top of the defect so that as much muscle as needed fills the underlying dead space. Most cases involve skin grafting a muscle flap, but, in some cases, a skin island can be designed on the muscle and may be part of the surgical planning in terms of strategic placement or for bulk over or, once de-epithelialized, inside the wound.

Postoperatively, skin grafts should be dressed with ointment and nonadherent gauze. The flaps are monitored hourly for the first 3 days with the cutaneous Doppler. The extremity is modestly elevated with the patient at bed rest for 5 days. At this time, with some of the edema of the thigh resolved, the leg is loosely wrapped with an elastic bandage over the flap area and the patient allowed to get up to a chair and to the bathroom with partial weight bearing, usually with crutches. The patient can generally be full weight bearing by the end of the second week, but maintain some assistance for walking as needed.

KNEE RECONSTRUCTION

Primary or recurrent tumors involving the distal femur, the proximal tibia, or the knee joint itself, once excised, require knee joint reconstruction with an allograft or endoprosthesis, if a multidisciplinary limb salvage approach is undertaken. In some cases, the region around the knee has been radiated, and local skin changes are obvious. However, function seems to be rarely significantly affected, unless excessive tumor characteristics, such as bulk, inflammation, or necrosis, are involved.

If tumors present either on the skin or subcutaneously, or if a large open biopsy has been taken (especially if the incision runs counter to the axial direction of the limb), a larger skin margin must be obtained with the tumor, and additional reliable coverage of the joint prosthesis must be obtained. On the other hand, in many cases minimal skin is excised, but much of the soft tissue surrounding the knee is excised to obtain clear tumor margins, and this extensive dissection tends to increase the ischemia of the skin flap margins. That a large prosthesis must be used, especially in cases of proximal tibial tumors, only complicates the subsequent skin closure over the prosthesis, which must not be under tension so as to minimize the potential for wound breakdown over the joint. Most of these patients also have been receiving chemotherapy, which can adversely affect the wound healing. In these circumstances, pedicled or free muscle coverage of the prosthesis provides an ideal protective interface that is well vascularized and contours appropriately for the leg (Fig. 2A–E). The muscle flap allows for minimal tension on the surrounding skin and provides an opportunity to simply remove any skin at the wound edges that appears ischemic. The gastrocnemius muscle, with a range of about 15 cm above the knee, suffices for many of the immediate coverage needs. However, for large or recurrent tumors or for many of the more extensive needs of delayed reconstruction, free tissue transfers of skin-grafted rectus abdominis or latissimus dorsi muscles is optimal for the coverage of prostheses and obliteration of dead space. Access to recipient vessels for the muscle transfers is relatively easy since the popliteal or superficial femoral vessels are nearby following the ablative procedure. The microvascular anastomoses can be completed either proximally or distally, depending on the ease of the inset and the availability of the vessels relative to the defect.

Insetting the flap is more critical in the knee area, because the bone or prosthesis present must be adequately covered with well-vascularized tissue, and the remaining native skin flaps must be assessed carefully for viability, since loss of any portion of the flaps can lead to exposure of the prosthesis and secondary infection and amputation. Drains are used liberally under flaps and removed when the wound drainage is under 30 cc for a 24-hour period, once the patient has begun mobilizing.

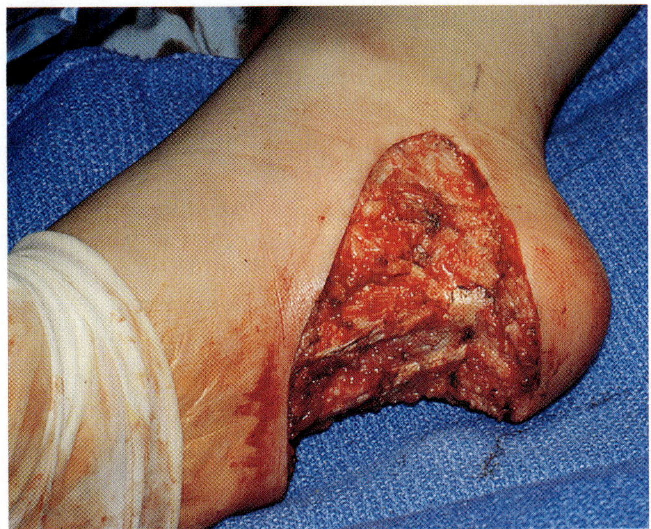

FIG. 4A. Large plantar defect following excision of an anaplastic tumor.

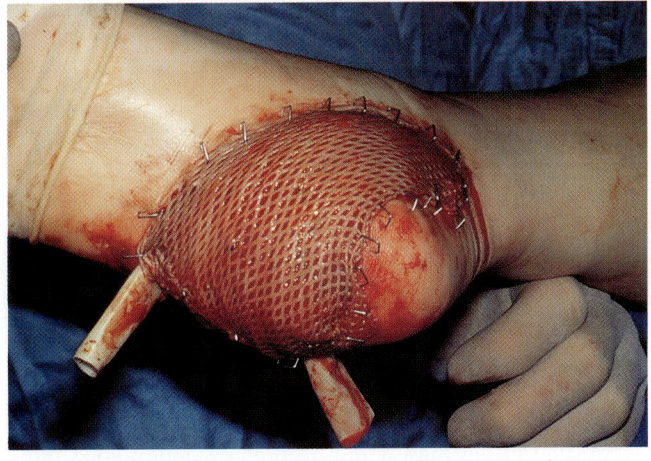

FIG. 4B. Revascularization and inset of a gracilis muscle free flap with skin graft.

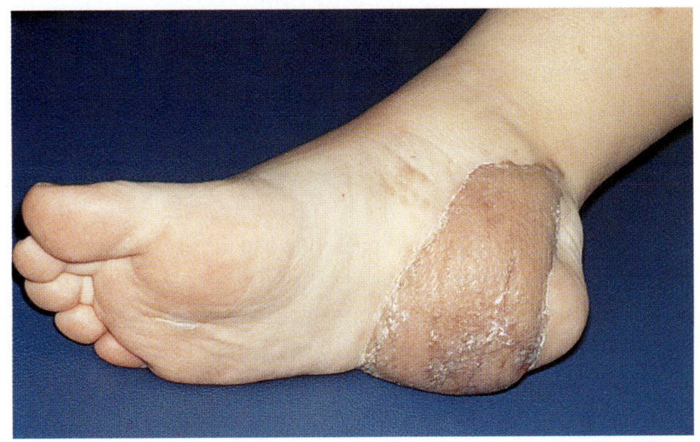

FIG. 4C. Healed muscle flap reconstruction of the foot at 2 months.

Many knee reconstruction patients require some form of straight-leg splinting in the postoperative phase. The first 3 days of flap monitoring are carried out without a splint to facilitate flap observation and the early manual care of the skin graft, which is placed without a bolster. The splint can then be secured on the leg for stability of the knee and an elastic wrap placed snugly around the knee and flap area to help reduce the local swelling and facilitate the patient's mobilization on about the fifth to seventh day in a non-weight-bearing fashion. The elastic bandage is recommended for at least a month to aid in contouring the flap. Full weight bearing then follows some weeks to months later at the discretion of the orthopedist.

In some reconstructions, a knee mechanical mobilizer is preferred by the orthopedist, which can be started at 30° in the same 5- to 7-day time frame if the wound healing is normal, and the angle increased gradually as the wound, flap, and patient tolerate it, with diligent daily wound inspection for any local problems.

LEG RECONSTRUCTION

For tumors involving areas of the leg other than the knee, the leg can be divided into thirds for the purpose of delineating the use of specific local flaps for reconstruction, much the same as in general reconstructive principles for extremity trauma. The pedicled medial and lateral heads of the gastrocnemius muscles provide abundant well-vascularized tissue to cover large defects located in the upper anterior third of the leg, while the soleus muscle can reliably reconstruct the middle third zone. Occasionally, one of the gastrocnemius muscles and the soleus muscle together are required for combined large defects bridging the middle and upper thirds of the leg, with minimal donor functional deficiency.

For smaller defects located anywhere on the leg, skin grafting and local fasciocutaneous flaps, such as rotational flaps or sliding bipedicle flaps, are useful in nonirradiated tissues. However, most tumor defects, especially those of recurrent tumors, are more extensive, usually beyond the application of local muscle flaps, in which free tissue transfer is the most reliable and expedient solution. This is especially true for the distal third of the leg, traditionally reserved for free flap applications, because of the paucity of reliable local tissues for reconstruction. The most common free tissue transfers for the distal third of the leg are the radial forearm fasciocutaneous flap, and the rectus abdominis, latissimus dorsi, and gracilis muscles, which would usually be skin grafted rather than being used as myocutaneous flaps in order to avoid the extra bulk (Fig. 3A–D).

The anterior and posterior tibial vessels are available as the primary recipient vessels, with occasional use of the peroneal vessels. The posterior tibial vessels are usually preferred to the anterior tibial vessels because they are larger in caliber and have a more consistent vein. Some additional soft tissue dissection may be necessary to reach the recipient vessels, especially in the proximal leg, but rarely enough to require vein grafts. An adequate-sized muscle or soft tissue flap, such as a radial forearm or scapular flap (especially in the distal third of the leg) should be planned for the defect and also for whatever additional dissection area is necessary to reach the recipient vessels.

Postoperatively, the patients are kept at bed rest for 7 days with the leg elevated, after which the extremity is dangled off the side of the bed, starting with 5 minutes out of the hour the first day and progressing to 15 to 20 minutes by the third day (waking hours only). The patient is then allowed non-weight-bearing ambulation on crutches or in a wheelchair with the flap area securely wrapped with an elastic bandage. The flap must be monitored for swelling or impending loss of the overlying skin graft (or congested skin of a fasciocutaneous flap) from prolonged dependence of the extremity. Patients must inspect and care for the leg and flap once they are out of the hospital, elevating the leg frequently, and maintaining the pressure wrap until the leg has developed more mature healing for weight bearing at 8 to 12 weeks. Patients who fail to do

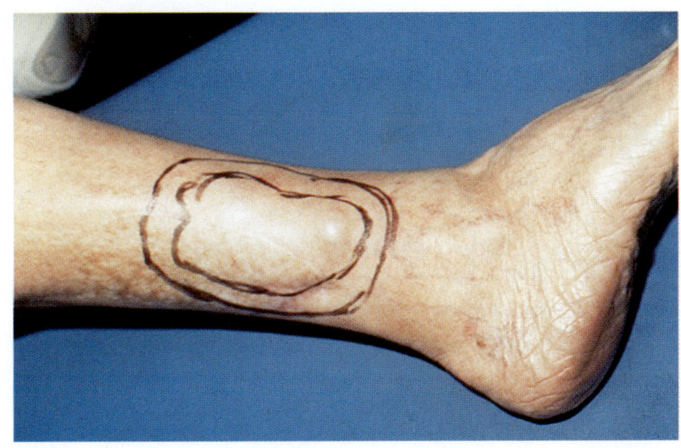

FIG. 5A. Recurrent sarcoma lateral aspect of the lower right leg.

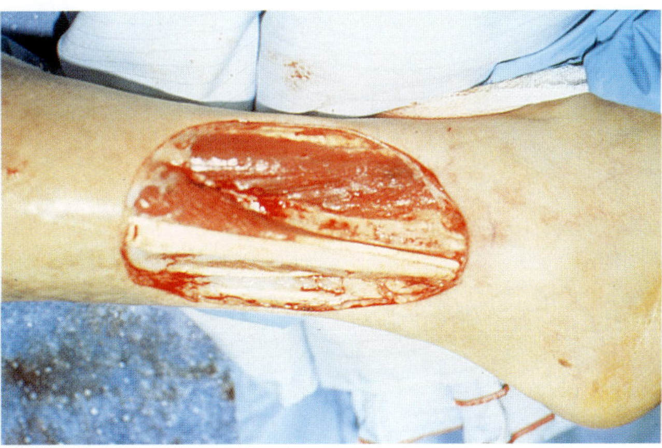

FIG. 5B. Defect following wide local excision of the recurrence.

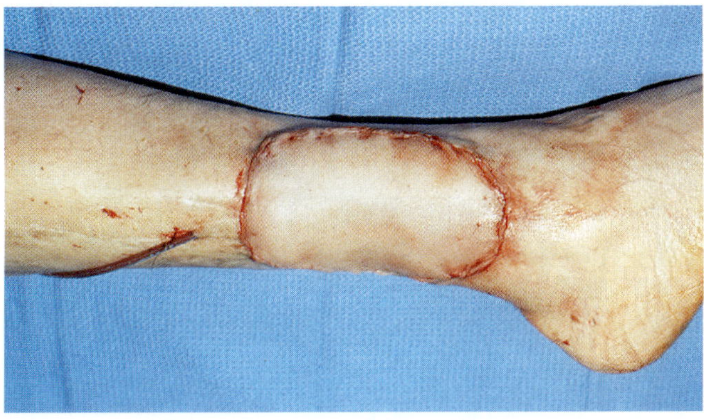

FIG. 5C. Revascularized free radial forearm flap inset into defect.

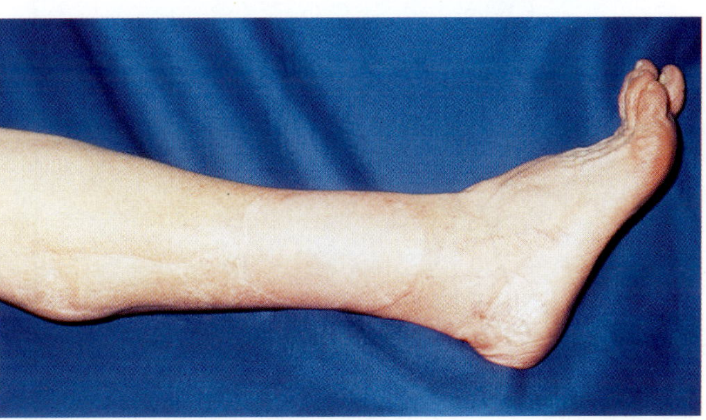

FIG. 5D. Healed flap right lower leg with normal extremity function.

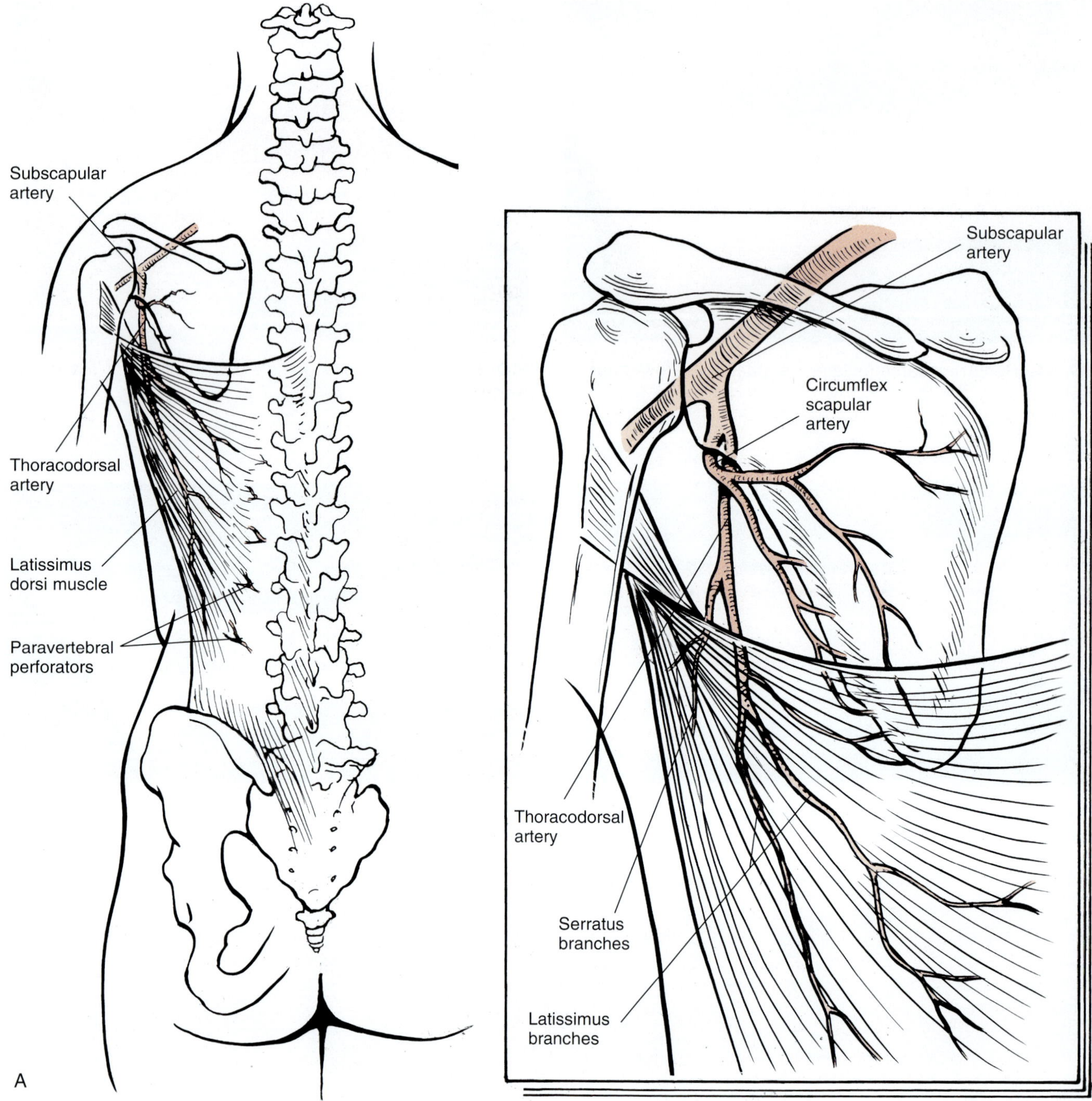

FIG. 6A–C. The latissimus dorsi muscle flap is based on the thoracodorsal vessels. It can be transferred as a myocutaneous flap, or a muscle flap that requires skin graft coverage.

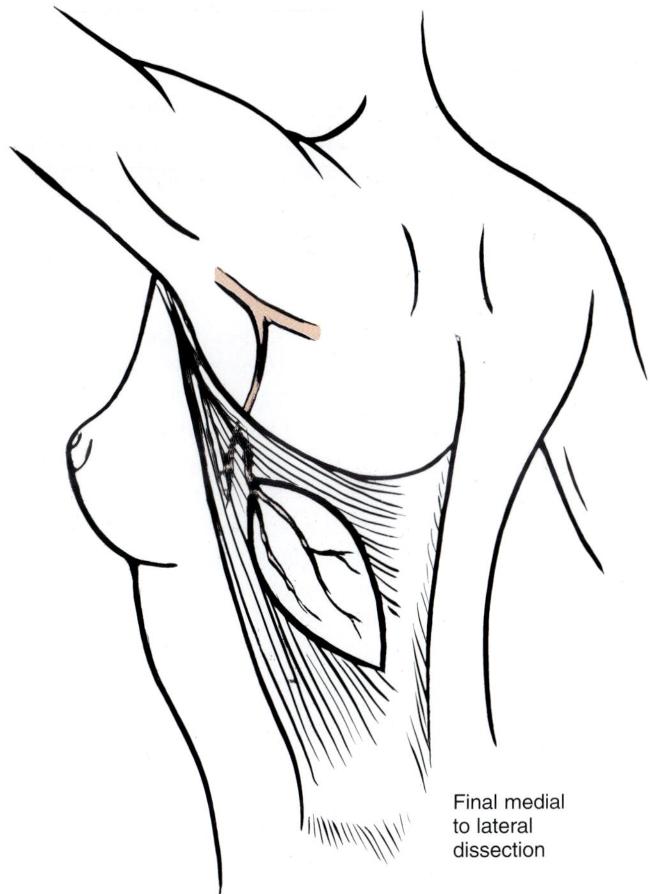

FIG. 6. *Continued.*

this can develop chronic edema and pain in the leg, with the high risk of permanent poor function and possibly even amputation.

FOOT RECONSTRUCTION

Malignant tumors of the foot often require amputation, but limb salvage procedures for the foot are more common now because of improved immediate reconstructive capabilities, especially in the application of free tissue transfers. The particular areas for potential reconstruction include (a) the heel and midplantar area, (b) the distal plantar area, (c) the non–weight-bearing posterior heel, and (d) the dorsum of the foot. Unfortunately, only sparse information is available on the overall success of foot reconstruction following surgery for malignancies, and even less on functional outcomes and quality of life for the limb-sparing procedures. However, our studies in these areas have demonstrated that often foot reconstruction offers the cancer patient a highly functional extremity and that daily activities are not significantly impaired.

For superficial or limited defects of any of the reconstruction areas of the foot listed above, skin grafts or local flaps such as plantar flaps, instep flaps, dorsalis pedis flaps, flexor digitorum muscle flaps, toe fillet flaps, and lateral calcaneal artery flaps can easily provide a satisfactory reconstructive solution without significant donor site morbidity or compromise of foot function. However, following wide local excision of large or recurrent tumors, the defects are frequently not amenable to the use of local tissue. In this situation, a free skin-grafted small muscle, such as the gracilis, internal oblique, or serratus anterior, can conform especially well to an irregular defect contour such as those common in the foot and also replace any dead space with well-vascularized tissue, which can be particularly helpful in irradiated defect sites (Fig. 4A–C). Larger reconstructions may require a rectus abdominis or latissimus dorsi muscle flap (which has the ability to be split for multiple surface applications) for an ample volume of well-vascularized tissue to fill the defect and provide appropriate contour for the foot. Too much flap bulk is usually a major disadvantage for ambulation and requires revision for the reconstructed foot to fit into shoes with reasonable ease, especially if orthotics are necessary.

Fasciocutaneous free flaps can also be used for specific foot reconstruction applications, such as the dorsum or forefoot, for which the radial forearm flap provides a thin, stable cover (Fig. 5A–D). The scapular flap, whether as a skin flap or as a thinner, skin-grafted fascial flap, is also useful around the heel and forefoot. Although these flaps can cover the heel and other weight-bearing surfaces well, shear of the flap fibrofatty layer over the deep defect surface seems to be a difficult flap stability problem for many patients. Both muscle flaps as well as fasciocutaneous flaps can develop pressure ulcerations at sites of redundancy of the flaps or at specific scar interfaces of the normal plantar skin and the flap. Patients must be vigilant for early flap breakdowns in any kind of reconstruction.

The dorsalis pedis and posterior tibial vessels are ideally located as recipient vessels for muscle and fasciocutaneous free flaps, allowing an extensive latitude in insetting the flaps from either the medial, lateral, or dorsal side of the foot. The inset of the flaps is more critical for the foot because of the necessary fit into shoes, if possible. Flaps should be inset tightly and well under the foot skin or plantar glabrous surface edge with prominent eversion to allow optimal final healing at the suture line and minimize tissue surface redundancy. Bulky flaps should be avoided or at least aggressively thinned at the time of surgery, and contouring of the flap postoperatively with a pressure elastic wrap is especially important. In some cases, a revision of the flap, especially of the thicker or bulkier pedicle area, is unavoidable in order to facilitate the patient wearing footwear. The pedicle area itself can be radically thinned, even with sectioning of the flap vessels, by 3 months, if the patient has not had radiation to the foot. In a patient with radiation, any significant manipulation or revision of the flap should be considered quite cautiously.

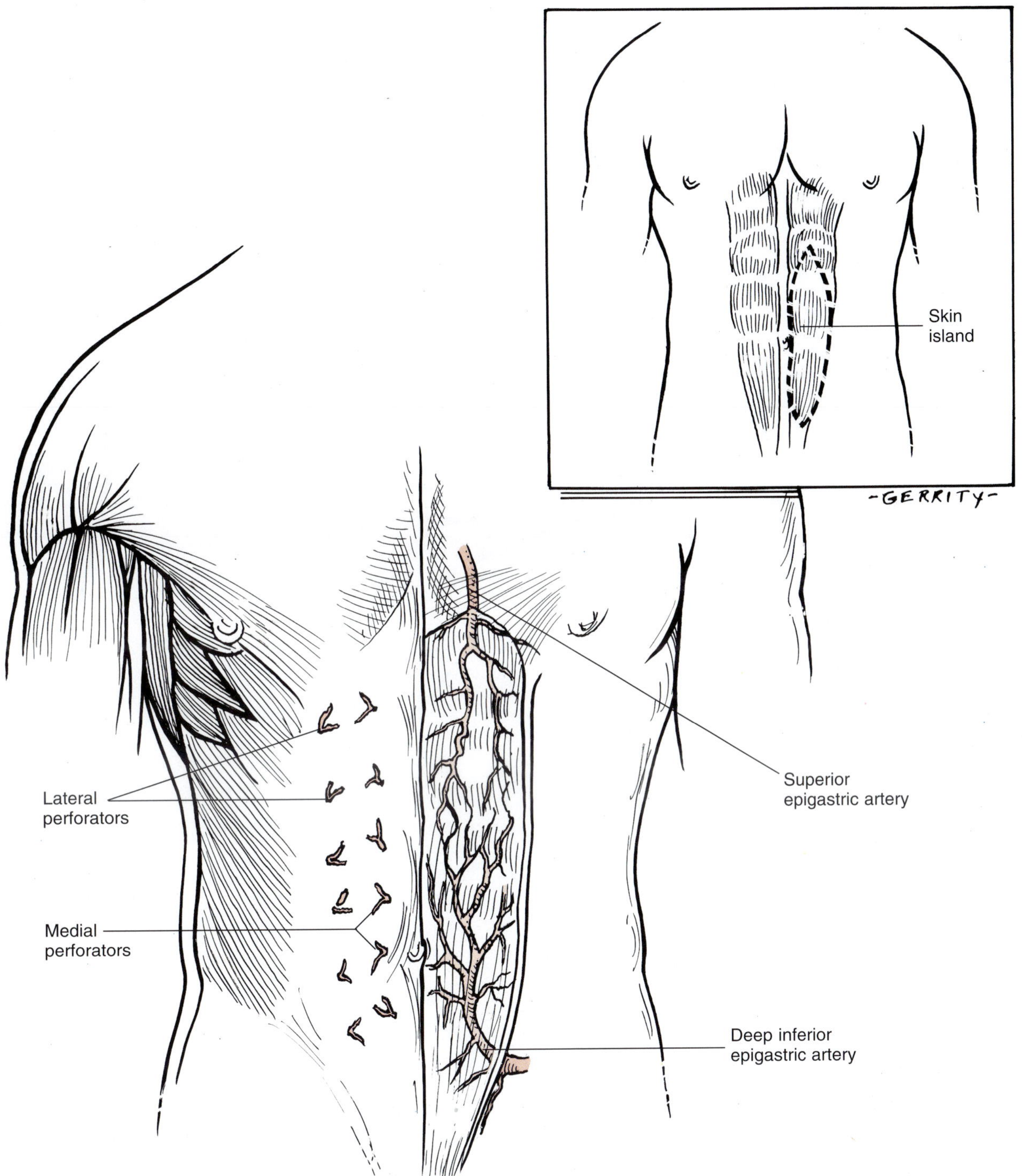

FIG. 7. The anatomy of the rectus abdominis muscle flap.

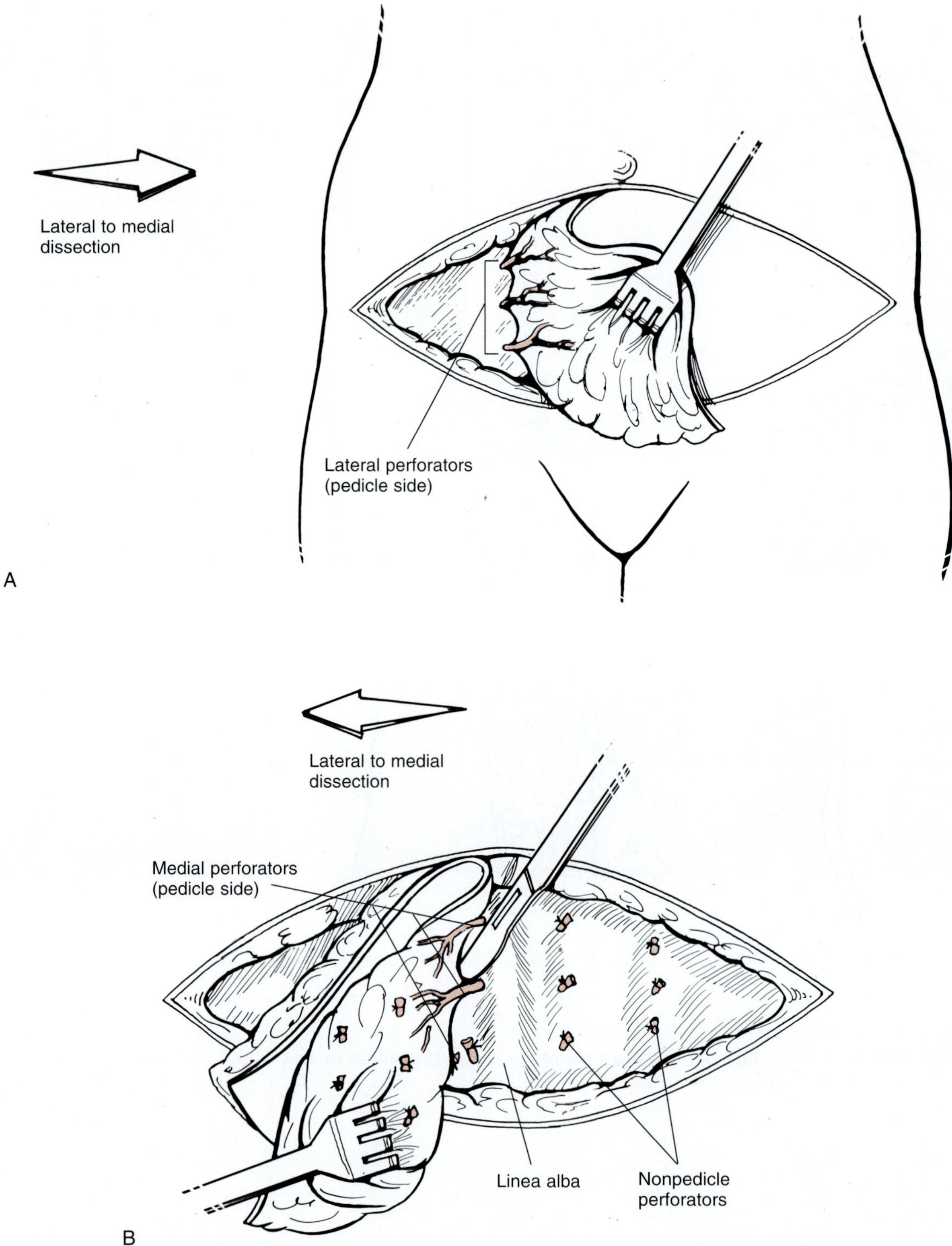

FIG. 8 A. Elevation of the rectus abdominis flap using the transverse rectus abdominis myocuaneous (TRAM) skin paddle. Lateral dissection to expose the lateral perforators **B.** Contralateral dissection to expose the medial perforators.

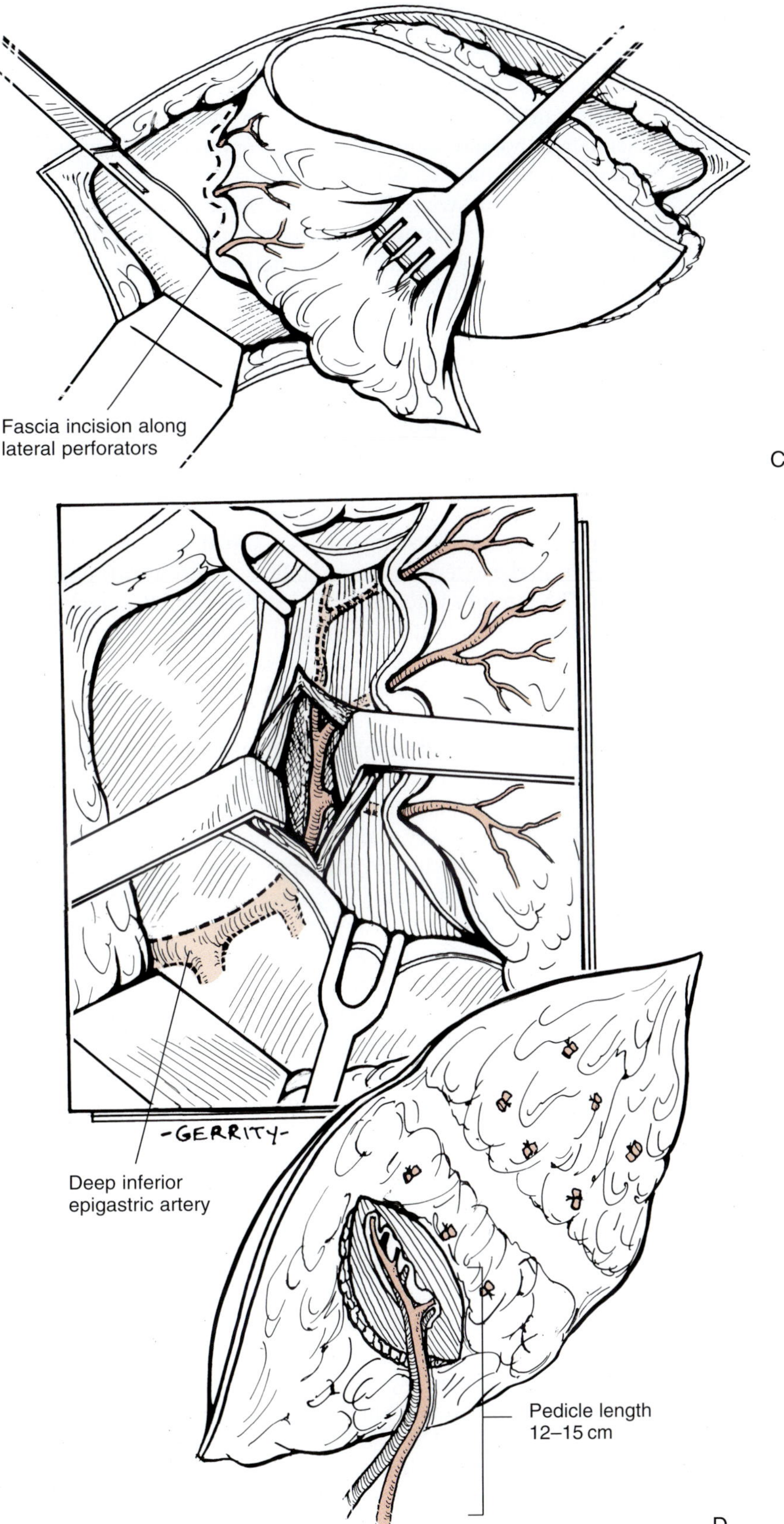

FIG. 8 C. Fascial incision around the perforators. **D.** Exposure of the deep inferior epigastric vessels and dissection to their origin.

BONE RECONSTRUCTION

If an extremity tumor originates in the femur, generally an amputation, segmental or otherwise, is carried out for maximum therapeutic effect. If the tibia is involved, other than proximally, especially after isolated radiation injury to the bone, where a segmental bone resection is a viable option, tibial reconstruction with soft tissue coverage can be obtained with a free fibula osteocutaneous flap from the contralateral leg. Occasionally, a swing or pedicled fibular flap is intercalated into the tibial defect. However, at our institution more commonly cadaver allograft is used for bone replacement, and the soft tissue reconstruction is paramount for graft coverage, protection, and revascularization.

DONOR FLAP HARVESTING TECHNIQUES

Latissimus Dorsi Muscle Free Flap

Anatomy

The latissimus dorsi muscle is a broad, thin, triangular-shaped muscle that originates from the external surface of the lower four ribs posteriorly, the spinous processes of the 7th through 12th thoracic vertebrae, and through the thoracolumbar fascia, from the posterior crest of the ilium and the spinous processes of the lumbar and sacral vertebrae (Fig. 6A–C). The muscle inserts anteriorly in the intertubercular groove of the proximal humerus. The size of the muscle varies but is generally about 40 cm in length and 20 cm in width near its base.

The primary blood supply to the latissimus dorsi muscle is the thoracodorsal artery and vein. These vessels are the terminal branches of the subscapular vessels, which arise from the axillary artery and vein just lateral to the tendon of the pectoralis minor. The subscapular artery and vein are approximately 2 to 3 cm long and give off the circumflex scapular and serratus anterior artery and vein before ending as the thoracodorsal artery and vein. The paravertebral portion of the muscle is supplied by perforating branches of the 9th through 12th intercostal and lumbar arteries and veins.

The latissimus dorsi muscle is innervated by the thoracodorsal nerve, which arises from the posterior cord of the brachial plexus and courses with the thoracodorsal vessels. Within the muscle and approximately 8 to 9 cm from the origin of the subscapular vessels, the thoracodorsal nerve and vessels bifurcate into a medial and lateral thoracodorsal neurovascular branch to supply the majority of the muscle. This anatomical division is the basis for splitting the latissimus dorsi muscle for two independent flap units.

Patient Positioning

The patient's position on the operating room table depends on the location of the tumor in the thigh and the availability of the latissimus dorsi donor site. When possible, the patient is positioned so that both the ablative and the reconstructive surgeons can work simultaneously. By working as a well-coordinated team, this approach decreases anesthesia exposure and total operative time.

If the tumor is located on the anterior, medial, or lateral side of the thigh, we prefer to use a VRAM or TRAM flap if possible so that the patient does not have to be turned during surgery. However, if the latissimus dorsi flap is preferred or required, the patient can be sterilely prepared and draped in the lateral decubitus position and then allowed to roll back into a semisupine position for the tumor resection. The patient is then rolled back to the lateral decubitus position for harvesting the latissimus dorsi flap on the ipsilateral side. To prevent postoperative nerve compression injury, a roll is always placed under the axilla on the side against the table. Alternatively, the tumor can be resected with the

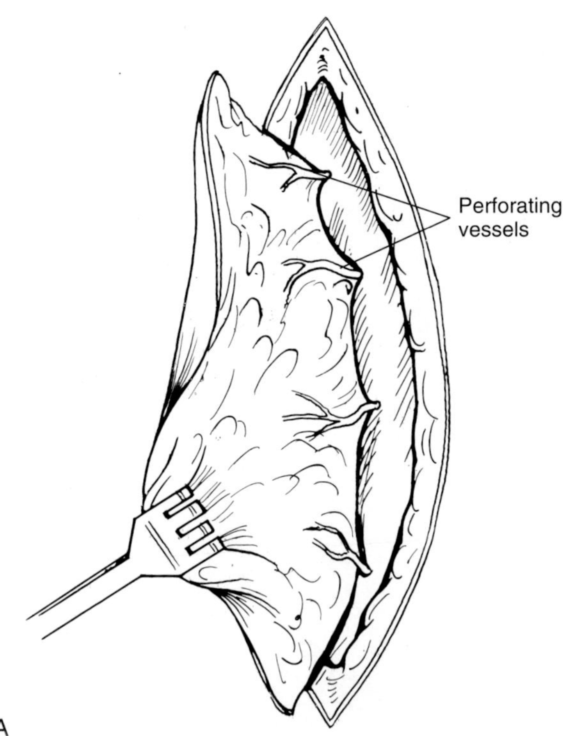

FIG. 9A. Elevation of the rectus abdominis flap using the vertical rectus abdominis muscle (VRAM) skin paddle design. The perforators are exposed laterally and medially.

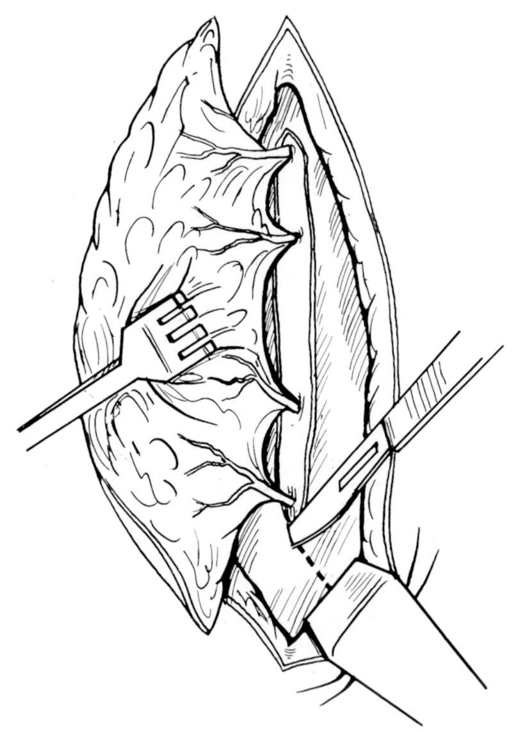

FIG. 9B. The fascia is incised circumferentially.

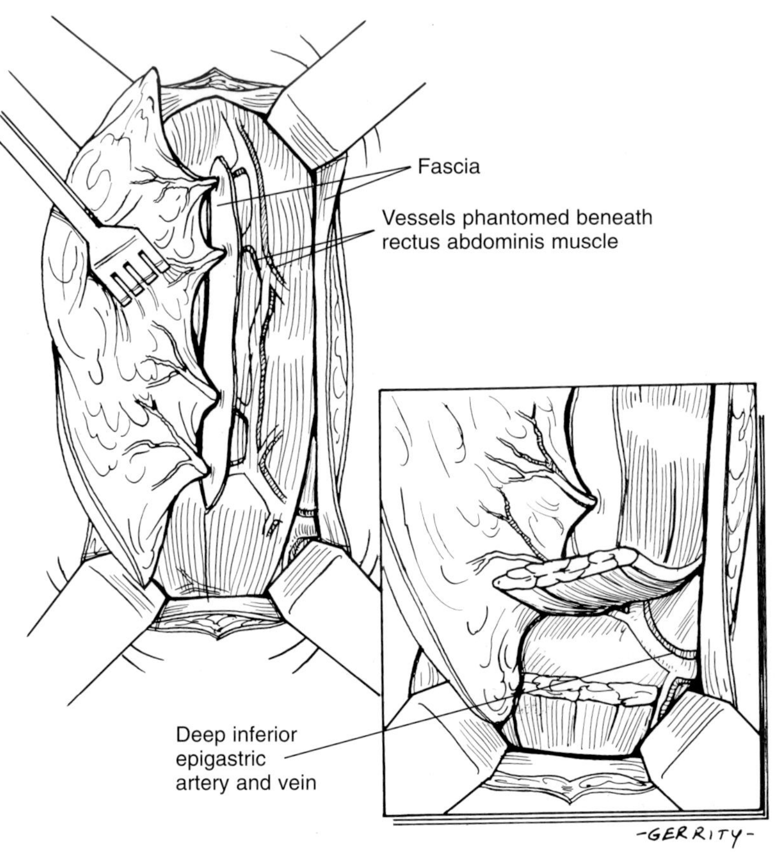

FIG. 9C. The deep inferior epigastric vessels are identified in the lower lateral aspect of the muscle. **Inset:** Once the lower aspect of the muscle is divided, the vessels are traced to their origin.

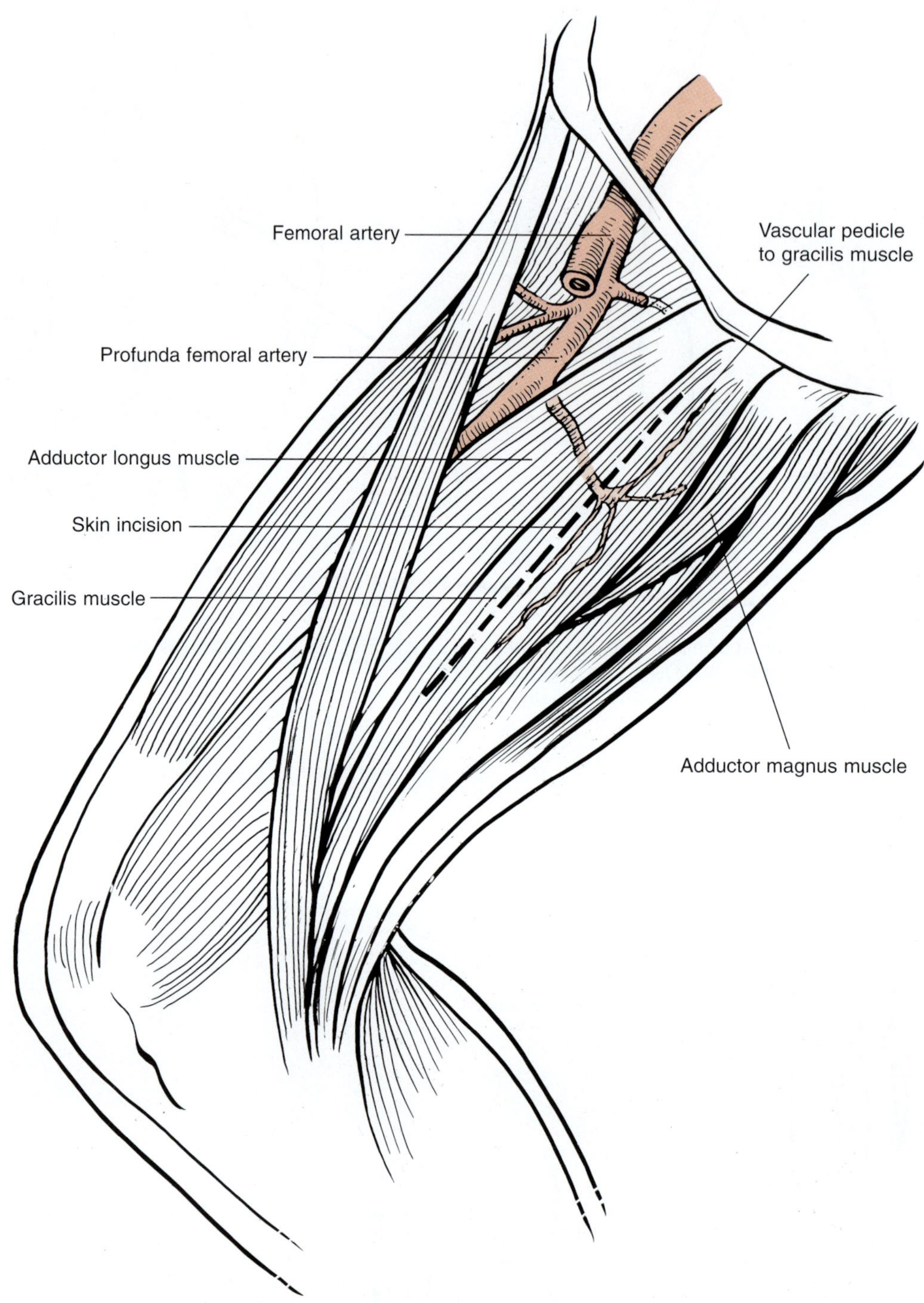

FIG. 10A,B. Anatomy of the gracilis muscle.

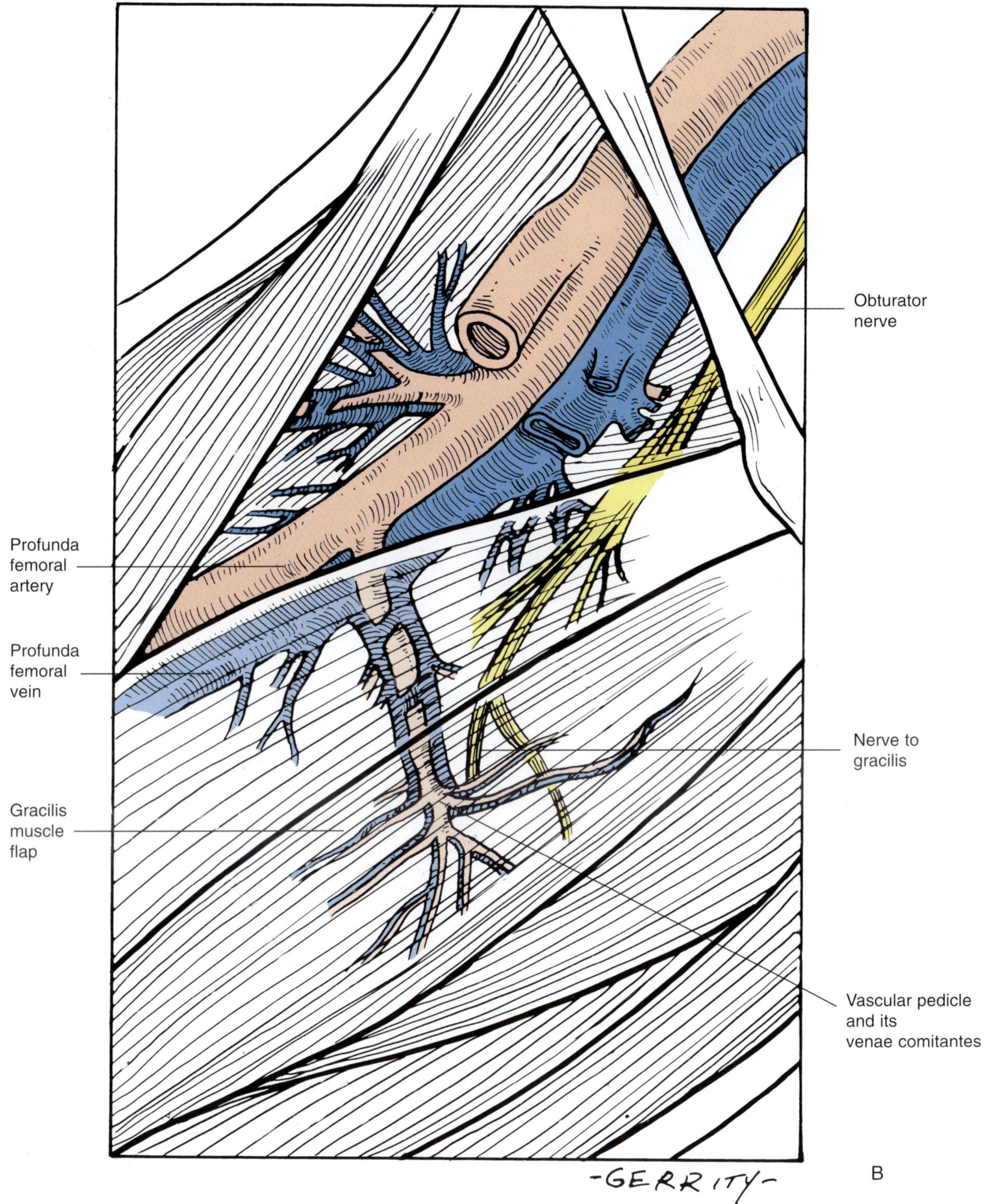

FIG. 10. *Continued.*

patient in a completely supine position, but this approach requires breaking down the sterile field to reposition the patient for flap harvest. Unless the ablative surgeon finds it necessary to position the patient in this fashion or the ipsilateral latissimus dorsi flap is not available and the contralateral flap must be used, we prefer to avoid this maneuver.

For tumors located on the posterior side of the thigh, patients also are sterilely prepared and draped in the lateral decubitus position but then rolled to a semiprone position for the tumor resection. The arm that is against the table is positioned with a roll placed under the axilla and the arm extended above the head.

Flap Design

If the size of the thigh defect is relatively small, that is, no wider than 8 to 10 cm, the latissimus dorsi flap may be harvested as a myocutaneous flap and the donor site closed primarily. For soft tissue defects that are wider than 10 cm, we prefer to repair the wound with a latissimus dorsi muscle free flap and a split-thickness skin graft. Harvesting a latissimus dorsi flap with a skin island wider than 10 cm generally requires closure of the donor site with skin grafts, unless the donor site was previously expanded. However, because the reconstructive surgeon must not interfere with any aspect of tumor treatment, we have not found it practical to expand a free flap prior to resection of malignant tumors.

Harvesting the Latissimus Dorsi Free Flap

After turning the patient to the lateral decubitus position, the initial part of the latissimus dorsi flap dissection varies with the type of flap required. If a myocutaneous flap is needed, an incision is made around the skin island and the dissection carried down to the muscle fascia. To prevent inadvertent undermining of the skin island, the dissection should be beveled away from the skin island. Although the rest of the flap can be raised through this incision, a counterincision in the axilla or an incision extending from the axilla to the skin island incision is usually required to facilitate the dissection of the vascular pedicle.

If a skin island is not required, the latissimus dorsi muscle flap is harvested through an incision extending from the posterior axillary fold to a point midway between the tip of the 11th or 12th rib and the spine. The skin and subcutaneous tissues are elevated from the superficial surface of the muscle posteriorly toward the spine and anteriorly toward the anterior margin of the muscle. These skin flaps are undermined cranially to the superior margin of the latissimus dorsi just above the tip of the scapula and caudally toward the iliac crest as far as is needed to provide a flap large enough to close the thigh defect. The descending part of the trapezius muscle, which covers the origin of the latissimus dorsi over the spinous processes of the lower thoracic vertebrae, must be reflected with the superior skin flap to avoid including this part of the trapezius muscle with the latissimus flap.

Starting at the anterior border of the muscle, the deep surface of the latissimus dorsi muscle is elevated from the serratus anterior muscle with care taken not to injure its neurovascular bundle. A retractor is placed under the latissimus dorsi muscle and dissection proceeds cranially toward the scapular tip. Once the cranial margin of the latissimus muscle is dissected free, attention is turned to elevating the remainder of the origin of the muscle near the spine and iliac crest. As this dissection proceeds, the intercostal and lumbar perforating vessels of the latissimus dorsi muscle are encountered. To obtain reliable hemostasis, these vessels should be ligated rather than cauterized. After the flap is elevated, the muscle is flipped up and out of the way for the axillary dissection of the vascular pedicle. Exposure of the vascular pedicle is facilitated by having an assistant hold the patient's arm in an extended position and by retracting the axillary portion of the muscle. The thoracodorsal artery and vein are dissected proximally toward the subscapular vessels, defining the serratus anterior and the circumflex scapular vascular

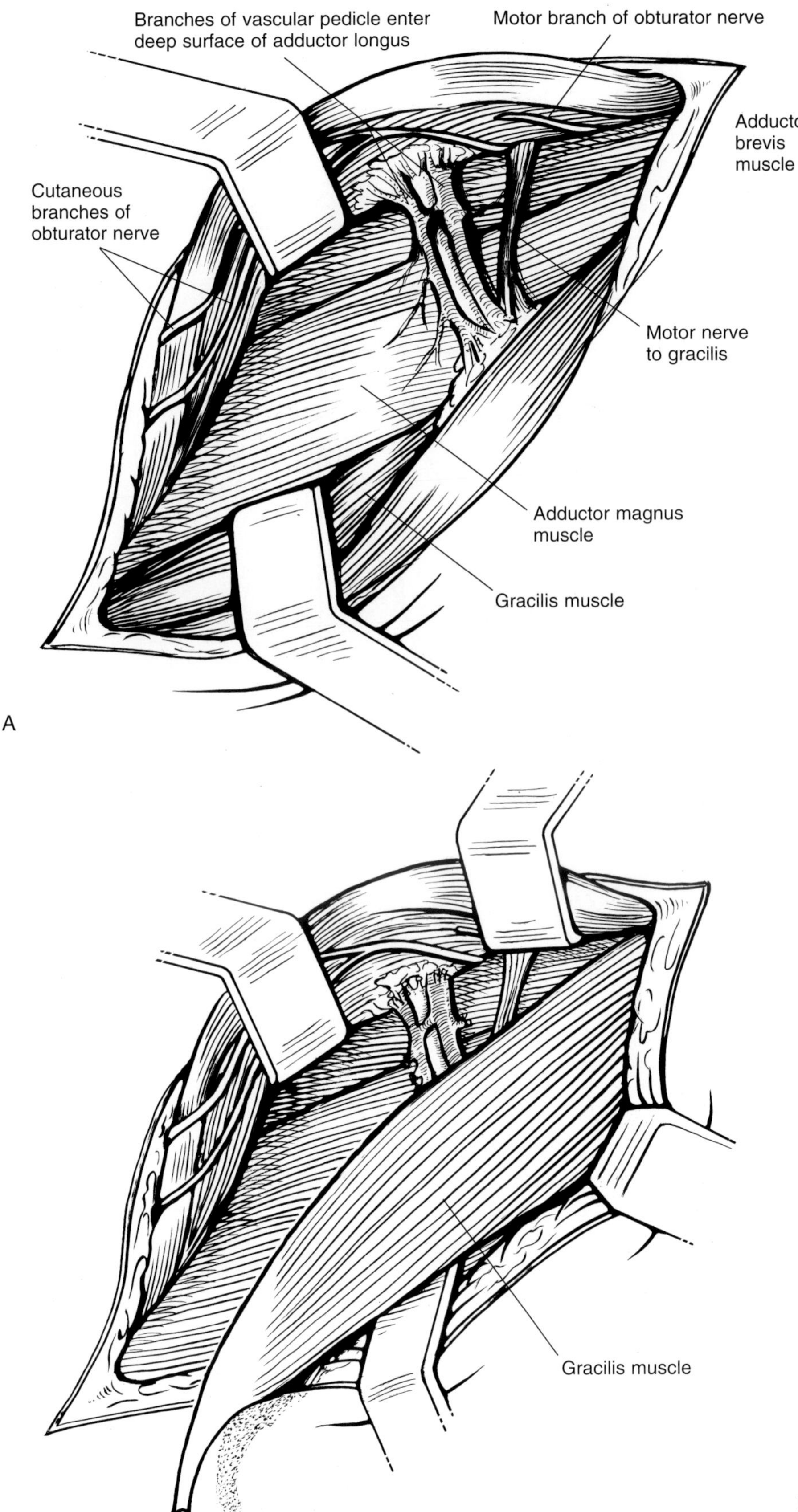

FIG. 11A,B. Dissection technique of the gracilis muscle.

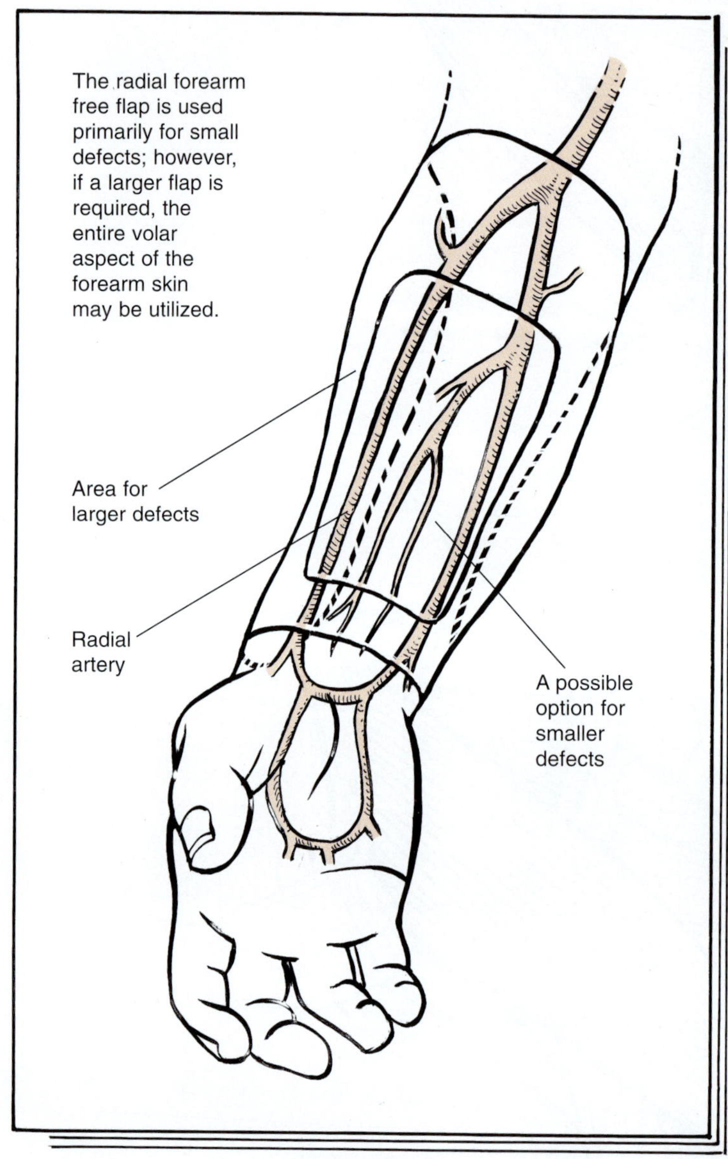

FIG. 12A. Anatomy of the radial forearm flap. Flap design over radial vessels.

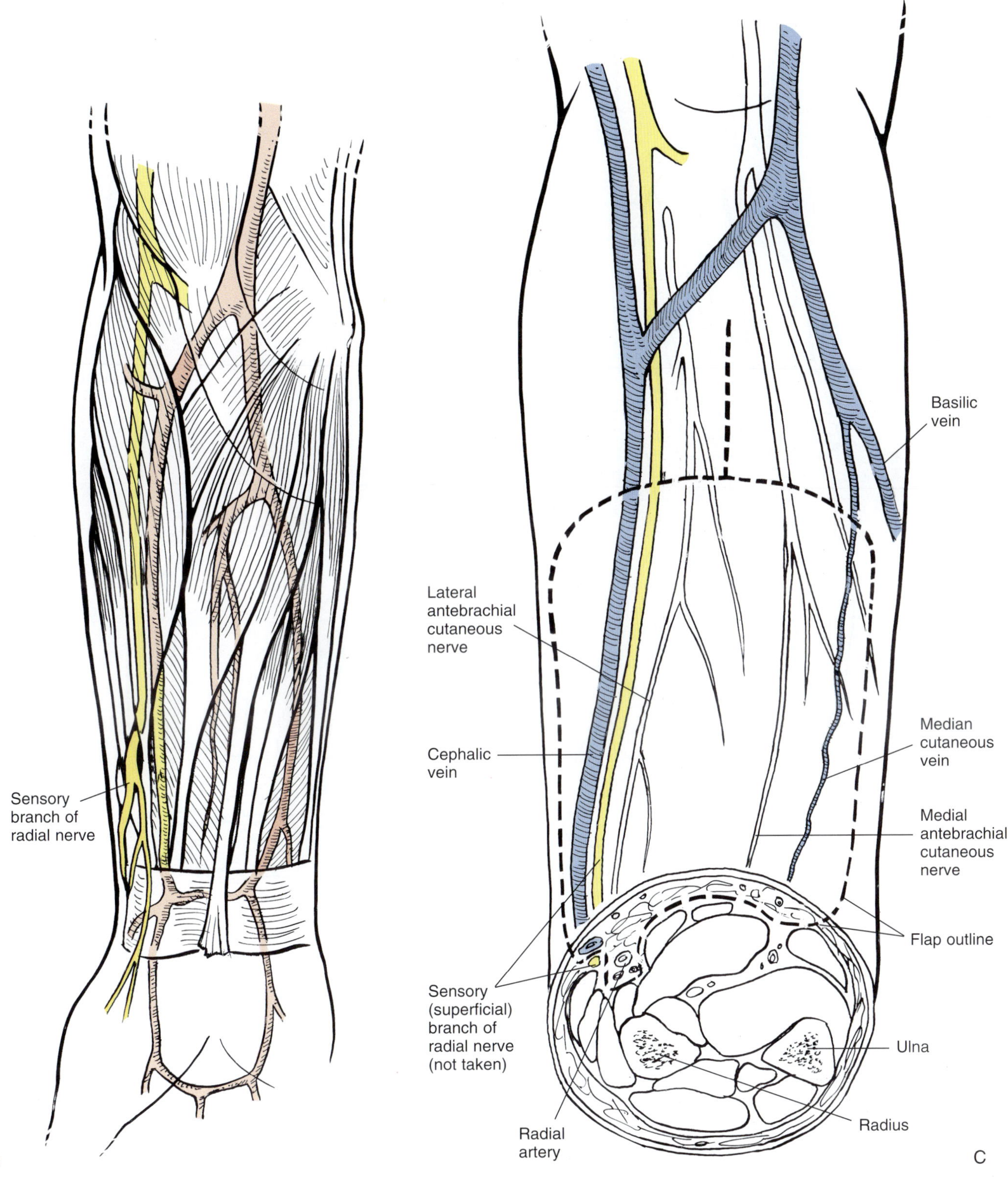

FIG. 12B. Vascular anatomy.

FIG. 12C. Cross-sectional anatomy of proposed flap elevation.

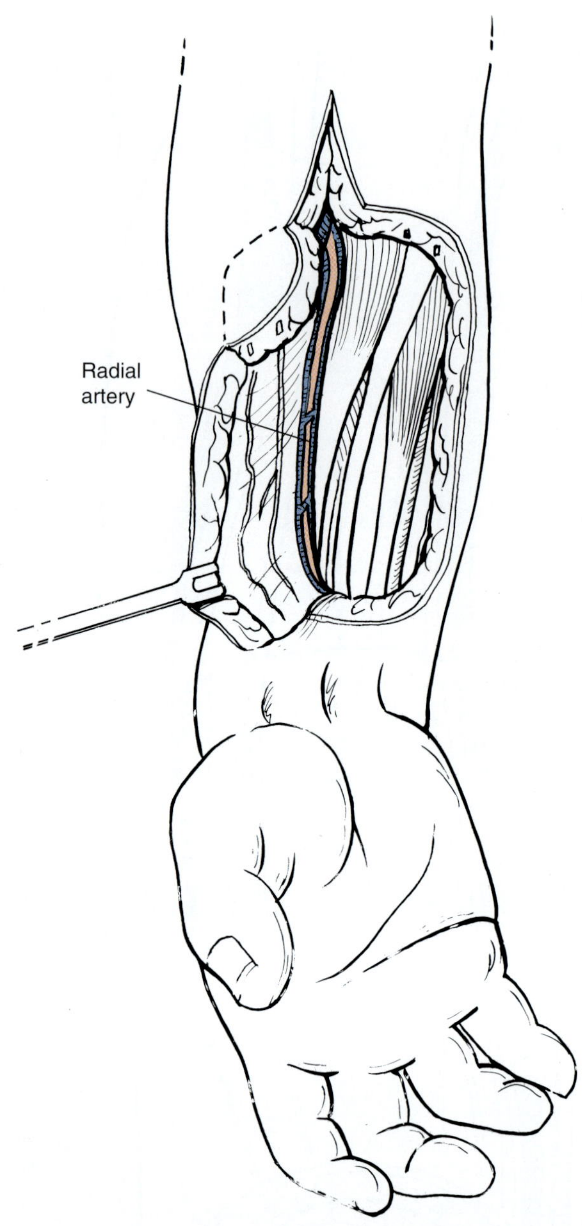

FIG. 13A. Radial forearm flap elevation. Medial incision and flap elevation with exposure of radial vessels.

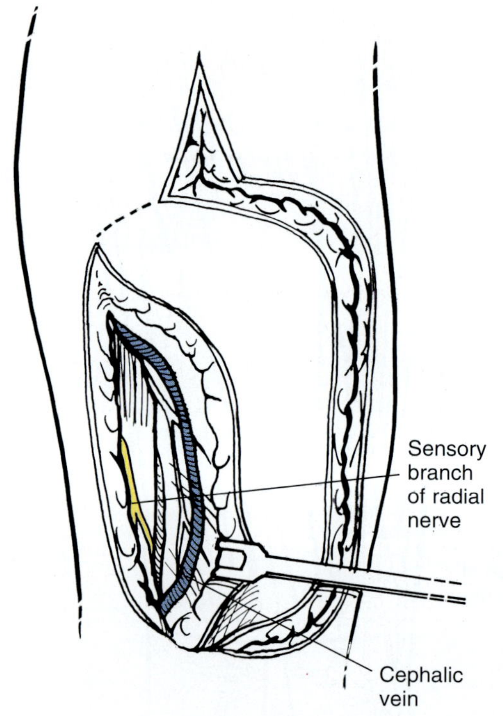

FIG. 13B. Lateral incision with exposure of cephalic vein, and identification and preservation of radial nerve.

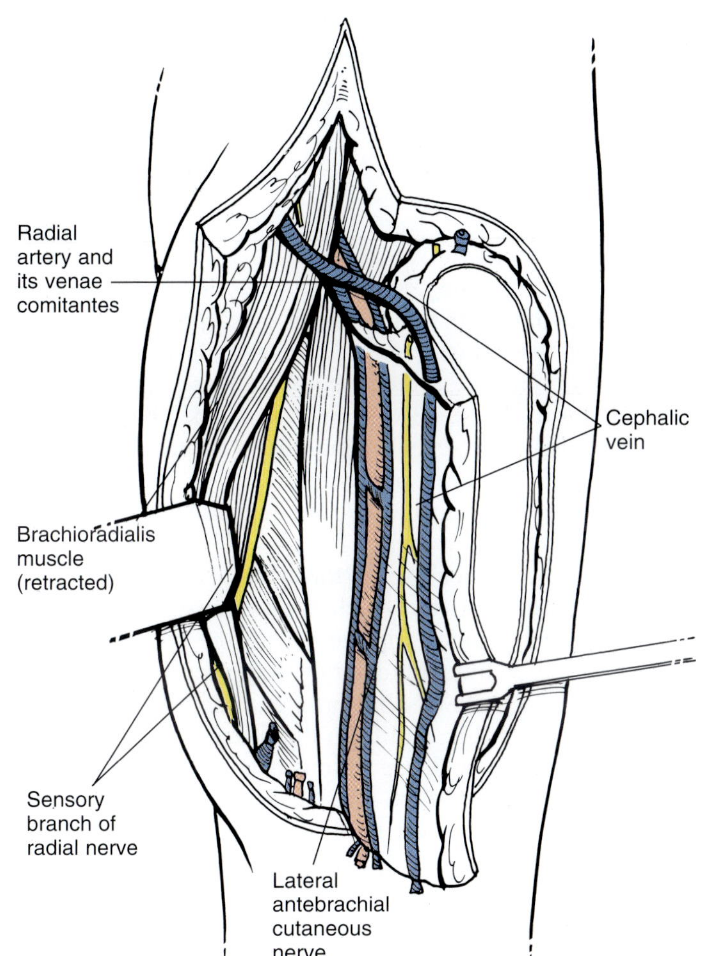

FIG. 13C. Ligation of vessels distally, with elevation of remainder of flap.

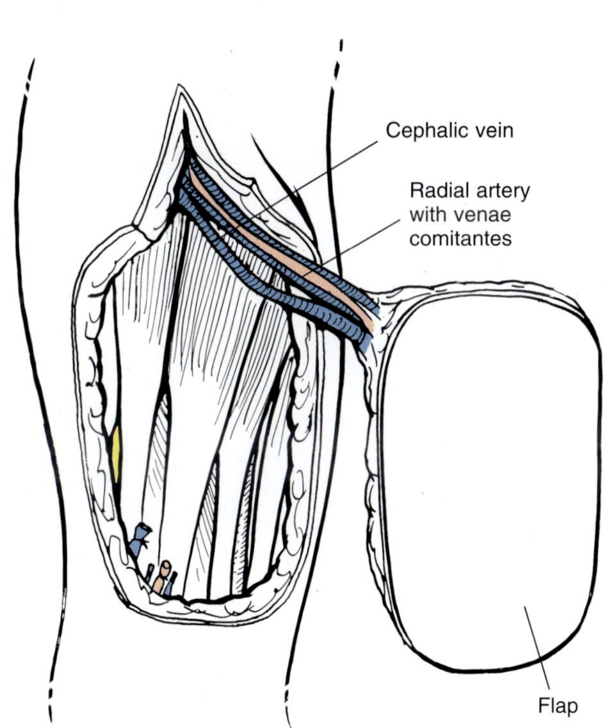

FIG. 13D. Donor vessels are then traced to their origin.

branches along the way. Upon completing this dissection, the branches of the serratus anterior and circumflex scapular artery and vein are clamped, ligated, and divided, leaving the flap perfused on a vascular pedicle approximately 10 to 12 cm long.

The thoracodorsal nerve is in close approximation to the thoracodorsal vessels and, unless a functional free flap is planned, must be dissected from the vascular pedicle and divided. The insertion of the latissimus dorsi muscle is dissected from the thoracodorsal vessels but is left intact to protect the vascular pedicle from accidental avulsion injury until the reconstructive surgeon is ready to harvest the flap. The flap is harvested by dividing the insertion of the muscle and then ligating and dividing the subscapular vessels near their origin from the axillary vessels. The donor site is closed in layers over two large drains.

Rectus Abdominis Muscle Free Flap

Anatomy

The rectus abdominis muscles are paired, long, narrow muscles that originate from the xiphoid process and the cartilages of the 5th to the 7th ribs on each side of the sternum, course caudally, and insert on the pubis (Fig. 7). Each muscle is segmentally innervated by intercostal nerves 8 through 12, which also contain the sensory nerve fibers to the skin of the abdominal wall. These nerves are accompanied by the terminal branches of the intercostal vessels, which enter the muscle on its posterior side at the junction between the lateral and medial thirds of the muscle.

The rectus muscles are almost completely ensheathed by the aponeuroses (fascial sheaths) of the transversalis and oblique abdominal muscles. The anterior rectus sheath is formed by a continuation of the aponeuroses of the external oblique and anterior layer of the internal oblique muscles. At the level of the arcuate line, a point halfway between the umbilicus and pubis indicating the end of the posterior rectus sheath, the anterior rectus sheath is formed by a continuation of the aponeuroses of the external oblique, internal oblique, and transversalis muscles. The fibers of these aponeuroses fuse from each side at the midline and form the linea alba. The anterior rectus sheath is firmly adhered to three to five dense fibrous bands (inscriptions) that cross the muscle just below the costal margin, at the umbilical level, and at a point in between these two locations. These fascial bands hold the anterior rectus sheaths firmly to the rectus abdominis muscles and each is often fused to the linea alba.

The posterior rectus sheath located posterior to the rectus muscle is formed by the posterior layer of the internal oblique abdominal aponeurosis, the aponeurosis of the transversalis, and the peritoneum. From the arcuate line to the pubis and inguinal ligament, the posterior rectus sheath is composed of only peritoneum.

The primary blood supply to the rectus abdominis muscles are the deep superior epigastric artery (DSEA) and the deep inferior epigastric artery (DIEA). (Each artery is accompanied by one or more veins with a similar name, i.e., deep superior epigastric veins and deep inferior epigastric veins.) The DSEA is a continuation of the internal thoracic artery and enters the muscle superiorly just under the costal margin on the muscle's posterior surface. It courses through the muscle toward the pubis branching into multiple vessels along the way that ultimately communicate with the terminal vessels of the DIEA via choke vessels. The DIEA originates from the external iliac artery and is usually larger than the DSEA. The DIEA courses in a superior-medial direction under the lateral border of the rectus abdominis muscle. Near the level of the arcuate line, the DIEA enters the muscle in its middle third and courses superiorly to anastomose with the choke vessels as described above.

As the DSEA and DIEA traverse the rectus musculature, they give off perforating branches that travel anteriorly through the rectus muscle and overlying anterior rectus sheath to supply the skin and subcutaneous tissue of the abdominal wall. Although some of these perforating branches are given off by the DSEA, most of the skin of the lower abdomen is supplied by the perforating branches originating from the DIEA.

These perforating branches are most commonly found from the level of the arcuate line to 1 to 2 cm above the umbilicus and usually exit the anterior rectus sheath in a medial and lateral row. The medial row of perforating vessels is usually found 1 to 2 cm lateral to the linea alba, whereas the lateral row of perforating vessels is usually 1 to 2 cm lateral to the medial row of perforators. Small lateral perforators that are within 2 to 3 cm of the lateral border of the rectus muscle are usually of intercostal origin.

Flap Design

The rectus abdominis free flap can be harvested with or without an overlying skin island. Because of the thickness of the subcutaneous tissue of the thigh and because most defects of the thigh requiring a free flap closure are usually large, a myocutaneous flap is usually preferred. The design of the myocutaneous flap as a TRAM or VRAM is determined by the size and location of the defect and by the location of scars on the abdominal wall from previous surgery. For example, the best flap design for closure of a relatively small thigh defect in a patient with a right paramedian abdominal scar may be a VRAM flap positioned over the left rectus abdominis muscle, whereas the best choice for closure of a much larger thigh defect in a woman without any abdominal scars would probably be a TRAM flap. The TRAM flap would not be a good option for wound closure in a patient with a posterior thigh defect because of the inability to place the patient in a prone or semiprone position after donor site closure. Although combination TRAM-VRAM flaps could be harvested, this type of flap is rarely needed. Irrespective of the choice of flap design, the vascular pedicle of the rectus abdominis free flap is always based on the DIEA and accompanying veins (DIEV).

When possible, the TRAM flap should be designed prior to surgery with the patient in a standing position. This approach allows the surgeon to obtain a better estimate of the amount of tissue available for transfer and permits the flap to be designed for the best cosmetic closure of the donor site. The TRAM flap is drawn in an elliptical shape with the long axis of the ellipse oriented transversely. The superior border of the flap is usually drawn at the level of the umbilicus or just above the umbilicus to include the perforating branches from the DIEA and DIEV. The inferior border of the flap is determined by having the patient flex at the waist and pinching the lower abdominal skin between the thumb (at the inferior border) and the fingers (at the superior border). If the mark indicating the position of the superior border can be brought to within 3 to 4 cm of the proposed inferior border, then the inferior border can be drawn at that level. The TRAM flap can extend several centimeters beyond the anterior superior iliac spine on each side, yielding flaps as long as the patient's waist line and 13 to 15 cm in width.

The VRAM flap can be designed over the entire length of the rectus muscle or just the superior portion between the umbilicus and costal margin. The width of the flap that can be taken depends on the surgeon's estimate of the ability to close the wound after flap harvest; in most cases, flaps 8 to 10 cm wide can be harvested.

Patient Positioning

Patients are placed on the operating table in the supine position for both the VRAM and the TRAM flap. The operating table must be able to flex at the waist level in order to close the TRAM flap without excessive tension. All pressure points, such as the shoulders, elbows, sacrum, and heels, must be adequately padded with foam cushioning to avoid pressure sores postoperatively.

Harvesting the TRAM Flap

An incision is made along the superior margin of the flap and the dissection beveled toward the costal margin as the dissection proceeds to the anterior rectus sheath (Fig. 8A–D). The abdominal skin above the TRAM flap is then elevated from the abdominal wall up to the xiphoid process and costal margin. After the superior dissection has been completed, an incision is made along the inferior margin of the flap and the dissection carried down to the fascial layer.

The lateral wings of the TRAM flap are then elevated from a lateral to medial direction up to the lateral row of perforating vessels. This part of the dissection is best accomplished under loupe magnification and by placing a traction suture in each end of the TRAM flap so that an assistant can pull the lateral wing of the TRAM flap upward while the surgeon pulls the abdominal fascia down and back. This maneuver demonstrates the areolar plane than must be dissected to raise the TRAM flap. Because hemostasis is easier to maintain and the perforators are easier to see if the tissues are not blood stained, we prefer to use the electrocautery (set at a low setting) for this dissection. As soon as the perforators are noted, the dissection up to the perforators is completed with tenotomy scissors.

After deciding which rectus abdominis muscle to use for the flap, a periumbilical incision is made and the umbilical stalk is dissected down to the anterior rectus sheath with care to leave a small cuff of fatty tissue around the umbilicus to maintain its blood supply. The TRAM flap is then elevated from the anterior rectus sheath on the side that will not be used for the flap. The perforating vessels are ligated with metal clips or sutures and divided. Dissection proceeds from medial to lateral direction across the linea alba until the medial row of perforating vessels on the flap are encountered. If these vessels are very small and the lateral row of perforating vessels are large, we sometimes sacrifice the medial row to save as much anterior rectus sheath as possible for closure. However, in most cases, the two rows of perforators are about the same size and every effort should be made to maintain both rows of perforating vessels.

After the cutaneous part of the TRAM flap has been isolated on its perforating vessels, the anterior rectus sheath is carefully incised around the exposed group of perforating vessels and fascial incision continued inferiorly and laterally to expose the DIEA and DIEV. After locating the vascular pedicle along the lateral border of the muscle, the anterior rectus sheath is elevated off the rectus muscle on both sides of the fascial perforators. The rectus muscle is then elevated from its bed and the vascular pedicle dissected down to its origin from the external iliac vessels. After the pedicle has been dissected free, the rectus abdominis muscle is transected above and below the perforators to the TRAM flap. When completing the inferior transection, the location of the vascular pedicle must be known at all times to avoid accidental injury.

The flap is harvested by ligating the DIEA and DIEV at their bases and transecting the vessels. While the flap is being inset and revascularized, other members of the reconstructive team close the donor site. This closure is accomplished by closing the anterior rectus sheath with a running 0 monofilament nonabsorbable suture and by placing two drains for drainage of the donor site. The abdominal skin flap is closed by flexing the table so that the superior skin edge can be approximated to the inferior skin edge. A new hole for the umbilicus is created, the umbilicus is inset, and the skin incision closed in layers.

Harvesting the VRAM Flap

The VRAM flap is harvested in a fashion similar to the TRAM flap. A skin incision is made around the skin island of the VRAM flap and the dissection is beveled out away from the skin island to avoid inadvertent undermining of the flap. After dissecting to the anterior rectus sheath, the dissection turns back toward the skin island to identify the medial and lateral rows of perforating vessels (Fig. 9A). If possible, both rows of perforators are saved and the anterior rectus sheath incised around the entire group of perforating vessels. The fascial incision is carried inferiorly to allow access to the DIEA and DIEV (Fig. 9B). The anterior rectus sheath on each side of the perforators is reflected away from the rectus muscle, and the vascular pedicle to the flap (DIEA and DIEV) is dissected from its investing tissue (Fig. 9C). If a long vascular pedicle is required, the intramuscular portion of these vessels usually can be dissected out for a short distance, effectively lengthening the pedicle by 2 to 4 cm.

The rectus muscle is then transected superiorly above the skin island and the flap elevated from its bed. The intercostal vessels and nerves are ligated and divided as the dissection proceeds toward the DIEA and DIEV. The rectus muscle is then transected 1 to 2 cm below the entrance of the inferior epigastric vessels into the rectus abdominis muscle. The flap is left attached by its pedicle to perfuse until ready for transfer. At the time of flap transfer, the DIEA and DIEV are ligated at their origin from the external iliac vessels.

The donor site is closed by undermining the abdominal skin on either side of the defect for some distance and closing the anterior rectus sheath with a running 0 monofilament nonabsorbable suture. The abdominal skin is closed in layers over one or two drains that exit the skin inferiorly.

Gracilis Muscle

Anatomy

Although the gracilis muscle does not provide bulk like the rectus abdominis muscle, the gracilis free tissue transfer does have the ability to provide function. The muscle originates from the pubis and the ischium, and inserts into the medial upper surface of the tibia, below the condyle (Fig. 10A,B). The muscle is thin and strap shaped, measuring approximately 42 cm in length. The gracilis tendon adds an additional 10 cm. The muscle is not wide, with an average width of 4 cm. There are two blood supplies to the gracilis muscle; the dominant vessel arises off the profunda femoris vessels, passing inferior medially between the adductor longus and the adductor magnus muscles and entering the upper third of the muscle consistently at 9 cm below the pubic tubercle. Several additional minor branches from the femoral vessel supply the distal muscle belly; however, only the dominant proximal vascular supply reliably nourishes the entire muscle. The anterior branch of the obturator nerve runs between the adductor longus and the magnus and splits into the motor and sensory nerves near the dominant vascular pedicle. The motor nerve enters the muscle with the dominant vascular pedicle and divides into two branches. The sensory branch crosses the gracilis muscle to innervate the overlying skin.

Flap Design

A cutaneous paddle can also be raised with the gracilis muscle; however, the distal third of the skin paddle does not receive sufficient blood supply from the muscle to be consistently reliable. Most often the flap is transferred as a muscle only and skin grafted. The patient should be marked in the standing position. This is critical, as difficulty delineating the boundaries of the gracilis can occur when the patient is supine. The anterior border of the gracilis corresponds to a line between the posterior border of the tendon of the adductor longus at the pubic tubercle. The muscle lies approximately 3 cm below the adductor longus. The distal end lies between the sartorius anteriorly and the semimembranosus posteriorly. The greater saphenous vein traverses the medial thigh and can be a source of vein grafts for this muscle.

Positioning the Patient

The muscle is harvested with the patient in the frog-leg position. If the flap is to be used for a distal leg or foot reconstruction, the entire leg should be prepped and draped. This allows for moving the extremity to better access the donor site, recipient site, and the recipient vessels. The muscle can be harvested from either leg, with some advantage to the leg opposite the defect when preparation of the recipient vessels near the defect requires special positioning. In some cases, such as in the elderly, confining all the surgery to one leg may help rehabilitate them to more effective ambulation earlier.

Harvest of the Gracilis Muscle Flap

The medial circumflex femoral vascular pedicle of the gracilis is isolated between the adductor magnus and the adductor longus after the gracilis muscle has been dissected free from all of the surrounding soft tissues (Fig. 11A,B). There is more friable, fibrofatty tissue around the neurovascular pedicle, which obstructs easy visualization of the vessels and makes isolation of the nerve and vessels more difficult. Careful dissection with tenotomy scissors and the bipolar cautery allows safe separation of the obturator nerve and the vascular pedicle close to the muscle. The vascular pedicle seems particularly prone to spasm with manipulation, so early and generous application of papaverine is a recommended preventative measure. The vascular pedicle runs between the adductor group of muscles and immediately gives off a very short pedicle to the adductor longus muscle. If the interval between the adductor muscles is aggressively opened above and below the circumflex pedicle as it goes under the adductor longus, the exposure of the more proximal portion of the circumflex pedicle as it branches from the profunda femoris vessel is vastly improved. The ligation of the short muscle pedicle into the adductor longus should be very gingerly performed so that the main circumflex vessels are not injured (Fig. 11A,B). The remainder of the pedicle is then further isolated down to the profunda vessels and then left to perfuse the muscle.

If the obturator nerve is not needed for a functional muscle transfer, it is isolated and divided. It is important to plan to harvest several centimeters of extra muscle and then trim any excess during the actual inset of the muscle, so that there is adequate pedicle length with some flexibility in the orientation of the muscle in the recipient site. The donor site is closed in layers over a suction drain. Once healing has begun, an elastic bandage can be applied over the thigh to improve the patient's comfort with ambulation.

Radial Forearm Free Flap

Anatomy

The radial forearm flap is supported by a fascial plexus that is supplied by multiple small perforators that stretch along its length and reach it from the radial artery passing along the fascial septum (Fig. 12A–C). The radial artery has 9 to 17 branches in the forearm with an average diameter of 0.5 mm that form a rich vascular plexus. The venous drainage of the radial forearm flap is based on both deep and superficial systems. The superficial system is composed of the cephalic and basilic veins. The cephalic vein arises from the radial border of the forearm and receives tributaries from the entire forearm. Medially it communicates with the basilic vein and below the elbow it communicates with the deep system through the median cubital vein. The deep system is usually composed of two venae comitantes accompanying the radial artery. Frequently, these veins are small (average diameter 1.3 mm), necessitating the elevation of one of the superficial veins with the flap.

Flap Design

A preoperative Allen's test is necessary to ensure the patency of collateral circulation, as absence of flow through the collateral system precludes the use of the flap or, at least, requires arterial reconstruction. The territory of the flap may be extended from the lower third of the anterior aspect of the proximal forearm to the proximal wrist flexion crease distally. The width of the flap can be taken from the lateral to medial humeral epicondyle. Proximal placement of the flap on the forearm allows for increased thickness of the flap and decreased pedicle length.

Patient Positioning

Patients are placed supine on the operating table for optimal harvesting of the radial forearm flap with the donor forearm on a standard extension table or a double arm board that is level with the operating table. From this position, any defect of the distal lower extremity can be well exposed by turning and padding under the patient's hips so that the lateral or posterior aspect of the extremity defect is optimally visible. Rotating the table (with the patient well secured) can also improve exposure when necessary for more posterior defects. This position also facilitates the closure of the radial forearm donor site, especially when grafting is necessary.

Harvesting the Radial Forearm Free Flap

Dissection is performed under tourniquet control, which is inflated to 250 mm Hg for 2 hours after the arm is exsanguinated with an Esmarch bandage. Our preferred method of elevation begins at the distal border (Fig. 13A–D). The flexor tendons, radial artery and vena comitantes, cephalic vein, brachioradialis, and median nerve are all identified, and initial ulnar elevation is performed, although radial elevation may be preferred by some. The antebrachial fascia is incised, and dissection proceeds just below the fascia along the flexor tendons. Preservation of the peritenon is critical for the adherence of a full- or split-thickness skin graft. Keeping the paratenon moist and avoiding desiccation during the remainder of the dissection is important.

The radial vessels are identified and care must be taken not to damage the fasciocutaneous perforating branches as they emerge from the intermuscular septum. The radial vessels are divided distally and the dissection continues toward the extensor carpi radialis longus muscle. Care must be taken not to injure the radial sensory nerve, which emerges between the tendons of the extensor carpi radialis longus and the brachioradialis tendon near the juncture of the distal and middle third of the forearm. The superficial vein is also divided distally, and the flap is elevated in a distal to proximal direction on its radial artery pedicle with the venae comitantes and the superficial vein intact. The incision along the forearm may extend to the antecubital fossa if a long pedicle is desired. The increased vessel diameter around the antecubital fossa (2 to 4 mm) facilitates microvascular anastomoses.

After dissection, the tourniquet is released and the hand evaluated for collateral circulation. The radial forearm free flap is transferred to the defect site by standard microvascular techniques. An end-to-end or end-to-side anastomosis is used. Full- or split-thickness skin grafting can be used for the donor site on those areas that can not be closed primarily. A volar splint is maintained for 5 days with the hand in position of function, and active and passive motion may then begin, if the graft appears to be viable.

The radial forearm free flap is ideal for three-dimensional defects; the thin and pliable skin is used for coverage of vital structures over the dorsum or plantar surfaces of the foot. The flap is inset with 3-0 absorbable suture along the dermis and 4-0 or 5-0 nylon sutures for skin approximation. The skin may also be taken off the flap and the fascia alone used for coverage. Split- or full-thickness grafts can be placed on the fascia if bulk is not desired, but the real advantage of this flap is the durable, yet thin, skin coverage achieved, which is ideal for many of the distal lower extremity defects. Completing sensory neurorrhaphies, if possible, to the antebrachial cutaneous nerves to possibly achieve better sensory return to the flap is controversial, since the sensory levels resulting do not seem consistently better than what is usually achieved in the flaps through ordinary peripheral neurotization in terms of protective sensation.

Summary

Treatment of tumors of the lower extremity often requires sacrifice of important functional tissue that significantly impacts ambulation and the patient's quality of life. The trend in the management of many tumors has now become limb salvage and microvascular reconstruction, if indicated oncologically and functionally. Effective rehabilitation following a successful extremity reconstruction thus remains the strategic focus in order to maximize the oncology patient's level of function and resultant quality of life.

SELECTED READINGS

Barwick WJ, Goldberg JA, Scully SP, Harrelson JM. Vascularized tissue transfer for closure of irradiated wounds after soft tissue sarcoma resection. *Ann Surg* 1992;216;591.

Bergman BA, Zamboni WA, Brown RE. Microvascular anastomosis of a rectus abdominis free flap into a prosthetic vascular bypass graft. *J Reconstr Microsurg* 1992;8:9.

Bostwick J III, Nahai F, Wallace JG, Vasconez LO. Sixty latissimus dorsi flaps. *Plast Reconstr Surg* 1979;63:31–41.

Boyd JB, Taylor GI, Corlett R. The vascular territories of the superior epigastric and deep inferior epigastric systems. *Plast Reconstr Surg* 1984;73:1–16.

Duchateau J, Declety A, Lejour M. Innervation of the rectus abdominis muscle: implications for rectus flaps. *Plast Reconstr Surg* 1988;82:223–227.

Gidumal R, Wood MB, Sim FH, Shives TC. Vascularized bone transfer for limb salvage and reconstruction after resection of aggressive bone lesions. *J Reconstr Microsurg* 1987;3:183.

Hidalgo DA, Carrasquillo IM. The treatment of lower extremity sarcomas with wide excision, radiotherapy and free-flap reconstruction. *Plast Reconstr Surg* 1992;89:96–101.

Karakousis CP, Emrich LJ, Rao U, Krishnamsetty RA. Feasibility of limb salvage and survival in soft tissue sarcomas. *Cancer* 1986;57:484–491.

Lindberg RD, Martin RG, Romsdahl MM, Barkley HT. Conservative surgery and postoperative radiotherapy in 300 adults with soft-tissue sarcomas. *Cancer* 1981;47:2391–2397.

McCraw JB, Arnold PG, eds. *McCraw and Arnold's atlas of muscle and musculocutaneous flaps.* Norfolk, VA: Hampton Press, 1986;157.

Milloy FJ, Anson BJ, McAfee DK. The rectus abdominis muscle and the epigastric arteries. *Surg Gynecol Obstet* 1960;122:293.

Moon HK, Taylor GI. The vascular anatomy of the rectus abdominis musculocutaneous flaps based on the deep superior epigastric system. *Plast Reconstr Surg* 1988;82:815–829.

Reece GP Kroll SS, Miller MJ, Schusterman MA, Baldwin BJ, Pollock RE, Romsdahl MM, Ross M, Janjan NA. Lower extremity salvage in cancer patients using free tissue transfer. *Riv Ital Chir Plastica* 1993;25(suppl 1):441–446.

Reece GP, Schusterman MA, Pollock RE, Kroll SS, Miller MJ, Baldwin BJ, Romsdahl MM, Janjan NA. Immediate versus delayed free-tissue transfer salvage of the lower extremity in soft tissue sarcoma patients. *Ann Surg Oncol* 1994;1:11–17.

Rosenberg SA, Tepper J, Glatstein E, Costa J, Baker A, Brennan M, DeMoss EV, et al. The treatment of soft-tissue sarcomas of the extremities: prospective randomized evaluation of 1) limb-sparing surgery plus radiation therapy compared with amputation and 2) the role of adjuvant chemotherapy. *Ann Surg* 1982;196:305–315.

Roswell AR, Eisenberg N, Davies DM, Taylor GI. The anatomy of the subscapular-thoracodorsal arterial system: study of 100 cadaver dissections. *Br J Plast Surg* 1984;37:574–576.

Shiu MH, Turnbull AD, Dattatreyudu N, Hajdu S, Hilaris B. Control of locally advanced extremity soft tissue sarcomas by function-saving resection and brachytherapy. *Cancer* 1984;53:1385–1392.

Steinau HU, Ehrl H, Biemer E. Reconstructive plastic surgery in soft tissue sarcomas of the extremities. *Eur J Plast Surg* 1988;11:99–108.

Tobin GR, Moberg AW, DuBou RH, Weiner LJ, Bland KI. The split latissimus dorsi myocutaneous flap. *Ann Plast Surg* 1981;7:272.

Tobin GR, Schusterman MA, Peterson GH, et al. The intramuscular neurovascular anatomy of the latissimus dorsi muscle: the basis for splitting the flap. *Plast Reconstr Surg* 1981;67:637.

Williams PL, Warwick R, Dyson M, Bannister LH, eds. *Gray's anatomy*, 37th ed. New York: Churchill Livingstone, 1989;610.

Subject Index

Subject Index